D1087185

# Malignant Medical Myths

**Why medical treatment causes 200,000 deaths in the USA each year, and how to protect yourself**

**by Joel M. Kauffman, PhD**

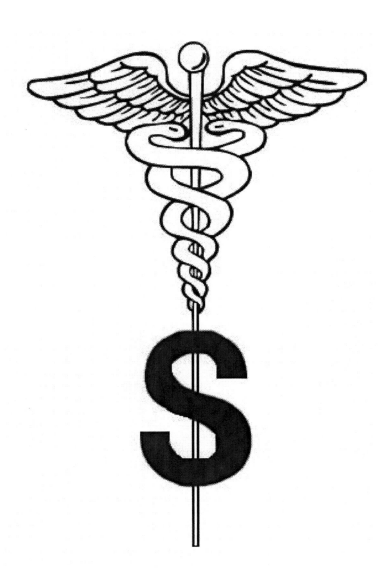

Copyright © 2006 by Joel M. Kauffman, PhD

*All rights reserved. No part of this book shall be reproduced or transmitted in any form or by any means, electronic, mechanical, magnetic, photographic including photocopying, recording or by any information storage and retrieval system, without prior written permission of the publisher. No patent liability is assumed with respect to the use of the information contained herein. Although every precaution has been taken in the preparation of this book, the publisher and author assume no responsibility for errors or omissions. Neither is any liability assumed for damages resulting from the use of the information contained herein.*

*Disclaimer: Any recommendations herein are based on studies published in peer-reviewed scientific journals, or reported by trusted clinicians. I am not an MD and I cannot engage in the practice of medicine. The content of this book is information to better enable people to judge the value of medical claims, a particular provider, and alternative treatments. Seek qualified professional advice.*

ISBN 0-7414-2909-8

Published by:

**INFINITY**
PUBLISHING.COM
1094 New DeHaven Street, Suite 100
West Conshohocken, PA 19428-2713
Info@buybooksontheweb.com
www.buybooksontheweb.com
Toll-free (877) BUY BOOK
Local Phone (610) 941-9999
Fax (610) 941-9959

*Printed in the United States of America*
*Printed on Recycled Paper*
*Published March 2006*

# Malignant Medical Myths

## Contents

# Acknowledgment

Sally Fallon of the Weston A. Price Foundation inspired the creation of this book. She also edited Myths 3 and 4 and Appendix B. Frances Eleanor Heckert Pane, MSLS, not only edited the whole manuscript several times, but provided information, citations, and was a wonderful source of encouragement. Her friend Eugene E. Sarafin, MSc, checked Myth 2, suggested inclusion of a glossary of useful medical terms, and provided other technical support. Duane Graveline, MD, MPH, ("Spacedoc"), provided inspiration and the synopses in most of the chapters. Many members of The International Cholesterol Skeptics, including its founder, Uffe Ravnskov, MD, PhD, were very helpful and supportive. Others are acknowledged at the end of the appropriate chapters, including Leslie A. Bowman, AMLS, who read much of the early versions. She also warned me that such a work would never be mistake-free. Please report mistakes to kauffman37@yahoo.com.

# Preface

Until about 1990, like most people, I believed that most medical and diet advice was reliable, especially from government agencies we pay so much to take care of us. About $30 billion annually goes to the National Institutes of Health alone. When medical brochures and advertisements referred to papers in peer-reviewed medical journals, I assumed that these papers were honest and complete, based on my own experience as the author of 80 journal papers myself, which were subject to rigorous peer review.

I took my baby aspirin, ate *trans* fat, drank fluoridated water and had my cholesterol measured in the belief that others were looking out for me by basing their recommendations on the best evidence from trials.

About this time I began to subscribe to alternative medicine newsletters from Drs. Julian Whitaker, William Campbell Douglass, Jr., and David G. Williams. I thought that some of their claims were nuts, and still do; but these MDs always had references to medical and nutritional journals. When I checked their references I usually found good support for many of their non-mainstream ideas. References that stand up to scrutiny show that an author is not merely pontificating, and can be trusted. *Malignant Medical Myths* has many references for the same reason. You can check on any of my claims and opinions. Believe it or not, some medical writers use references to fool the reader into acceptance of false data, where the papers cited do not say what the writer claimed for them, or do not actually address the topic, or are even contradictory. An actual example is given in Myth 3.

Around the year 2000 I decided to find the truth about daily aspirin for preventing heart attacks, since the recommendations were strongly contradicted by dissenters. It was quite a shock to find that long-term daily aspirin is of no overall benefit (see Myth 1). This was the start of checking up on other medical and nutritional dogma that led to this book.

Determined to understand medical papers, I struggled with jargon and slowly caught onto the tricks of the trade, such as incomplete and misleading abstracts. The abstract of a paper is supposed to summarize the purpose, choice of subjects, trial protocol, and results. When key results are left out of the abstract, such as all-cause mortality and side-effects, they remain left out of any press release, newspaper article and sales literature. Often we can only get the abstracts by searching PubMed, Free Medical Journals, or individual journal websites. The cost of complete papers of $20-30 each is reasonable if it relates to your employment, but not if the dollars come out of your own pocket. When the whole paper is examined, shocking cover ups come to light, in many cases, such as excess cancer deaths even when some easily measurable stuff, like cholesterol, is lowered, which is supposed to be a benefit, but is not. People who would most benefit from a diet intervention are often excluded from the chosen subjects. Very high dropout rates because of treatment side-effects usually do not find their way to the abstract.

*Malignant Medical Myths* is written to make some concepts, such as the randomized placebo-controlled clinical trial, understandable. The trick in advertising: "do this and your risk of so-and-so will go down by 50%" is shown to be a relative and not an absolute number, worthless on its own.

Another of my awakenings was finding that promoters of alternative treatments were sometimes even less scientific than the mainstream promoters. And that debunking of all alternatives (some are valuable) was carried out routinely by more powerful commercial interests and the government agencies they control. Websites that appear to be those of self-help groups with certain ailments can be owned by corporations making products for those ailments.

However uplifting it may be to read about individual health successes, anecdotes are avoided when possible in favor of observational or clinical trials with large numbers of subjects.

In the USA you have the last word on what medical or diet advice you will act upon. *Malignant Medical Myths* provides you with the power to *evaluate* this advice, and shows how to find reliable sources of medical and diet information.

# Introduction: How good is mainstream medical advice?

*The main obstacle to progress is not ignorance, but the illusion of knowledge.*
--Daniel Boorstin, Librarian of Congress

## You Do Not Have To Trust Your Doctor

In the United States, as this is written, you have the right to decide which medical tests and treatments to accept, if any. Physicians are supposed to present the risks and benefits of these possible tests and treatments so that you may decide, a decision which includes the choice of *no* tests or treatments. Patients usually recognize that the physician knows a great deal more, and they usually ask the physician to make the decision. While many physicians and other medical providers mean well, the information they use to make their recommendations for many common conditions is often outdated, biased, flawed and sometimes is based on outright fraud. Your doctor cannot be blamed for using medical guidelines based on bad science, because failure to do so might result in fewer referrals or even de-licensing. Many medical tests and treatments are not based on sound research, including some very common ones discussed in this book, but on the pitches of opinion leaders paid by those who would profit from their use. Thus the level of trust between medical doctor and patient that has been so important over the years, even taken for granted, is now seriously threatened.

How are doctors subverted? On 27 June 2004, Gardiner Harris reported in *The New York Times* that "The check for $10,000 arrived in the mail unsolicited. The doctor who received it from the drug maker Schering-Plough said it was made out to him personally in exchange for [executing] an attached 'consulting' agreement that required nothing other than his commitment to prescribe the company's medicines. Two other physicians said in separate interviews that they, too, received checks unbidden from Schering-Plough, one of the world's biggest drug companies." Johnson & Johnson, Wyeth and Bristol-Myers Squibb have also been implicated in similar enticements to subvert the prescribing habits of physicians.

How are patients subverted? When people hear and see a white-coated figure on television give a pitch for a test, a drug, or some other procedure, whether as an actor in a drug advertisement, or as a real medical expert on a news program, some people will ask their physicians to provide the product. Other people may be skeptical, but this often vanishes when their physicians support the information from the media by recommending the advertised test or drug without being asked. This may not only be the effect of Big Pharma salespeople with biased information on drugs or tests, but the aim of Continuing Medical Education programs often sponsored by Big Pharma. Respected reporters and commentators often owe portions of their salaries to advertising by corporations whose products they endorse during what are supposed to be non-advertising segments of programs on radio and TV or articles in newspapers called Press Releases.

## A Brief History of Medicine

Medical myths are as old as medicine and are based on remedies often used for centuries. They include leeches for bleeding, mercury compounds as purgatives, and powerful cathartics, most of which had no proven benefits. The common belief that supported the practice before the 20th century was that they did indeed cause vomiting or diarrhea, which supposedly removed toxins from the body,. However, it was not possible then to measure the amount of almost any toxin in the body before and after treatment, so there was no evidence that treatment effected a cure. Old-time docs would point to improvement in their patients as evidence, knowing that many would have recovered without treatment.

Real progress in medicine, sanitation and diet has taken place in the last 200 years. For example, in the eighteenth century the need for essential nutrients was recognized, with citrus fruits or sauerkraut adopted to prevent or reverse scurvy. Cowpox vaccination was found to immunize against smallpox. In the nineteenth century, the germ theory of infectious diseases was developed, then vaccines for the prevention or treatment of more diseases. So also were slow, sterile surgeries performed under general anesthetic, eliminating deaths from shock or infection. Then in the twentieth century, the rational development of insulin, thyroid extract, antibiotics, Xrays and other medical imaging techniques, and superior prosthetics occurred. This was followed by hundreds of other drugs for chronic conditions as well as automated tests for dozens of substances in serum, all made possible by huge expenditures for medical research. One would think that most of the commonly used procedures, drugs, and tests in the twenty-first century are results of what is now called "evidence-based medicine". Sadly this fine ideal has been compromised because so much of the "evidence" has been compromised, as you will see.

Many of our chronic conditions and later-life ailments are not curable or reversible, yet these chronic afflictions cost the most for tests and treatments whose effectiveness and safety are exaggerated. Examples are annual mammograms, cholesterol assays and drugs, blood pressure drugs, cancer chemotherapy drugs, coronary artery bypass surgery, and stenting, to name a few. The exaggerations have relegated what "everybody knows" to be "true" about these common medical topics to the level of myth.

## Medical Myths Exposed

Each chapter in this book is an in-depth examination of one of the common medical myths still prevalent. Most of the myths reviewed are promoted by articles that cite randomized clinical trials (RCTs) in medical journals, position statements from powerful organizations, and pervasive advertising. Each has lasted for at least 15 years, thus each may be considered malignant. Each has caused false hope, unwanted side-effects, other forms of worse health, and $billions in wasted expenditures on health care. Wasted $billions lower standards-of-living for those of us not employed as medical providers, medical researchers, or malpractice and class-action attorneys, because of the exploding cost of health insurance premiums and out-of-pocket medical expenses. Wasted $billions (from about $2 trillion per year spent on healthcare in the USA) threaten the solvency of the federal and some state governments, if the present promises of health insurance, Medicare, and Medicaid are fulfilled.

## Why the Randomized, Placebo-Controlled Clinical Trial?

The randomized clinical trial (RCT) was needed to show that the minor beneficial effects of drugs for chronic conditions did more than a placebo (sugar pill) did over long periods of time. It became the gold standard of medical research in the 1970s. The RCT is carried out by selecting two identical groups of subjects by age, sex, race, health status, socioeconomic status, etc. The treatment group gets the drug, test, or operation. Ideally the control group gets a fake drug (placebo), test, vaccination, or operation. There is a powerful psychosomatic effect of believing that, if you are being treated, you must benefit. This placebo effect often shows up as positive results in 30-50% of subjects in the placebo group. If the treatment group is really benefiting from treatment, the positive results must be significantly higher than 30-50%, or whatever the placebo group did.

You may find it amusing that some of the most effective treatments were adopted without any RCT, simply because the results were so obvious, for example, rabies and yellow-fever vaccines, insulin, thyroid extract, sulfa drugs and many later antibiotics, such as penicillin, tetracycline and streptomycin. Conversely, RCTs with thousands of subjects may be needed to show a statistically significant, yet minor effect of a typical drug for a chronic condition (see Myths 1, 3 and 4).

Many common tests fall into the same category, or had defective RCTs, such those for mammograms (see Myth 9) or the PSA test (see Myth 10). Many surgical procedures from tonsillectomies, now thought useless and contributing to allergies or asthma, to radical mastectomy, were carried on for long periods before studies showed how damaging and useless these surgeries had been.

So the RCT, valuable as it can be, is *not* the the only or even the best criterion for success. Clinical observations, if done honestly, can be of equal value. The *British Medical Journal* recognized this fact by publishing a paper reminding us that the use of parachutes for surviving free-fall from aircraft has never been subjected to a RCT (Smith & Pell, 2003).

<u>Too Much Testing and Treatment</u>

When your physician, surgeon or nurse tells you that you need a test, or an operation, or that you should take a prescription drug, you would assume that the advice was based on the best medical science as found by controlled studies and medical trials (RCTs). You would be wrong. A number of the most commonly done tests, such as the digital rectal examination and the PSA test for prostate cancer (Welch, 2004, 18ff), and annual mammograms (Kauffman & McGee, 2004; Welch, 2004, 19ff) are poor diagnostic tools. Many diagnostic tests are done which give too many false positives or false negatives.

Aggressive diagnosis (too many tests) is not prevention, merely early detection. Often there is no cure for the condition for which the test is done, so the only outcome of early diagnosis is early mental distress (Robin, 1984, pp28-45). Equally often, treatments in very common use may be of no value. For example, there is no evidence that radical or total mastectomy gives a better outcome than lumpectomy (Fisher et al., 2002) or that the effects of angioplasty or stenting last more than a few months (McGee, 2001, pp20-38; Bogaty & Brophy, 2003).

There is considerable evidence that treatment with some of the best-selling classes of prescription drugs fail to prolong life or improve its quality (Kauffman, 2004) in many of the people who take them. This includes anticholesterol drugs, blood pressure drugs, and most anticancer drugs used for chemotherapy (Kauffman & McGee, 2004; Moss, 2000). Allen Roses, MD, worldwide vice-president of genetics at GlaxoSmithKline, said that fewer than half of the patients who were prescribed some of the most expensive drugs actually derived any benefit from them. "The vast majority of drugs - more than 90 per cent - only work in 30 or 50 per cent of the people," Dr Roses said. "I wouldn't say that most drugs don't work. I would say that most drugs work in 30 to 50 per cent of people. Drugs out there on the market work, but they don't work in everybody." He cited some response rates for specific therapeutic areas as drug efficacy rate as the per cent of patients who benefit:


Alzheimer's: 30%
Analgesics (Cox-2, i. e. Vioxx™, Celebrex™): 80
Asthma: 60
Cardiac Arrhythmias: 60
Depression (SSRI, i. e., Prozac™): 62
Diabetes: 57

Hepatitis C (HCV): 47
Incontinence: 40
Migraine (acute): 52
Migraine (prophylaxis)50
Oncology (chemotherapy): 25
Rheumatoid arthritis: 50
Schizophrenia: 60

## Follies at the AMA, FDA and USDA

More than ever, most individual medical providers, including mainstream ones, cannot use their own judgment or experience, because they can be threatened with lawsuits for malpractice if "official" guidelines for diagnosis and treatment are not followed. Failure to follow procedures based on myths, or using an alternative treatment not sanctioned by the American Medical Association (AMA) can lead to ostracism by peer physicians or even de-licensing (Carter, 1992, xv ff). Some guidelines appear to have the sanction of the US government. One example is the "New Cholesterol Guidelines" which appear to be promulgated by the National Heart, Lung, and Blood Institute (NHLBI), a branch of the National Institutes of Health (NIH). These guidelines, which promote more and more aggressive use of cholesterol-lowering drugs, were prepared by drug experts, many involved with drug manufacturers, with no government supervision or approval. Yet these guidelines are being promoted nationally as official guidelines of the NHLBI utilizing government funds (your taxes) and facilities (Ottoboni & Ottoboni, 2002). Conversely, lack of official guidelines may be used as a ruse by an insurer to refuse to pay claims even for treatments of proven benefit (see Myth 7).

The US Food & Drug Administration (FDA) is charged with judging the safety and efficacy of drugs, tests, and devices. Most people believe that the FDA actually tests drugs and devices. The FDA does not; it examines the test results the manufacturers choose to offer (Cohen, 2001, pp176-197). Most people believe that the FDA is relatively independent of the manufacturers and not unduly influenced by them; this is not so (Moore, 1998). At least a dozen drugs were recalled by the FDA in the 1990s just a few years after the FDA approved them. Others have side-effects that were underplayed in the trial results presented to the FDA. Or we are supposed to ignore the side-effects because the main beneficial effect is purported to be so dramatic, especially in the press releases and advertising of Big Pharma.

The FDA, medical providers, and the public are easily fooled by the effect of drugs on some easily measured symptom whose significance has reached the level of folklore (myth). Many interventions are justified on conveniently measured parameters, such as bone density, cholesterol level, EKGs, and blood pressure. In all of these cases, examples exist in which the intervention improved the easily measured symptom, called the surrogate endpoint, such as lowering blood pressure, yet worsened the primary endpoint of heart attack, bone fracture, or death. One extreme example was the use of antiarrhythmic drugs. "Success" was shown by altered EKGs (electrocardiograms), but the drugs caused sudden cardiac death (Fleming & DeMets, 1996; McGee, 2001, pp9-11). Conversely, the FDA has sometimes been a ferocious obstructor of effective and non-toxic alternative treatments, while accepting toxic drugs merely based on surrogate outcomes in RCTs (Kauffman, 2002, 2003).

4

> You are probably suspicious of drug advertising. Based on the problems at the FDA, you should be almost as suspicious of drug instructions and package inserts. At the least you should look at the package insert, or its equivalent in a PDR (Physicians's Desk Reference, also available online) before taking a drug. A warning in a black rectangle, as shown around this paragraph, always spells toxicity, and is called a Black Box Warning. But surely articles in peer-reviewed medical journals, often cited in the package insert, and the press-releases based on them can be trusted? The referees or reviewers, usually 1-4 in number, are supposed to be anonymous to the authors and independent of the financial sources of the authors, yet be their peers in expertise. Many are, but considerable trading of favors and behind-the-scenes pressures must occur to lead to the publication of so many poorly written, or well-written yet misleading papers (Kauffman, 2004).

One reason for poor performance at the FDA is known. "The Food and Drug Administration yesterday...held advisory committee meetings to discuss the safety and efficacy of two new drugs for diabetes. In each case, one-third of the committee's nine members had financial ties to the drug manufacturers that submitted the new drug applications, or their competitors. Why does the agency persist in inviting conflicted scientists to serve on its panels? Last June, [2005,] Rep. Maurice Hinchey (D-NY) attached a rider to the FDA appropriations bill that would ban the practice. Nearly three dozen Republicans joined with most Democrats to pass the measure 218-210. The bill is slated to come before the [US] Senate, probably next week. Aides to Sen. Richard Durbin (D-IL), its sponsor, hope that the concern on both sides of the aisle about the agency's safety record will translate into a positive vote." (Goozner, 2005).

If not the FDA, surely the US Department of Agriculture (USDA) recommendations, as in their Food Pyramid, can be trusted. Alas, theirs, too, will be shown in Myth 2 to be flawed advice.

### Independent? Research at the NIH

But surely the various Institutes of the National Institute of Health (NIH) in supporting medical research in universities and in-house to the tune of $30 billion per year are independent of manufacturers and untainted by financial conflicts of interest? Maybe more than 25 years ago this was so, but in 1980 a change in the rules on who could obtain patent rights on new medical treatments lowered the objectivity at NIH, as did the initiation of permission for staff members to engage in private consulting deals. According to The Los Angeles Times, Dr. Stephen I. Katz of the National Institute of Arthritis and Musculoskeletal and Skin Diseases collected over $1 million in consulting fees in the last decade, including $170,000 from Schering AG, which in, turn, received $1.7 million in grants from this Institute. At least 5 other researchers and directors at NIH received large fees or stock options from commercial firms who received preferential treatment (Willman, 2003). While the NIH's policies are open to public scrutiny, its actual practices are not. Of the 2,259 current consulting deals made by NIH employees in the upper salary brackets, only 127 are subject to full public disclosure. The rest fall through an administrative loophole that allows these employees, who are already receiving substantial salaries from taxpayers, to file minimal details of their outside agreements, and these are for internal use only (Anon., 2003).

Dr. Charles B. Nemeroff, Chairman of the Department of Psychiatry and Behavioral Science at Emory University, reviewed two dozen treatments for psychiatric disorders in an article in *Nature Neuroscience*. He favored three of the treatments he stood to profit from, based on his ties to Eli Lilly, AstraZeneca, Wyeth-Ayerst and others as a consultant or grantee. Seeing this, Drs. Bernard Carroll and Robert T. Rubin wrote to the Editor of *Nature Neuroscience* pointing out the journal's failure to

disclose Nemeroff's financial ties. After 5 months of fruitless waiting for their letter to appear, Carroll and Rubin gave *The New York Times* the story. In his defense, Nemeroff told the *Times* that he would have been happy to list his ties, if only the journal's staff had asked.
(http://www.washingtonmonthly.com/features/2004/0404.brownlee.html)

So bad had the situation become that the NIH announced that all consulting deals by its staffers had to be reported to the Director of the NIH, as reported on the Public Broadcasting System on 8 Jun 04. These staffers have salaries over $100,000 per year, comparable to what they would make if they were directly employed by drug companies. Yet by accepting about $60,000 per year in addition to their salaries, they provide conduits that allow the drug companies to influence the research carried on at NIH, and learn of its progress long before regular peer-reviewed publication of it, or even before talks at scientific meetings. One can even imagine that dissemination of valuable discoveries at the NIH funded by federal tax dollars might be delayed by the drug, test or device makers by their influence on the income of NIH staffers.

Bill Moyers showed in his TV program NOW on 30 Apr 04 that drug manufacturers now have the most numerous lobbyist force in Washington, about 600 of them. Other segments of the health care industry have hundreds more. These people are major sources of "information" for Congress and its staffers.

Can university or medical school faculty or researchers be trusted? When you hear them on radio or see them on television, or they are quoted in print, you are not told who their sponsors are. Only when their their sources of funding are revealed, as in a medical paper in a peer-reviewed journal — and assuming that the required disclosure is complete even there — only then might you have enough information to make a decision. The sellout of universities has reached such proportions that researchers who need to publish for career advancement may be prevented from doing so by confidentiality agreements with the sponsor, sometimes hidden in the employment agreements the faculty or staff member must sign (Robinson, 2001, pp70-82). Researchers who go ahead to publish findings unfavorable to the sponsor have been threatened with loss of all funding, lawsuits, or blacklisting from future contracts or even employment (Cohen, 2001, pp130-138). University officers themselves, enjoying the indirect costs and capital equipment from contracts, are behaving as though they are running for-profit companies (Press & Washburn, 2000). By 1989 the situation with medical school research was so corrupt that the NIH began to operate the Office of Scientific Integrity (Anderson, 1992, pp133-134).

## Examples of Phony Evidence

A world-famous diet expert told me that microwaving food in general was dangerous, and that there was a journal paper on this topic. Asked to provide evidence, she sent a copy of a newspaper article that told of a finding in *The Lancet,* a respected journal, as well as the "paper" in *The Lancet.* The article claimed that Austrian researchers found that the proteins in babies' milk heated in a microwave oven were turned into poisons that attack the brain (Anon., 1990). The "paper" in *The Lancet* turned out to be a letter to the editor. A letter is not seen by peer-reviewers, and does not have the status of a paper.

The letter gave experimental evidence that microwaving samples of babies' milk formulae for 10 minutes produced an unnatural isomer (different geometric form) of amino acids, while heating the formulae at 80°C in a water bath for 10 minutes did not. One of the "toxic" isomers found was of the common amino acid called D-proline, found at 1-2 parts-per-million (ppm), (Lubec et al., 1989). It is easy to remember that 1 ppm is 1 milligram per liter (mg/L), less easy to remember that it is 0.03 ounces per ton. This would provide an exposure of 0.5-1.5 mg per day, or about 0.1 mg per kg for a 10-kg infant. Since the effect of a dose of anything depends on the weight of the dosee, this general use of "mg/kg" allows us to compare doses among animals of different weights. The researchers found no actual evidence of harm, and cited only a 1978 paper on D-proline involvement with lethal convulsions in chicks, which had nothing to do with microwaving food. This was the only basis for claiming neurotoxicity. *The Lancet* authors simply advised further research. They did not use the words of the newspaper reporter: "brain damage".

A more recent study was found on feeding D-proline (the natural isomer being called L-proline, a mirror-image of the D) to rats at 50 mg/kg for 28 days. The organs suspected of damage, including the brains, were inspected in several ways, including microscopically. No signs of damage whatever were found at 500 times the mg/kg exposure likely from microwaved milk (Schieber et al., 1997).

Perhaps microwaving will some day prove to be a danger, but a search on PubMed in 2005 did not provide an example. Any type of cooking can be carried too far and cause unwanted chemical changes in food.

One of the favorite types of phony evidence results from what is called "selection bias". This is simply the inclusion of all studies that support one's biases, and omission of some or all that do not. The 2005 report in *Annals of Internal Medicine* on the "dangers" of vitamin E is an example given in Myth 1.

The most spectacular example I have seen is from one of most influential fat-bashers, Prof. Ancel Keys, for whom the US Army K-ration is named. He made a plausible case for the unwary in 1953 with his Six Countries Study, in which he tried to show that the higher the proportion of diet calories consumed as fat, the greater the incidence of cardiovascular disease (CVD). He published a graph of CVD incidence vs. % calories from fat, obtaining a smooth curve, thus demonstrating a solid correlation. Case closed? Not so fast. At the time there was data available for 16 other countries he did not use because most of the data points did not fall on his curve! No correlation after all. On top of this, he could not explain how CVD rates vary by a factor of 5 in Italy and Finland depending on the location within each (Ravnskov, 2000, pp17-19).

One of the favorite tactics of the "fear industry" we all hear too much from is ignoring relevant studies that *others* have already done. Nowhere is this more blatant than with mercury in fish. Warnings abound that eating even canned tuna will cause us to ingest the mercury in the fish and suffer from its neurotoxic effects. Yes, there is mercury in fish at 1-1.5 ppm in tilefish (white snapper), swordfish, king mackerel and shark; but only 0.2 ppm in canned tuna, about 0.03 micrograms in a 6 oz (150 g) can. Fresh tuna and lobster contain twice as much; but scallop, catfish, salmon and shrimp only 1/5 as much (PCD, 2003). Yes, a high enough dose of mercury in any form is toxic. Case closed? Not so fast. There are long-term observational diet studies on fish by researchers who were not trying to scare anyone about mercury, and, in fact, ignored it (Kauffman, 2004).

The Chicago Western Electric Study followed the effects of fish consumption in 2,107 men aged 40-55, and followed for 30 years. Those who ate an average of ≥35 g daily (about 1 big fish dinner every 5 days) had only 9/10 of the all-cause mortality rate of men who ate no fish. The Nurses' Health Study on 84,688 women aged 34-59 years and followed for 16 years for outcomes vs. fish and omega-3 fatty acid intake, had the following findings: women consuming fish five times weekly had only 7/10 the all-cause mortality rate of those eating fish once a month. (See Myth 1, Part B for references.)

Pregnant women have been cautioned to restrict their intake of fish (http://www.cbc.ca/storyview/CBC/2002/10/21/Consumers/mercuryfish_021021) despite evidence that children receive most of their mercury from vaccines. Hepatitis b vaccine carries 12.5 micrograms per dose; influenza and other common vaccines carry 25 micrograms per shot, over 830 times the amount in a can of tuna. It has been reported that vaccines said not to contain the mercury compound, thimerosal, still might have it (PCD, 2003). The long duration of the diet studies makes it very clear that the mercury content of fish, in general, is not shortening life.

## Medical Journals Perverted

Decisions on what treatment guidelines to recommend are often made by committees composed of MDs considered to be reliable and loyal by their peers, and also to be opinion leaders. Their guidelines can become, in effect, mandatory, because physicians who do not follow them risk censure, lawsuits and loss of medical license, as noted above. The decisions are often represented as being based on studies in major medical journals. Brochures for tests, procedures and drugs, as well as the TV and magazine advertisements often quote articles in these same medical journals. Press releases usually contain any or all of the flaws in medical papers listed below. How appalling then, that so many papers have flaws, that many are deliberately misleading (Kauffman, 2004), and that press and public, as well as many practicing physicians, still need to be made aware of the problems. Typical perversions of medical papers:

• Key findings in the body of the paper do not appear in the abstract, which is all that physicians, reporters, insurers and others may ever read.
• References may be selected to include only the ones that support the paper's conclusions.
• Relative risks are given in the absence of absolute risks; more on this later.
• Reduction in death rates of only one type are given without all-cause death rates.
• Trials and studies may not have a control or placebo group.
• Trials often fail to compare the new drug with the "best" older drug or with supplements.
• Drop-out rates in trials are often omitted from abstracts or in counting adverse effects. This is facilitated by a "run-in" period early in a trial, which allows that subjects with the most serious side-effects to be eliminated early.
• Adverse effects are usually deprecated.
• Trials are run only as long as the outcome favors treatment.
• Unfavorable trial results are not published.
• End-points may make use of changes in easy measurements, such as cholesterol or blood pressure, and fail to include real end-points, such as all-cause death.
• Real end-points are often combined with non-fatal outcomes to make the overall outcome look better.
• Data for men and women are often combined, concealing adverse results for one or the other, as is the case for aspirin (see Myth 1) and at least one statin (anti-cholesterol) drug (see Myth 3).
• Subjects 20-60 years old are usually selected for trials, then the outcome is used to make recommendations for children and the elderly as well.
• Bell-curve statistics for the statistical significance (shown by a $p$ value) of trial results are usually presented with no indication of whether the trial results really follow a bell curve.

Examples of all these expensive and potentially deadly transgressions of good medical science appear in all the individual Myths. Here is an introduction to some of these transgressions.
Since the use of Medline and other online search engines, such as PubMed, often yields only abstracts of articles in medical and nutritional journals, it is vital for authors to include all the important findings in the abstract. When press releases based on imminent or actual publications in medical journals are distributed to reporters, the press release is likely to include only the results in the abstract of the paper. Even medical reporters of large news organizations are easily fooled. Reporters feel they have done enough if they quote an "expert". You would be appalled to find how often only

favorable results are cited in an abstract (Kauffman, 2004); many examples are given in the individual chapters that follow.

The use of unnamed ghostwriters and figurehead authors in papers on drug research has been well documented, along with directions from sponsors to authors about what key phrases to include, and what findings to de-emphasize (Cohen, 2001, pp129-165). At least two recent cases of biased selection of references in support of a predetermined position have been exposed (Ravnskov et al., 2002; Ravnskov, 2003). By these methods, incomplete or misinformation from highly-regarded medical journals is used to support promotion of drugs, tests, or devices.

Why should you care? Most of you do not read medical papers as a hobby the way I do. Because these papers are held up as the best possible and honest authority on medical trials, and quoted as authoritative.

## Deception with Relative Risk?

Most medical claims usually use a presentation of treatment results based on lowering a relative risk (RR) for some condition. "Take this test or treatment and your chances of a heart attack will drop by 50%." This is the same as saying that the RR = 0.5 if one has the test or treatment compared with similar people who do not. The presentation of RR is a major method used to perpetuate today's medical myths on diet, blood pressure control, cholesterol control, annual mammograms and many other subjects. Because "everybody knows" or claims that the accepted test or treatment is worthwhile, "everybody" is ready to accept a lowering of RR. After all, such claims often reinforce what "everybody knows" already to be true.

A significant fraction of medical papers still report outcomes of epidemiological studies or trials in terms of the relative risk (RR) of a certain condition, such as cardiovascular deaths, or non-fatal heart attacks, without giving the absolute risk. As favorable as the selective endpoint may appear to be for undergoing treatment, it is not possible for either you or your doctor to make any personal or policy decisions unless the absolute change in the death rate with treatment is known. Furthermore, any reduction in the RR of some condition, however large, may be insignificant when the absolute risk is considered. Suppose you were told by your physician that taking a certain drug would cut your risk of acquiring some affliction by 50%. Would you take it? There is not enough information for you to decide. Suppose taking the drug for 10 years cut your absolute risk of acquiring the sickness from 2 in a million to 1 in a million, a 50% drop in RR. Would you take it based on such odds? Think of your co-payments of as much as $2400 per year in the USA ($24,000 in 10 years) and the almost inevitable side-effects of drugs. People do buy lottery tickets on worse odds.

An example of failure to give absolute risk, cited in at least two books, appeared in one of the medical papers on the West of Scotland Coronary Prevention Study Group (WOSCOPS) on 6,595 men 45-64 years old with initial mean serum cholesterol level of 272 milligrams per deciliter (mg/dL, the same as 7.0 millimoles per liter, or 7.0 mmol/L).

Half the men in the WOSCOPS trial were assigned 40 mg pravastatin (Pravachol™) daily, and the other half were assigned placebo, and all were followed for a mean of 4.9 years. Results in the Abstract included the statement, "We observed a 22% reduction in the risk of death from any cause in the pravastatin group (95% CI = 0-40%, $p = 0.051$)" (Shepherd et al, 1995). Sounds good — after all a mortality rate was actually given.

The CI is the "confidence index" obtained by assuming (it is almost never proven) that the data from both the active treatment group and the placebo group follow a bell curve (or gaussian, or normal curve). The 95% CI gives the range that 95% of the data would fall into, if the data followed a bell curve. In this case, it means that there was a 95% chance (19/20ths) that the 22% reduction in the risk of death from any cause observed in the pravastatin group was actually somewhere between 0% and 40% based on the laws of chance. This also means that there was about 1 chance in 20 that there was no reduction in mortality due to the use of pravastatin, but that the reduction happened by chance.

In this case the *p*-value of 0.051 was supposed to show that there were only 5.1 chances in 100 that the actual RR of death did *not* fall between 0 and 40% reduction of RR by chance alone, rather than because of the drug. By convention, this would be called "barely significant". Since the 1920s, the convention has been to call results with a *p*-value of under 0.05 "significant"; but this is completely arbitrary.

The actual absolute percentage of the men alive after 4.9 years in the placebo group was 95.9%, and in the pravastatin group it was 96.8%, an absolute difference of just 0.9%; the difference amounts to only 0.18% per year! (Gigerenzer, 2002, pp34-36; Ravnskov, 2000, pp200-202). This simple representation of the outcome, the % still alive, was not seen in either the abstract or the discussion of this paper, or given the slightest consideration in the online Physicians Desk Reference (PDR) Family Guide to Prescription Drugs on pravastatin: (http://www.pdrhealth.com/drug_info/rxdrugprofiles/drugs/pra1344.shtml).

Still another simple way to look at the result of this trial is to note that the reciprocal of 0.18% is 556. This is the "number needed to treat" (NNT) of people to prevent 1 death for just 1 year! Looking at 4.9 years for the whole duration of the trial, the NNT was 111, because 9 deaths among 1,000 patients (about 1 in 111) were prevented by the drug. So 110 people of 111 had no benefit of not dying, but all suffered the side-effects and the costs.

Myths 1, 3 and 4 will show that this very minor benefit is the norm, at best, for most of the drugs sold to treat common chronic conditions.

## The Operation was a Success, but the Patient Died

Still another misleading ploy is the failure to report *all-cause* death rates for some treatment or drug, instead giving only the reduction in some non-fatal condition, such as the lowering of blood pressure or serum cholesterol. The chapter on aspirin (Myth 1) describes an example of this game, where aspirin significantly reduces the rate of non-fatal heart attacks, but increases the all-cause death rate slightly. Since all-cause death rates are always available and not subject to medical examiner bias, there is no ethical reason not to include them (Gigerenzer, 2002; Ravnskov, 2000).

An especially egregious failure to give changes in the all-cause mortality rates is in the use of cancer treatments, where radiation or chemotherapy really does lower cancer death rates, yet with no real effect on all-cause mortality (Kauffman, 2002, 2003), because these treatments change the cause of death, typically to heart attacks, new cancers or infection (see Myth 10).

## More Ways to Subvert Medical Trials

Expensive randomized clinical trials (RCTs) may also have flaws in design or be subject to the impossibility of double blinding, as in the case of anti-cholesterol and anti-cancer drugs, because of their unmistakable side effects, which provide a strong placebo (favorable mental) effect. Even the lack of placebo controls is sometimes falsely justified by a perverted medical ethic, the often false assertion that the standard treatment is actually beneficial, and that failure to provide it is unethical (Kauffman, 2004). Sometimes clinical observations depict outcomes in chronic diseases more accurately than RCTs (O'Brien, 2003).

Yet another game played in designing trials reported to the FDA or in papers in medical journals is failure to compare trial results with earlier work, or with competitor's drugs (Kauffman, 2002, 2003), which is bad science. This is compounded when reports of trial results do not make comparisons with over-the-counter drugs or supplements or generic drugs. A generic drug has exactly the same active ingredient as its prescription ancestor.

The subjects selected for trials may often be of middle ages, say 20-60, who frequently will metabolize a drug faster than children or the elderly, yet lower doses of the drug for slow metabolizers are rarely worked out (Cohen, 2001).

What many physicians and insurers do not realize is that only the studies with the most favorable results on tests, devices and drugs are sent to the FDA or published. Trial results sent to the FDA do not have to be peer-reviewed, which is worthwhile when done honestly. Companies routinely delay or prevent publications that show their drugs to be ineffective. For instance, it is said that a majority of studies on Zoloft™, one of the antidepressant drugs called an SSRI, showed it to be no better than placebo: (http://www.washingtonmonthly.com/features/2004/0404.brownlee.html).

In 1990, more than a decade after antiarrhythmic drugs had been introduced, it was estimated that they were killing more Americans every year than had died in action in the Vietnam War. No such data indicating lethality had been published as a result of clinical trials (Chalmers, 2004). The journals are also to blame, often refusing to publish on "treatment has no effect" trials and studies (Houston, 2004). Legislation in Spain, to have taken effect on 1 May 04, obliges drug companies to publish in peer-reviewed journals all the results of trials carried out in Spain. Also, all papers on drug trials are to give the sources of financial support for the trial and all of the papers' authors (Shashok, 2004).

Even in 2004 it was necessary for a law student to use the Freedom of Information Act along with congressional intercession to obtain information from the FDA on the true incidence of side-effects of a common anti-cholesterol drug. The details are in Myth 3.

Many of the class-action lawsuits about damaging drugs have actual merit, and are not merely the antics of greedy attorneys (www.DrugIntel.com).

Perversions of clinical trials by Big Pharma became so outrageous that 11 of the most read general medical journals agreed that, as of 1 Jul 05, no results of clinical trials would be published by these journals unless the goals and design of the trial was pre-registered in an accessible form on the internet. This substantiates my contention that medical papers on trials that appear very well done are, even so, overstating the benefits of drugs, imaging, tests, etc., by changing the duration or endpoints of a trial on the fly to favor a product.


## Perversion of Peer Review

Peer Review has been the class act for making scientific papers in journals, not just medical ones, more accurate and balanced. The editor of the journal sends the manuscript to 1-3 anonymous (to the authors) reviewers or referees for comment. If the comments are very negative, the paper will not be published. Often a rewrite or more work will make a paper acceptable. However, reviewers have their biases, too, and sometimes flaunt their anonymity by unwarranted criticism or sloppy review. Or they are selected because the editor knows they will provide a favorable review.

Writing in *New Statesman,* Colin Tudge opined: "Peer review? Well, it has never been quite what it was made out to be. There has always been bias. Much worse, however, is the state described by Richard Horton, editor of the *Lancet,* in *The New York Review of Books* last month [March, 2004]. Drug companies now pay academics to give papers at international conferences, reporting favourable results from trials. (The companies also pick up all the other delegates' expenses, including evening concerts and day trips, and generally shower them with gifts. I have picked up the odd diary myself over the years.) These papers are then published, and commonly appear as supplements in respectable scientific journals, often with little or no peer review and with no direct input from the editor. This is public relations, but it is solemnized by the reputation of the journal, in turn built up by the honesty of others."

(http://www.afr.com/articles/2004/04/29/1083224511201.html) There is no reason to believe that the results of clinical trials submitted to the FDA are any less biased than what is published in journals. Nor is there any reason to think that the trial results submitted include the ones with the poorest results.

While the *Journal of the American Medical Association*, the *British Medical Journal*, *The Lancet*, and the *New England Journal of Medicine*, among others, are to be commended for publishing devastating exposés of conflicts-of-interest and tips on spotting misleading presentation of data, the sad truth is that every medical paper, even in these journals, must be judged on its own merits and sources of funding. "The predominance of positive results in published reports might also be associated with the income journals receive from drug-company advertising. As a result, some editors might find it difficult not to comply with industry's wishes to publish material, no matter how poor the study [report] might be..." (Collier & Iheanacho, 2002). According to Durmond Rennie, MD, when he was Senior Editor of the *Journal of the American Medical Association*, "...There seems to be no study too fragmented, no hypothesis too trivial, no literature citation too biased or too egotistical, no [trial] design too warped, no methodology too bungled, no presentation of results too self-serving, no argument too circular, no conclusions too trifling or too unjustified...for a paper to end up in print" (Anderson, 1992, p101). On the other hand, some papers are paragons of brilliance, teamwork, persistence (some studies have followed subjects for up to 50 years), and clear, complete, and honest reporting. No other system for vetting research reports has been any better.


## A Medical Mutiny

Appendix A lists a number of other books and some websites which also may be considered accurate exposés of malignant medical myths, along with the ones already cited. All you can do is learn the "usual" tricks, make judgments with care, and study about what tests or treatments you will accept — even those your medical provider says you must undergo or die. A perfect example is that of Michael Gearin-Tosh, a teacher of English Literature at Oxford University. When he was 54 years old, he was diagnosed with multiple myeloma, and told to begin chemotherapy within a week. "Refuse our treatment and you will be dead in less than a year" he was told. He asked how much longer he would live if he accepted chemotherapy. "Nobody knows, but longer...2-3 years at most." After seeking other opinions on the value of chemotherapy, Gearin-Tosh refused in favor of a combination of alternatives. Eight years later Gearin-Tosh was still alive and employed (Angier, 2002).


## Summing Up

So the "shocking" revelations of Dr. Allen Roses on the minimal benefits of common drugs are only the tip of the iceberg. As you will find in some of the chapters, several of the best-selling classes of drugs are of no benefit at all where it really counts — making you live longer or feel better. The figures Dr. Roses cites for effectiveness probably refer to some surrogate or mixed endpoints, so even his figures for benefit are probably exaggerated.

Some drugs would be of greater benefit if used at lower doses than are prescribed or in which they are available (Cohen, 2001). Many create nutritional deficiencies, and many of those can be counteracted by taking vitamins and supplements. This advice almost never appears in the physicians or manufacturers instructions for the drug, and is almost never added to the label on a prescription by the pharmacist (Pelton & LaValle, 2000).

Widely used screening tests are often of no value in symptomless populations in extending lifespan because early treatment of some conditions is no more effective than later treatment. Because of the great number of false positives in many tests, great costs for further testing are mostly wasted. Excessive treatment based on false positives damages patients.

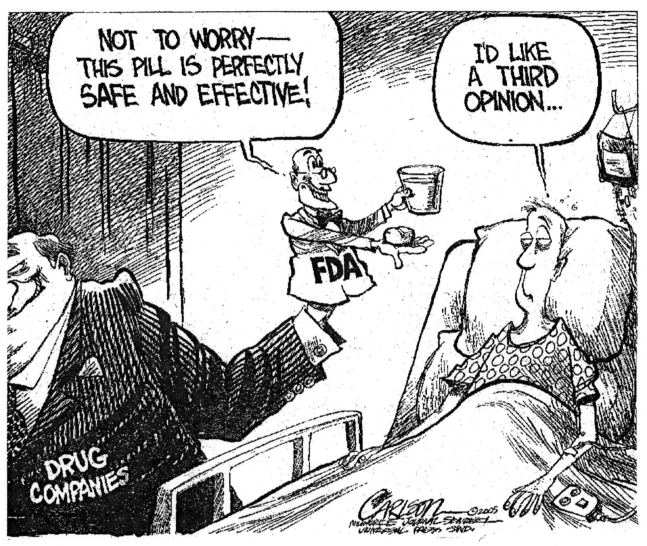

AGENCY CAPTURE

*The Trentonian,* Trenton, NJ, 9 March 05, p24

Most of you are skeptical about advertising claims, but you should be shocked at the lack of reliability of claims by many academic researchers or government officials. You should be shocked at the perversion of RCTs as reported in medical journals, a theme that will be pursued throughout this book. Despite the serious flaws in the medical peer-review system, there are many valuable and accurate medical papers. Flaws in trials or flawed reporting of trials is important to understand because these reports are the sort of evidence the FDA uses to judge drugs, devices and tests. Press releases and advertising are based on the same sort of evidence, as is the direct promotion of drugs, devices and tests to physicians by armies of "detail women".

What if you cannot follow medical papers or you do not have the time? By reading this book, you will have a good introduction to the games played in advertising, press releases, package inserts and even medical papers in peer-reviewed (refereed) journals. You will be shown that the Physicians Desk Reference (PDR), the Family PDR Online and the AHFS Drug Information compendium put together by pharmacists all perpetuate many of the Malignant Medical Myths.

On the other hand, a sure sign of quackery or junk medicine is a radio or television announcement, a book, a report, or a newsletter claim of medical progress in which no RCTs, or even clinical observations on patients are cited, preferably ones which have been published in peer-reviewed journals. Anecdotes usually are not worth much. Often in print media there is a list of references, but without individual citations in the text, as done in this book, making it almost impossible to find which reference supports a given statement. This is compounded when the titles of the references are left out. The authors of such things are saying: "trust me". That is why this book contains a lot of references and a lot of data. You do not have to trust me, because you can look up my sources. You should ultimately be able to decide which authors or websites you trust, either on specific issues or in general.

In the USA you are the final judge of what medical care you will accept. By avoiding useless testing and treatment, your medical insurance, which may have a lifetime dollar limit, may actually last your lifetime. With the help of this book and other sources cited, you ought to be less likely to fall victim of a Malignant Medical Myth.

Introduction Acknowledgement

Fred Ottoboni, PhD, MPH, Alice Ottoboni, PhD, and Frances E. H. Pane, MSLS, edited the Introduction.

Introduction References

Anderson M (1992). *Impostors in the Temple,* New York, NY: Simon & Schuster.

Angier N ( 2002). *New York Times Book Review. Physician, Take a Hike,* of *Living Proof, A Medical Mutiny,* by Michael Gearin-Tosh, 5 Jun 2002.

Anon. (1990). Super-heated babies' milk can lead to brain damage. *Examiner* 13 Feb:21.

Anon. (2003). Secrecy damages the NIH. *Nature,* 426(6968):739.

Bogaty P, Brophy J (2003). Increasing burden of treatment in the acute coronary syndromes: Is it justified? *Lancet,* 361:1813-1816.

Carter, James P., *Racketeering in Medicine: The Suppression of Alternatives.* Norfolk, VA: Hampton Roads Press, 1992.

Chalmers I (2004). In the dark. *New Scientist,* 181(2437):19 (6 Mar 04).

Cohen JS (2001). *Over Dose. The Case Against the drug Companies.* New York, NY: Tarcher/Putnam.

Collier J, Iheanacho I (2002). The pharmaceutical industry as an informant. *The Lancet* 360:1405-9.

Fisher B, Jeong J-H, Anderson S, Bryant J, Fisher ER, Wolmark N (2002). Twenty-Five Year Follow-Up of a Randomized Trial Comparing Radical Mastectomy, Total Mastectomy, and Total Mastectomy Followed by Radiation. *New England Journal of Medicine,* 347(8):567-575.

Fleming TR, DeMets DL (1996). Surrogate end points in clinical trials: are we being misled? *Annals of Internal Medicine,* 125:605-613.

Gigerenzer G (2002). *Calculated Risks: How to Know When the Numbers Deceive You.* New York, N.Y: Simon & Schuster, p34.

Goozner, M (2005). GoozNews Update: FDA Once Again Packs Its Advisory Committees September 09. http://www.gooznews.com/archives/000187.html

Houston R (2004). Publish or be damned. *New Scientist,* 182(2442):32 (10 Apr 04).

Kauffman JM (2002). Book Review of "The Burzynski Breakthrough" by Thomas D. Elias, *Journal of Scientific Exploration,* 16(3):514-521.

Kauffman JM (2003). Book Review of "The Burzynski Breakthrough" by Thomas D. Elias, *Journal of American Physicians and Surgeons,* 8(1):30-31.

Kauffman JM, McGee CT (2004). Are the biopositive effects of Xrays the only benefits of repetitive mammograms? *Medical Hypotheses,* 62(5):674-678.

Kauffman JM (2004). Bias in Recent Papers on Diets and Drugs in Peer-Reviewed Medical Journals. *Journal of American Physicians and Surgeons,* 9(1):11-14.

Lubec G, Wolf C, Bartosch B (1989). Aminoacid isomerisation and microwave exposure. *The Lancet* 2(8676, 9 Dec):1392.

McGee, CT (2001). *Heart Frauds: Uncovering the Biggest Health Scam in History,* Colorado Springs, CO: HealthWise Pubs.

Moore TJ (1998). *Prescription for Disaster. The Hidden Dangers in Your Medicine Cabinet.* New York, NY: Simon & Schuster.

Moss RW (2000). *Questioning Chemotherapy,* Brooklyn, NY: Equinox Press.

O'Brien LJ (2003). Misplaced notions of simplicity, denial of complexity (i.e., value of randomized controlled clinical trials). *BMJ Rapid Response* ; July 11, 2003.

Ottoboni A, Ottoboni, F (2002). *The Modern Nutritional Diseases: heart disease, stroke, type-2 diabetes, obesity, cancer, and how to prevent them.* Sparks, NV: Vincente Books.

PCD (2003). Madness. Physicians for Civil Defense, *Civil Defense Perspectives* 19(2):2.

Pelton R, LaValle JB (2000). *The Nutritional Cost of Prescription Drugs,* Englewood, CO: Perspective/Morton.

Press E, Washburn J (2000). The Kept University. *The Atlantic Monthly,* March, 39-54.

Ravnskov U (2000).*The Cholesterol Myths: Exposing the Fallacy that Saturated Fat and Cholesterol Cause Heart Disease,* Washington, DC: New Trends Publishing.

Ravnskov U, Allen C, Atrens D, et al. (2002). Studies of dietary fat and heart disease. *Science,* 292:1464-1465.

Ravnskov U (2003). Retreat of the diet-heart hypothesis. *Journal of American Physicians and Surgeons,* 8(3):94-5.

Robin ED (1984). *Matters of Life & Death: Risks vs. Benefits of Medical Care.* Stanford, CA: Stanford University Lumini Association.

Robinson J (2001). *Prescription Games. Money, Ego, and Power Inside the Global Pharmaceutical Industry.* Toronto, Ontario: McClelland & Stewart.

Schieber A, Bruckner H, Rupp-Classen M, et al. (1997). Evaluation of D-amino acid levels in rat by gas chromatography-selected ion monitoring mass spectrometry: no evidence for subacute toxicity of orally fed D-proline and D-aspartic acid. *Journal of Chromatography B: Biomedical and Scientific Applications* 691(1):1-12.

Shashok K (2004). Publish or be damned. *New Scientist,* 182(2442):32 (10 Apr 04).

Shepherd J, Cobbe SM, Ford I, et al. (1995) Prevention of coronary heart disease with pravastatin in men with hypercholesterolemia. *New England Journal of Medicine,* 333:1301-7.

Smith CS, Pell JP (2003). Parachute use to prevent major trauma related to gravitational challenge:the systematic review of randomised controlled trials. *British Medical Journal,* 327:1459-1461.

Welch, H. Gilbert, *Should I Be Tested for Cancer? Maybe Not and Here's Why,* Berkeley, CA, USA, University of California Press, 2004.

Willman D (2003). Stealth Merger: Drug Companies and Government Medical Research. *The Los Angeles Times,* 7 Dec 03, p1.

# Myth 1: Taking an Aspirin a Day Forever Will Make You Live Longer

*"Nothing is Simple." --Harry Rowe Mimno, Professor of Applied Physics, Harvard University*

<u>An Overview by an Enlightened Family Physician</u>

You would think by now the aspirin issue had been put to rest long ago. Yet the debate still continues with the primary care physician pinioned right in the center, trying to decide which tune to follow. Three decades ago, right in the middle of my 23 year "tour of duty" as a family doctor, the general consensus, the tune to which we all danced, was that for all males over the age of 50 (and probably women as well), the benefits of a baby aspirin daily far outweighed possible risks. It seemed logical that inhibition of platelet clumping to make blood clots, the proven mechanism of action of aspirin in men, would be helpful in both primary and secondary prevention of myocardial infarctions (MIs or heart attacks) and, although women may come from Venus and men from Mars, I never saw any strong reason to withhold this medication from women.

You give 81 mg of "baby" aspirin to 1,000 people and 25 of them will likely bleed excessively into their tissues and return to the office looking like victims of physical assault. Another 25 will have no observable effect on platelets whatsoever, demonstrating complete insensitivity to aspirin at that dose. That is what makes medicine an art rather than a science. Our DNA mandate is such that no two of us are alike and that goes for reactions to medicines of all kinds. So in public health as in primary and secondary prevention of MIs, you try to find the middle road when sometimes there is no such thing.

And now we find that the results of longitudinal studies of large numbers of people are not nearly as supportive of aspirin as we once thought. I have heard doctors say as they go off for their year of self-sacrifice into third world countries, "You give me all the salt, penicillin and aspirin I need and I can practice medicine anywhere." How much can you do with salt? "They" have now taken away penicillin with threats of dire sensitivity reactions and a limited spectrum of effectiveness. What if they take away our aspirin?

First of all, the buffer in aspirin has proven to be critical for its vital magnesium content. Secondly, after critical appraisal of side effects and all cause death rates, the use of low dose aspirin in primary prevention can no longer be supported. Secondary prevention is quite another matter with very favorable outcomes for limited periods of times after the thrombotic event (clot). Thankfully, this still fits with our knowledge of relevant pathophysiology - the inhibition of platelet stickiness by aspirin. In secondary prevention you are dealing with an endothelial wound — damage to an arterial wall — and aspirin during the healing period seems reasonable. In primary prevention there is no wound – this is a different kind of problem. So our challenge for rational aspirin use seems to be one of identifying those patients at risk, those with open endothelial lesions or those very likely to have them.

Since we now better understand the vital role of inflammation in atherosclerosis we are in need of better markers of inflammation to guide our identification of those at risk. Our C-Reactive Protein (CRP) is a weak step in that direction, but a much better marker is necessary. With such a marker we physicians would have little doubt in determining which patients to place on aspirin and the super-aspirins, which surely will follow, now that we are focusing on the true etiology of inflammation and unwanted blood clots. On this subject of inflammation, we are indebted to Kauffman's suggestion of such aspirin substitutes as oils with omega-3 fatty-acids, coenzyme Q10, magnesium, and even vitamin E, all of which address inflammation or other aspects of heart health at least as effectively as aspirin, if not more so, and they do so with near absence of side effects.

-------Duane Graveline, MD, MPH, astronaut, flight surgeon (Spacedoc)


## Part A: The Aspirin Controversy


### Introduction

The most common advice about aspirin given in books and articles for general audiences is to take a daily aspirin forever for fewer heart attacks and the promise of a longer life.  Most physicians in the USA and elsewhere give similar advice. Many practicing cardiologists and other physicians still do not understand the findings in clinical studies, and believe that this was all settled 15 years ago, when the results of the Physicians Health Group Study (PHS 89) were published in *The New England Journal of Medicine.* The press releases on this study were quite simplistic in reporting that daily aspirin led to fewer *first* heart attacks, which it did. Most MDs make use of the findings they think were reported in that study to recommend daily aspirin, typically 81 mg and enteric coated (see below).

A few MDs and others claim that flaws exist in some of the largest and formerly best-regarded studies, including PHS 89. They cast doubt on whether what was taken that was supposed to be aspirin was actually aspirin alone, and that the other compounds mixed with the aspirin produced some or all of the beneficial effects. They noted that the implied promise of longer life was not fulfilled, and that the side-effects of aspirin are not negligible.

This chapter will show that careful examination of original peer-reviewed papers will allow us draw our own conclusions about who could benefit by taking aspirin. These may be at odds with some strongly-held opinions and advertising.  The following skeptical examination of the benefits of aspirin, as broadcast by many sources, and attributed to trials in the peer-reviewed medical literature, shows frequent misinterpretation or worse by writers for lay audiences. Purveyors of aspirin exaggerate its value. Yet you will be shown that aspirin does have some merit in prevention of *second* heart attacks. So the whole story is not simple, but you will understand it.

As a result of the controversy, studies of the supposed benefits of aspirin in preventing heart attacks continued during the 1990s and to the present day.


### What is Aspirin?

What chemists call the "structural formula" for aspirin is shown in Figure 1-1.  The most common chemical name for this organic compound is acetylsalicylic acid (ASA).  The acetyl part is

Figure 1-1:  Structural Formula of Aspirin (Acetylsalicylic Acid or ASA)

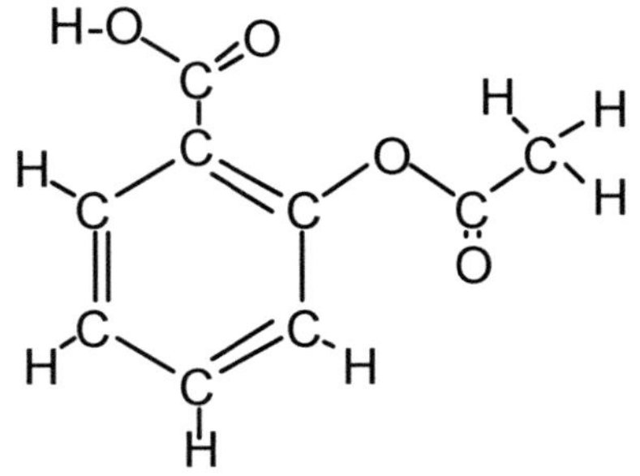

-(C=O)CH$_3$, and the acid part is -CO$_2$H. There are at least 32 other names for it, mostly trade names (Windholz, 1976). It is an early example of a synthetic drug, since this particular compound is not found in nature.

It was first synthesized (constructed from other compounds) by Carl R. Gerhardt in 1853 (Mustard, 1982). Aspirin was not "invented" in 1897 as stated in the book *The Aspirin Wars* (Mann & Plummer, 1991, p7 and cover). The major therapeutic use of aspirin in providing relief from the pain of rheumatoid arthritis was recognized by Felix Hoffman, an employee of Bayer AG, in 1897, who administered aspirin to his father, who tolerated aspirin much better than other salicylates already in use, such as sodium salicylate made from plant sources. This simple compound, aspirin, was difficult to purify, and would decompose during storage if not very pure by reaction with water. The odor of old, impure aspirin is that of acetic acid (CH$_3$-CO$_2$H), the active compound in vinegar.

First trademarked in 1899 by Bayer AG (Vane & Botting, 1992), Leverkusen, Germany, the name Aspirin™ became a generic term for ASA in the manner of xerox, kleenex and frigidaire. For most of a century aspirin has been used as the preferred treatment for arthritis pain, and has been used for headache, fever, and, in the past 15 years, for prevention of heart attacks. It has been called the most successful drug in history. A decade ago 1 in 5 Americans took aspirin every day (*The Aspirin Wars,* cover; Lemaitre et al., 2003). In 2003, 40 million pounds of aspirin were produced in the USA — 200 tablets for each person in this nation. (http://www.newswithviews.com/Howenstine/james10.htm)

Bayer was luckier with aspirin than with its older best-selling drug, which was also made by acetylating a natural product, morphine, to make diacetylmorphine, said to be non-addicting and to have fewer side-effects than morphine. The diacetylmorphine was sold as a key ingredient in cough medicine, for pain relief, and many thought it was a fine tranquilizer, until side-effects, finally recognized, led Bayer to take this drug off the market after about 15 years. Bayer wanted a catchy name for secrecy about the content, and to match the -in ending of several other drugs of the late 19th century, so they called it heroin (Jeffreys, 2004, pp71-72).

Not until the 1970s was the mystery solved of how aspirin worked to relieve arthritis and headache pain! Sir John Vane was awarded a Nobel Prize for uncovering the mode of action of aspirin (Feinman, 1993). Aspirin inhibits the enzyme cyclooxygenase, preventing the cells of the body from making certain prostaglandins (a class of 20-carbon compounds that send signals around the body), such as thromboxane A2, that cause inflammation, thus easing the pain of arthritis or headache. Aspirin also limits the amounts of other prostaglandins your body can produce, ones which cause the clumping of blood platelets to form clots. The clots, or thromboses, are responsible for "ischemic events", which are the local anemias, strokes, or blood shortages, caused by blockage of arteries. When these are coronary arteries, the blockages are called "heart attacks" of the myocardial infarction (MI) type. The common slogan "aspirin thins the blood" is not strictly true; aspirin prevents clot formation by platelets, thus preventing heart attacks. These are two separate and desirable drug actions. Like most drugs, aspirin has still other actions which are undesirable, and are called side-effects. Some will be discussed later.

The aspirin content of a standard aspirin tablet is 325 milligrams (mg). Extra-strength or arthritis-strength tablets contain 500 mg. For other uses tablets containing 160 and 81 mg are available. The 81 mg size is often called "baby aspirin" and is now the most commonly recommended dose size to prevent heart attacks.

Enteric-coated aspirin tablets resist the acidic environment of the stomach; the aspirin is absorbed in the alkaline small intestine, avoiding damage to the lining of the stomach. You would not expect "fast, *fast*, FAST relief of headache" with these, but some studies showed that stomach erosions and ulcers were less frequent (McDonald, 1982).

"Buffered" aspirin is no faster than plain aspirin (*The Aspirin Wars,* p164) and only slightly less irritating, if at all (www.mayohealth.org). Besides containing 325 mg of aspirin, a Bufferin™

tablet has an actual alkali (anti-acid) content of 158 mg of calcium carbonate, 63 mg of magnesium oxide and 34 mg of magnesium carbonate; Bayer Aspirin with Stomach Guard is the same. Either brand of tablet provides a total of 48 mg of magnesium, which may also be important for preventing heart attacks. These details are important in trying to unravel the conflicting claims about aspirin. In chemical terms, not just with drugs, a "buffer" is some reagent or combination of reagents that will resist a change in acidity. However, it is not clear that the irritating effects of aspirin on the stomach are due to its acidity, which is why combining it with common alkalies to neutralize the acidity of aspirin does not eliminate all of its irritating effects.

## Primary vs. Secondary Prevention of Heart Attacks

One must be skeptical about any recommendation for or against aspirin that does not distinguish between primary and secondary prevention of heart attacks. Primary means that people not at any particular risk of heart attack may prevent a fraction of potential *first* heart attacks from occurring by taking small doses of aspirin for a long period. Any of the side effects of aspirin can be serious if people begin taking it at age 45-50 and continue for 30-40 years. Secondary prevention means that actual victims of heart attack or unstable angina, a high-risk group, may prevent a fraction of *second or further* cardiovascular problems by taking aspirin. Any recommendation you see for or against aspirin that does not make this distinction can be disregarded as superficial.

*The Aspirin Wars* distinguished between primary prevention of first heart attacks and secondary prevention of subsequent heart attacks on p11 quite well, and described the U. S. Food and Drug Administration (FDA) decision to allow advertising for second heart attacks, but not for first heart attacks, due to an unusual number of strokes in the aspirin-using group in a large study on primary prevention, a prescient decision. The FDA reaffirmed its position in December, 2003. But by p334 in *The Aspirin Wars:* "...aspirin is the drug of doctors' dreams. It is hugely effective. One aspirin a day, or every other day, will save hundreds of thousands of lives a year. It can be taken safely by more people than almost any other drug... It is likely to remain the only heart attack preventive sold in grocery stores for years to come." You will be shown that this later fit of enthusiasm in *The Aspirin Wars* is unwarranted.

## Surrogate End Points in Clinical Trials: Are We Being Misled?

This is the title of an unusual medical paper (Fleming & DeMets, 1996). Randomized clinical trials (RCTs) are now the standard scientific method for evaluating a new drug or a new use for an old drug. The true endpoint in most trials should be cure of a disease or condition, as indicated by longer lifespan (lower all-cause death rate, also called mortality) of good quality (fewer adverse side-effects) or, at least, reduction of symptoms. A surrogate endpoint is a laboratory measurement or a physical sign used as a convenient substitute for a clinically meaningful endpoint that measures survival or well-being directly. Changes induced by a therapy on a surrogate endpoint are supposed to reflect changes in a clinically real endpoint; but all too often, they do not. Examples of surrogate endpoints are reduction of cholesterol level (see Myth 3) or blood pressure (see Myth 4), two parameters easy to measure in the short term.

A meta-analysis (summation of results) of 50 cholesterol-lowering interventions examined by clinical trials, including diet, resins and lovastatin (the first statin drug, Mevacor™), showed that cholesterol levels were lowered an average of 10%, but there was a 1% *increase* in overall mortality. This should not have been a surprise, since high blood cholesterol levels are only loosely correlated with cardiovascular trouble, not an actual cause of it, as homocysteine is (see Myth 3), (McCully & McCully, 1999). Cholesterol levels rise with age naturally, as does cardiovascular trouble, so many researchers were fooled by claims of a greater correlation than there really ever was (see Myth 3). And this was truly a correlation without a cause, as those who study health statistics are always taught.

A meta-analysis of trials of early calcium channel blockers, even though they really do lower blood pressure, showed harmful effects overall, including more fatal heart attacks (see Myth 4). Here again, the surrogate endpoint of blood pressure was misleading. In addition, two antiarrhythmia drugs approved by the FDA in the 1980s, encainide and flecainide, clearly suppressed arrhythmias, as seen by electrocardiograms (EKGs), the surrogate endpoint. However, in trials of antiarrhythmia drugs, it was found that 3 times as many patients in the drug group died as in the placebo group!

In evaluating aspirin, it is, therefore, not enough to show reduction in the rate of non-fatal heart attacks or other undesirable vascular events, such as clots; one must determine total (all-cause) death rates (mortality) for a period of many years in order to find whether some toxic effect of aspirin is countering its positive effect on preventing non-fatal heart attacks. On the other hand, one does not want to carry on trials for *too* many years since the ultimate death rates of treatment and placebo groups converge — to 100%. It turns out that prevention of non-fatal heart attacks does not necessarily lead to lower all-cause death rates. Aspirin and other drugs can and do prevent clots, but they also can cause side-effects that lead to hemorrhagic stroke or sudden cardiac death due to an arrhythmia. The actual results of trials on aspirin will be given later.

## Whisper Down the Alley

This is one name for a grade-school game in which someone in a classroom whispers a phrase of a few words to the nearest student, who whispers the same phrase (supposedly) to the next student. The output of the 30th or so student is compared with the input and all have a good laugh, since the two are never equal.

Adult scientists are not supposed to scramble the input — but some do. Here is an example beginning with a publication of combined results of 25 clinical trials on aspirin. A massive meta-analysis (this is a weighted combination — more subjects means more attention to the bigger trials) of 25 completed clinical trials of *secondary* prevention of MI was reported in the *British Medical Journal (BMJ)* in 1988 (*BMJ*, 1988, adapted with permission). The title: "*Secondary* Prevention of Vascular Disease by Prolonged Antiplatelet Treatment" [italics added] makes clear that most of the patients involved had *already* suffered from MI, transient ischemic attack, unstable angina, or minor stroke. "Antiplatelet Treatment" indicates that aspirin was not the only drug tested; these facts are, of course, confirmed in the text and tables, of which one of the key tables is reproduced here as Figure 1-2. It is important that you take some time to understand this Figure, since it is a typical example of how medical interventions, not just with drugs, are presented in medical journals, and how such a presentation can mislead even experienced professionals.

The vertical print at the far left explains that the top group of trials "Cerebrovascular" were done to find the effect of drugs on hemorrhagic stroke rates. The next group down "Myocardial infarction" is for trials that were done to find the effect of drugs on heart attack rates. The final group of two trials were done to find the effect of drugs on angina pain. The next column gave the name, usually an acronym, or location of the trial. Citations to the original reports of each trial were in the text of the *BMJ* article. The next column gives the names of the drug(s) used. Note that only 12 of those 25 trials employed aspirin alone, and note also that only 6 of the 9 trials on the effects of drugs on heart attack, which is all we are considering here, used aspirin alone.

# Figure 1-2. Meta-Analysis of Antipatelet Treatments (BMJ, 1988)

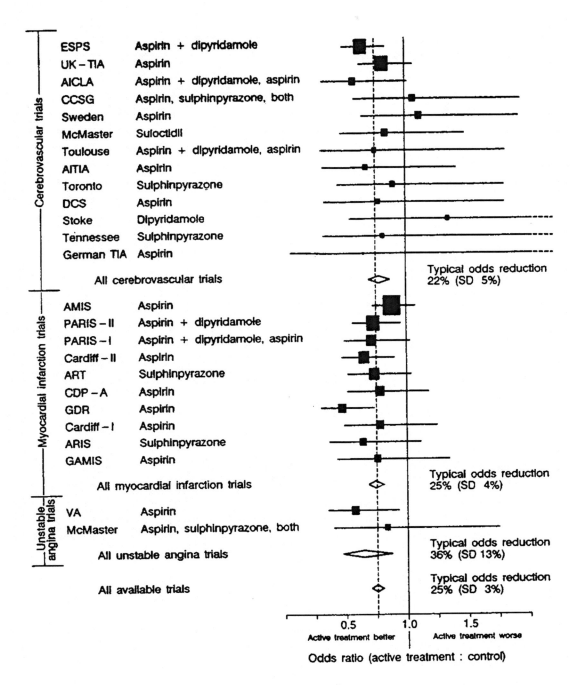

Odds ratios (active treatment:control) for first stroke, myocardial infarction, or vascular death during scheduled treatment period in completed antiplatelet trials. ■—■=Trial results and 99% confidence intervals (area of ■ proportional to amount of information contributed). ◇=Overview results and 95% confidence intervals. Dashed vertical line represents odds ratio of 0·75 suggested by overview of all trial results. Solid vertical line represents odds ratio of unity (no treatment effect).

The results are shown compared with the solid vertical line which corresponds to no difference in results between the treatment and control groups. When the results of treatment were better than those of the controls, the data square is to the left of the vertical line. The area of the square is proportional the the number of subjects in each trial. Note that the largest trial by far, the AMIS trial, showed only about a 10% lower "odds reduction", which is similar to relative risk.

Overall odds (risk) reduction in any vascular death, non-fatal heart attack, and any stroke (combined) was about 25% lower than in the control groups, mostly in the first 2 years of treatment. Also, overall reduction in heart attacks, mostly non-fatal, was 25%. Here is a typical problem with medical papers — all-cause mortality was not reported in Fig. 1-2, even though it had to have been available to the researchers in each trial. All of this Figure uses relative risk (RR), not absolute risk. As will be made clear later, a 25% lower RR of mostly non-fatal heart attacks amounts to only about a 0.1% lowering of absolute risk per year of treatment! Yes, this means that only 1 in 1000 men taking aspirin for 1 year will miss having a heart attack, and probably a non-fatal one at that.

A special note was made that men aged 55-74 with no history of vascular disease for whom aspirin treatment was actually *primary* showed no difference in mortality. Yes, the early aspirin trials were carried out only on men!

This *BMJ* article was cited in *Science*, a publication of the American Association for the Advancement of Science, with reproduction of that same figure, as an excellent example of how to do a meta-analysis, along with an explanation of how to do one (Anon., 1990). The secondary nature of the trials was indicated only by the word "recurrence" and the endpoint was implied to be only "heart attack", omitting strokes and angina. This differs from the legend in Figure 1-2, which includes as endpoints all heart attacks, all strokes, angina, and other vascular deaths.

The *Science* article was cited by Dean Radin in the book *The Conscious Universe* as an example of the power of meta-analysis (Radin, 1997). Here Radin wrote implying that *only* aspirin was involved in the trials covered by the meta-analysis, and that the outcome was *only* for "heart attacks", and he ignored the *secondary* nature of the treatment, which led me to believe, when I read *The Conscious Universe,* that I should have continued using aspirin myself after all, as recommended in *Consumer Reports* (see below).

By the time the perverted information from sources other than the original *BMJ* and *NEJM* articles were picked up in the magazines and newsletters quoted in the next section, in which aspirin was recommended, all balance and important details in the articles were lost. Relative risks were repeated with no conception of the meager changes in the absolute risks of heart attacks. The non-fatal nature of most of the heart attacks prevented was lost. Aspirin's lack of effect on mortality was ignored.

### Recommendations for You to Take Aspirin for *Primary* Prevention of Heart Attacks

Besides the almost universal recommendations for daily aspirin from physicians in the USA, there are a great number of sources of advice in publications for the general public to take aspirin for primary prevention of heart attacks.  Here are a few:

#### Consumer Reports magazine

*Consumer Reports (CR),* with about 5 million subscribers and about 20 million readers, recommended that postmenopausal women, men over 35 with risk factors such as smoking cigarettes, and possibly men over 45 without risk factors all take aspirin daily.  No dose level was given, although the study quoted was based on "one 'aspirin' tablet every other day", and the use of enteric coated aspirin was advised only "if uncoated aspirin caused damage to the stomach". *CR* does not explain how would one know before the damage has already occurred.  "The...[PHS 89] study found that one aspirin tablet every other day cut the rate of initial heart attacks almost in half... The implications were stunning." But then *CR* was very cautious, noting that the clinical study they were citing showed significantly more hemorrhagic strokes (ruptures of blood vessels in the brain), ulcers and allergic reactions, and that no benefit was observed in another trial on healthy male physicians in the UK (*CR,* 1988). While the studies used did not get any citations, the first was certainly the Physicians Health Study (PHS 89) in which 22,071 male physicians were studied for 5 years (PHS 89, 1989), and the second was probably the Medical Research Council study in the UK (BMJ, 1988). *CR's* inclusion of women in its recommendation was irresponsible at best, since women were not present in the trials then. *CR* failed to notice that PHS 89 used Bufferin, not aspirin.

*Health & Healing newsletter*

In his popular newsletter, Julian Whitaker, MD, properly referenced PHS 89, and recommended that everyone take aspirin for primary protection from MI, but at the rate of 162 mg every other day, or 81 mg every day, half the dose used in PHS 89, and Whitaker failed to include the fact that PHS 89 used Bufferin. While the study involved only male physicians, Whitaker did not restrict his recommendations to males. Whitaker wrote that the usual side-effects of aspirin could be avoided by taking the low dose he recommended with a meal, but he gave no evidence for this from trials (Whitaker, 1996).

*Life Extension magazine*

In the February, 2000, issue of *Life Extension* magazine, the recommendation for taking 81 mg of aspirin per day with food is unequivocal: "A lot of people in alternative medicine criticize The Life Extension Foundation for recommending the daily use of low-dose aspirin, but The Foundation stands firm on the recommendations it made in 1983: most healthy people should take low-dose aspirin to specifically reduce their risk of heart attack. Aspirin may protect in ways that supplements do not." (Knorr, 2000) Of the 34 references cited at the end of the article, just 9 were to articles in peer-reviewed journals. The citations were done in such a way that one cannot tell which aspect of the article each one backs, that is, there were no numbers to citations in the text. PHS 89 is not cited, nor is any peer-reviewed paper that shows lower total mortality in low-risk subjects. The article is cleverly laid out with a large space taken up by art work so that it ends on the top half of its last page. The bottom half of the last page is an advertisement for Life Extension Foundation's brand of aspirin. Does this fact make you skeptical of their recommendation?

<u>Recommendations for You *Not* to Take Aspirin for *Primary* Prevention of Heart Attacks</u>

A Linus Pauling website

From an anonymous author on a website trying to bask in the fame of Linus Pauling (www.internetwks.com/pauling/lie/mag.html): "We have been told that all the aspirin studies that 'prove' an aspirin a day keeps a heart attack away -- were with buffered aspirin, i. e., with added magnesium. Our sources point out that it is unlikely that further studies using 'plain' aspirin will be undertaken because preliminary studies always show 'plain' aspirin does not show the same protective effect against heart attacks. So if you still believe what you read in the mass media, make sure that your daily aspirin is buffered! (Or much better yet, take a magnesium tablet instead!)"

*What Doctors Don't Tell You* newsletter

"Possibly the largest collaborative study ever performed in medicine, this meta-analysis (ATC, 1994) pooled the results of some 174 clinical trials from around the world, testing an aggregate of 110,000 patients... The overview was designed to determine whether medium-dose aspirin (75 mg to 325 mg per day) ...could prevent...nonfatal heart attacks, strokes, or deaths in [mostly] high-risk patients... The researchers reckoned that this sort of therapy reduced the risk of [premature] death [a solid endpoint] from one of these causes by one-sixth... This isn't the case with low-risk patients; the study showed that among those taking aspirin as 'primary prevention', although heart attacks were reduced by a third, there was a 'non-significant' increase in nonfatal strokes. However, that increase was cited as 21% (hardly a 'non-significant' increase in our view)... However, the study makes quite clear that for low-risk people or for those with so-called risk factors like high cholesterol, hypertension, or smoking, but without vascular disease, there is no evidence that this so-called preventive therapy does any good. In fact, the risks (particularly of hemorrhage or stroke) may outweigh the benefits. Therefore, there is no scientific justification for your doctor's view that you should start taking aspirin just in case." Thus wrote the editors of the newsletter *What Doctors Don't Tell You* (McTaggart, 1995).

*Second Opinion* newsletter

And from William Campbell Douglass, Jr., MD: "I'm sure you've heard about the study [PHS 89] showing that an aspirin a day prevents heart attacks. In that study, men who took a daily aspirin had 47% [*sic*] fewer heart attacks than men who didn't. What you *haven't* heard, and what I'm sure the aspirin companies don't want you to know, is that the subjects in that study took *buffered* aspirin — aspirin mixed with *magnesium.* Numerous studies have proven that magnesium has a powerful protective effect on your heart. It dilates blood vessels...aids potassium absorption into your cells (preventing heartbeat irregularities)...acts as a natural blood thinner...and keeps your blood cells from clumping together [the anti-platelet effect]; indeed autopsies of heart attack victims almost always find a magnesium deficiency! ...Not only that, but recent studies link aspirin to macular degeneration — the #1 cause of blindness in people over the age of 55! But the biggest strike against aspirin may come from the very study touting its heart benefits. If you read the study's fine print, you'll find that even though the group taking aspirin had 47% fewer heart attacks, there was *no* difference in the death rates of the two groups. That means that death from *other* causes was 47% higher in the aspirin group! So stop taking that daily aspirin! Stick to magnesium instead." (Douglass, 1998) But note Douglass's fractured logic: his assumption that all the heart attacks prevented by "aspirin" were fatal; in fact, most were not.

James Howenstine, MD, website

James Howenstine, MD, posted an aspirin report on his website on 21 Apr 04, in which he notes that 20,000,000 people in the USA are taking daily aspirin to prevent heart attacks and strokes, mostly because of encouragement from their physicians. He noted that the evidence for such a recommendation is not very solid. He also noted that the PHS 89 study showed no decrease in fatal heart attacks, and no improvement in the all-cause mortality rate. He thought that the decrease in non-fatal heart attacks resulted from the presence of magnesium in the Bufferin used in PHS 89. He wrote that aspirin can cause gastrointestinal bleeding, blindness through cataract formation, and liver damage.
(http://www.newswithviews.com/Howenstine/james10.htm).

*Are these people crazy?* Not entirely. Now we know enough to divide the original question that is the subject of this chapter into two separate questions: on *primary* as distinct from *secondary* prevention of heart attacks. Let us go to the original peer-reviewed literature to answer the first of the properly posed questions:

<u>Should You Take Aspirin to Prevent *a First* Heart Attack?</u>

Antiplatelet Trialists' Collaboration, 1988

In the Antiplatelet Trialists' Collaboration (ATC, 1988) there were some low-risk men aged 55-74 for whom aspirin treatment was actually primary. The paper concludes with the opinion that the absolute benefits in *primary* prevention of MI were uncertain because they might be outweighed by a small increase in cerebral or other serious hemorrhagic disease. "Thus only for patients with an appropriate history of vascular disease is there at present clear evidence that antiplatelet treatment [with aspirin] reduces the overall incidence of fatal or disabling vascular disease." This opinion recognizes that the most important endpoint is life extension, not merely minimizing heart attacks, most of which are non-fatal.

Physicians Health Group Study, 1989

Now it is time to take a serious look at the Physicians Health Group Study (PHS 89), from which Figure 1-3 is reproduced. This massive study on 22,071 male physicians in the USA, half taking 325 mg of "aspirin" every other day, and the other half taking placebo, showed that total deaths in the aspirin group over the 5-year period of the study were 4% fewer than in the placebo group (RR = 0.96, $p = 0.64$), thus the difference was not even close to being statistically significant. The reduction in heart attacks was seen only in those aged $\geq 50$. Using the endpoint of life extension, not just non-fatal heart attacks, there was hardly any benefit from taking aspirin. With respect to non-fatal bleeding of several types the aspirin group had a relative risk of 1.32 ($p = 0.00001$). Furthermore, 48 in the aspirin group and 28 in the placebo group required blood transfusions ($p = 0.02$). There really was a significant ($p < 0.00001$) reduction in non-fatal heart attacks of 44% (RR = 0.56). But what did this mean in real benefit? It meant that in a 1-year period the chance of having a non-fatal MI was cut from 0.44% to 0.26%, just a 0.18% per year lower chance to have a non-fatal MI, or just 1 in 555 physicians per year. This had to be calculated from data in the text of PHS 89, since all its Figures were in terms of relative risk.

There is no doubt that PHS 89 used Bufferin, not aspirin. Monthly calendar packs containing either Bufferin or placebo were provided by Bristol-Myers Products. Domenick Mellace of Bristol-Myers was acknowledged for his logistic support. Bristol-Myers contrived to have a 1.5 page advertisement placed just ahead of this paper in the journal. They were careful to advertise Bufferin only for *secondary* prevention as directed by the FDA.

Press releases and the Abstract of PHS 89 grossly exaggerated the benefits of "aspirin". This was the main source of blanket recommendations of physicians that everyone over 50 take daily aspirin, women included, despite the trial protocol of every other day, and the lack of women in the trial.

Is it possible that the reduction in heart attacks was due to the magnesium present in the Bufferin and not the ASA content? The only scientific way to make certain was to run a trial with plain aspirin.

Figure 1-3. Actual Deaths and Causes in the
Physicians Health Group Study on Bufferin (PHS 89).

| Cause* | Aspirin Group | Placebo Group | Relative Risk | 95% Confidence Interval | P Value |
|---|---|---|---|---|---|
| Total cardiovascular deaths† | 81 | 83 | 0.96 | 0.60–1.54 | 0.87 |
| Acute myocardial infarction (410) | 10 | 28 | 0.31 | 0.14–0.68 | 0.004 |
| Other ischemic heart disease (411–414) | 24 | 25 | 0.97 | 0.60–1.55 | 0.89 |
| Sudden death (798) | 22 | 12 | 1.96 | 0.91–4.22 | 0.09 |
| Stroke (430, 431, 434, 436)‡ | 10 | 7 | 1.44 | 0.54–3.88 | 0.47 |
| Other cardiovascular (402, 421, 424, 425, 428, 429, 437, 440, 441) | 15 | 11 | 1.38 | 0.62–3.05 | 0.43 |
| Total noncardiovascular deaths | 124§ | 133 | 0.93 | 0.72–1.20 | 0.59 |
| Total deaths with confirmed cause | 205 | 216 | 0.95 | 0.79–1.15 | 0.60 |
| Total deaths¶ | 217 | 227 | 0.96 | 0.80–1.14 | 0.64 |
| Person-years of observation | 54,894.6 | 54,864.2 | — | — | — |

*Numbers are code numbers of the *International Classification of Diseases*, ninth revision.

†All fatal cardiovascular events are included, regardless of previous nonfatal events.

‡This category includes ischemic (3 in the aspirin group and 3 in the placebo group), hemorrhagic (7 aspirin and 2 placebo), and unknown cause (0 aspirin and 2 placebo).

§This category includes one death due to gastrointestinal hemorrhage.

¶Additional events that could not be confirmed because records were not available included 23 deaths (12 aspirin and 11 placebo), of which 11 were suspected to be cardiovascular (7 aspirin and 4 placebo) and 12 noncardiovascular (5 aspirin and 7 placebo).

Antiplatelet Trialists' Collaboration, 1994

The Antiplatelet Trialists' Collaboration (ATC) in the UK were doing just that, and by 1994, they published a meta-analysis that was now up to 100,000 patients of whom 30,000 were in the low-risk category. The doses were 75-325 mg of plain aspirin per day, but the exact source of the aspirin was not given. "There was no clear evidence on the balance of risks and benefits of antiplatelet therapy in primary prevention in low-risk subjects." (ATC, 1994) In fact a graph was shown with "% free from a vascular event", including fatal, as the ordinate, and "years to first vascular event" as the abscissa. For low risk subjects after 4 years the treated group had 0.4% fewer events, that is, 4 per 1000. This is only 0.1% per year, mostly non-fatal. But this graph included all of the antiplatelet treatments, including 2 trials with drugs that were more effective than aspirin, so it is likely that aspirin was of no benefit in low-risk subjects — no value in *primary* prevention of heart attacks.

UK Physicians Study, 1998

And reported in 1998, a study on about 5500 physicians in the UK on primary prevention of ischemic heart disease (clots in coronary arteries, which cause heart attacks) was carried out with 75 mg of plain aspirin daily in a controlled-release formulation, and for a median time of 7 years. The main effect of aspirin was a 32% reduction in non-fatal heart attacks (less effective than PHS 89 which used double the dose and contained magnesium), but there was an increase of 12% in fatal heart attacks leading to an overall rise in death from all causes of 6%, which was not considered significant (Meade, 1998). The *absolute* reduction in *all* heart attacks per year was only 0.23%, not that different from PHS 89.

Note that there is a 10% absolute increase in overall death rate in the aspirin group in this study compared with the Bufferin group in PHS 89 (+ 6% vs. -4%). Could this spread of 10% of between the two "non-significant" findings have been due to a lack of the beneficial effect of the magnesium in Bufferin? Another difference from PHS 89 is that the men in this UK study were recruited from the quintile considered to be at highest risk for heart attacks based on heredity, smoking, blood pressure and obesity; but this is still a lower-risk group than the one composed of actual victims of heart attacks.

Aspirin in the elderly, 1998

Gender bias in aspirin trials did not end until a paper published in 1998. Randomized clinical trials testing aspirin in 5011 elderly people of average age 72 years, 58% of whom were women, followed for a mean of 4.2 years, showed that use of aspirin caused a 4-fold increase in hemorrhagic stroke ($p = 0.003$) overall, and a 1.6 to 1.8-fold increase (RR = 1.6-1.8) in ischemic stroke in women, but not in men (Kronmal et al., 1998).

Nurses' Health Study, 1999

Based on the Nurses' Health Study involving 79,319 women aged 34-59 years at the beginning (baseline), the role of aspirin in primary prevention of stroke was uncertain (Iso et al., 1999). This was based on a questionnaire, so the reduction, mostly in older women, of large-artery occlusive infarction (another name for ischemic stroke or blocked arteries) by half (1 to 6 aspirin per week) or a doubling of the risk of hemorrhage (15 or more aspirin per week) might have included the use of a large fraction of buffered aspirin. This was not thought important. Total death rates were not included.

Cleveland Clinic cohort study, 2001

The authors of a recent paper in *JAMA* on all-cause mortality according to aspirin use in a prospective*, observational, 3.1-year study came to the conclusion that aspirin use was strongly protective, cutting the death rate from 8% to 4% absolute (Gum et al., 2001). This *JAMA* study was among the first to include women, and the raw data for women should not be ignored: 3.8% of female" aspirin" users died vs. 3.4% of non-users, a mortality risk of 1.12 (Kauffman, 2002).

For the study population as a whole, many of whom were only suspected of having cardiovascular disease (CVD), the raw data showed that 4.5% of "aspirin" users died vs. 4.5% of non-users. The extreme manipulation of data carried out in the form of patient matching to produce a positive result for "aspirin" might have been warranted if the obvious confounding variables had been considered, and a much longer time-frame adopted.

The conclusions of this study contradict both the conclusions of a recent review (Kauffman, 2000) and the arguments of JGF Cleland (Cleland 2002a, 2002b). In the *JAMA* paper, Gum et al.

---

*A prospective study is one whose participants and end-points are selected beforehand. It is considered less biased than a retrospective study in which a population is selected and examined after it has been exposed to its treatment or risk factors (hindsight).

continued to perpetuate the myth that the PHS trial used aspirin (their Ref. 1), when, in fact it used buffered aspirin containing magnesium and calcium. Because Gum et al. did not have the attending physicians distinguish between plain and buffered aspirin in their subjects, the results of their study are inadequate to make a recommendation for treatment, or to draw the conclusions they did on the effectiveness of "aspirin".

Another flaw in their study is that Gum et al. did not match patients for use of either magnesium (Ford, 1999) or vitamins C (Enstrom et al., 1992) or E (Stephens et al., 1996), all of which are more protective against cardiovascular disease than plain aspirin. It is quite plausible that subjects conscientious enough to take "aspirin" on their own might have taken any or all of these, as well as other supplements, since this study did not involve dispensing aspirin to be taken while the subject was observed by a medical person, or checked later for compliance. Nor were patients matched for alcohol or nut consumption. High nut consumption in one study reduced the rate of cardiovascular death  (RR = 0.61), and of all-cause death  (RR = 0.82) in a very old population (Fraser et al., 1997).

The duration of the trial by Gum et al. was much too short at 3.1 years to reveal long-term adverse effects, as shown by the greatly increased risk of cataracts in subjects $\geq$ 55 years old who took aspirin for $\geq$ 10 years (Cumming & Mitchell, 1998).

Gum et al. wrote that "It is less clear if aspirin reduces long-term all-cause mortality in *stable* populations." This was already resolved for men, at least, by the study on 5,500 male physicians in the MRC trial — it does *not*  in a 7-year trial (Meade, 1998), which was available to Gum et al.

## A meta-analysis of 5 aspirin trials, 2002

The results of a meta-analysis of "aspirin" in 5 large trials for primary protection, whose duration was 3-7 years (too short), showed little effect on thrombotic stokes or *all-cause mortality,* but that both non-fatal and fatal myocardial infarction *taken together* were reduced (RR = 0.72). Combining endpoints is a common trick in medical papers to exaggerate a benefit of treatment. These results are quite similar to the raw results of all the earlier studies above.  An involved risk-benefit calculation was recommended (Pignone et al., 2002) in order to decide which future patients should take aspirin; but in view of the unchanging all-cause mortality and very real side-effects in earlier trials, such as the UK Physicians Study reported in 1998, this does not make sense.

## Another meta-analysis of 5 aspirin trials, 2003

And the most recent meta-analysis of 5 trials of aspirin for *primary* prevention which obtained half its data from the ATC and PHS trials described above, and the rest from trials that verged on *secondary* prevention, concluded that: "For apparently healthy individuals whose 10-year risk of a first coronary event is 10% or greater...the benefits of long-term aspirin therapy are likely to outweigh any risks." (Eidelman et al., 2003)   In this meta-analysis there is no distinction between aspirin and buffered aspirin. There is no indication of all-cause death rates; the only mortality event  data are combined with non-fatal events. For hemorrhagic stroke the "aspirin" groups had a RR = 1.69 based on my calculation, not 1.56 as reported, and it is significant.  For vascular death the "aspirin" group had RR = 1.09 based on my calculation, not 0.98 as reported.  The number needed to treat (NNT) to prevent even 1 *non*-fatal MI is 143 for a 5-year period, seemingly an even worse outcome than in the ATC and PHS 89 trials. Therefore, the conclusion by Eidelman et al. quoted above is not supported, especially when one accepts the fact that there is no way to predict a 10-year risk of first heart attack in a given individual. Even the PHS 89 trial whose results were so ballyhooed reduced non-fatal heart attacks by just 0.11% per year absolute (see Fig. 3-7 in Myth 3).

Women's Health Study, 2005

The National Heart, Lung and Blood Institute of the NIH was the major sponsor of the Women's Health Study, whose actual results on aspirin for the primary prevention of heart disease were exaggerated (Nabel, 2005). Its Press Release of 7 Mar 05 followed the Abstract of the article in the *New England Journal of Medicine (NEJM),* (Ridker et al., 2005). In this largest and longest trial on aspirin in women ever, half of 40,000 healthy women 45 or more years old at the start were assigned to 100 mg of aspirin every other day, and half to placebo of like appearance; the duration of the trial was 10 years. Note that this was the lowest dose and longest duration in any of the trials.

It was honestly reported that aspirin did NOT prevent first heart attacks or death from cardiovascular causes. However, neither the press release nor the Abstract of the NEJM paper mentioned that there was no significant difference in all-cause mortality (RR = 0.95, NS), surely the most important end-point.

Stroke was said to be 17% lower with aspirin; this was emphasized as an important benefit. First, note that this is a relative number. The absolute reduction was not given, and it was 0.22% for the 10-year period (for an NNT of 500), or about 0.022 % per year, a trivial benefit. Second, note that this was non-fatal ischemic stroke (clots) only; fatal and hemorrhagic stroke were unchanged. The 26% reduction of ischemic stroke in women 65 or older was also trivial in absolute terms. The actual number of "strokes" supposedly prevented was 46!

Both the Press Release and the Abstract minimized the side-effects of increased incidence of several types of bleeding caused by aspirin. In fact, 2067 (10%) more women on aspirin reported easy bruising; 480 (2.4%) more reported nosebleed (epitaxis); 160 (0.8%) more reported blood in urine (hematuria); 129 (0.65%) more reported peptic ulcer; 159 (0.8%) more reported gastrointestinal bleeding; and of these 36 more on aspirin required transfusions. What may be the most serious problem caused by long-term aspirin use, doubling of cataracts, was not even mentioned.

The Press Release said that "The bottom line is that many women, especially those 65 and older, may benefit from taking aspirin every other day to prevent stoke." The analysis given above shows this advice to be flawed, since the risks far outweigh the benefits.

The aspirin and placebo pills were provided by Bayer HeathCare. Several of the authors of the NEJM paper cited financial ties with Bayer.


Bottom line on primary protection with aspirin

"No conventionally used prophylactic aspirin regimen seems free of the risk of peptic ulcer complications... Alka-Seltzer may be associated with higher risk (2X) and enteric-coated aspirin with lower risk (0.5X) compared with plain aspirin." (Weil et al., 1999) But: "No evidence exists that reducing the dose of aspirin or using slow-release formulations would reduce the incidence of gastrointestinal haemorrhage" (Derry et al., 2000). Users of aspirin for long periods to relieve arthritis pain have suffered so badly from side-effects that a multitude of alternates, such as ibuprofen (Motrin™) and naproxen (Aleve™), then later celecoxib (Celebrex™) and rofecoxib (Vioxx™) were introduced, whose side-effects were at least as serious (Wolfe & Sasich, 2002). Vioxx causes nearly double the rate of congestive heart failure that aspirin does (Mamdani et al., 2004), and was taken off the market by Merck before it could be recalled by the FDA. Both aspirin and acetaminophen (Tylenol™) can cause kidney or liver failure (Fored et al., 2001).

If delaying death is the real end-point, not reduction in non-fatal heart attacks, then it seems pointless to take aspirin for *primary* protection, with its certainty of obnoxious side-effects, which may include gastritis, peptic ulcer, other internal bleeding, hemorrhagic stroke, fatal heart attacks, and sudden death, to which has been added macular degeneration (in 1988) and twice the risk of cataracts.

In the Australian Blue Mountains Eye Study, subjects taking aspirin of unspecified dose more than once per week for over 10 years had RR = 2 for cataracts (Cumming & Mitchell, 1998). This was in people who were ≤ 55 and then took aspirin for ≥ 10 years, *in trade* for a probable reduction of only 0.2% absolute per year in *total* (mostly non-fatal) MIs. This is not sensible, especially when safer alternatives exist, such as magnesium and omega-3 fatty acids (see Part B). The prevalence of cataracts in Australians in 1997 was 5.5% (McCarty & Taylor, 2001). About 70,000 Australians undergo cataract surgery each year. In the USA cataract surgery cost $3.4 billion in 1995, where the prevalence of cataracts is 17% in those 40 or older (NIH, 2005). Around 1991 1/5 of Americans took aspirin. If all did, the prevalence of cataracts might climb to 30%.

Aspirin is known to cause excretion of calcium, and to deplete levels of vitamins B5 and C, and of iron, sodium, potassium and folic acid (Pelton & LaValle, 2000, p51-52). Perhaps some of the side-effects of aspirin are related to these depletions. No clinical trials investigating supplementation of any of these during aspirin use have come to my attention.

Now it is time to ask the more difficult question...

## Should You Take Aspirin to Prevent a *Second* Heart Attack?

Early studies, mostly in UK

Five earlier studies on *secondary* prevention of heart attacks of the myocardial infarction type (MIs) by aspirin were reported from 1974-1980. There was said to be no beneficial effect overall (Gent & Carter, 1982). One multicenter study, nevertheless, the earliest of this type I have seen, had positive results. A single daily dose of 300 mg of aspirin in a gelatin capsule or a similar-looking placebo was to be taken before breakfast to ensure rapid absorption by each of 1,239 men who had had a recent heart attack. The aspirin group showed a reduction in total mortality of 12% at 6 months, 25% in 1 year, and 28% at 2 years. The authors modestly acknowledged that the results were statistically inconclusive, but they were in the range of what was observed in later larger trials (Elwood & Cochrane, 1974). The much larger size of the later trials was needed to obtain results that would be statistically solid, at least by the widespread convention of looking for $p < 0.05$.

Second International Study of Infarct Survival, 1988

Reported in 1988, the second International Study of Infarct Survival (ISIS-2) Collaborative Group in the UK determined the effect of aspirin *vs.* placebo in 17,187 people entering 417 hospitals after the onset of suspected acute MI. The aspirin used was clearly stated to be 162.5 mg in an enteric coated tablet given daily for *1 month.* All-cause mortality was said to be similar to vascular mortality. After 5 weeks aspirin produced 23% fewer vascular deaths (heart failure and strokes combined) overall ($2p$ <0.00001), cut total heart attacks from an absolute value of 2% to 1%, cut non-fatal stroke from 0.6% to 0.3%, and did not cause any increase in cerebral hemorrhages. Survival rates after 2 years were 81.7% in the aspirin group *vs.* 80.0 % on placebo (ISIS-2, 1988). Here is an example of reporting a trial result by giving absolute rates that are easy to understand, statistically very significant, yet fairly minor in absolute terms. You should note carefully that 2-year mortality was improved by under 1% absolute per year! NNT = 59 for the 2-year period.

Antiplatelet Trialists' Collaboration, 1994

In 1988 the Antiplatelet Trialists' Collaboration (ATC), (BMJ 88, 1988) on 29,000 patients, a majority with a history of transient ischemic attack, stroke, unstable angina, or MI, were treated by a variety of methods, including with ≥300 mg ASA daily, which did not differ greatly in results from other drug regimens employed in the trials, as shown by a meta-analysis (see Figure 1-2 above). The authors thought that vascular (blood-vessel related) mortality was reduced by 1/6, and non-fatal vascular undesirable events by 1/3 in high-risk patients. By 1994, now with up to 70,000 high-risk patients under study, the Antiplatelet Trialists' Collaboration (ATC, 1994) found similar results; but now the daily aspirin dose was 75-325 mg.

Second International Study of Infarct Survival, 1998

By 1998 ISIS-2 was still following 6,213 high-risk patients in the UK of the 17,187 originally in the trial. During the first 35 days of follow-up, the use of aspirin during the first month reduced the death rate by 22%. Hence all of the survival benefit of an early, one-month course of oral aspirin (162.5 mg enteric coated, daily) seemed to accrue during the first month, with little further benefit between day 36 and the end of year 10, by when the death rate was down 1% absolute relative to placebo (Baigent et al., 1998).

North of England Aspirin Guideline Development Group's recommendations, 1998

This then was the background of the North of England Aspirin Guideline Development Group's recommendations to physicians: Aspirin should be used in patients with acute MI at 150 mg daily for one month, then 75 mg daily for several years. In patients with MI, anginas, ischemic stroke (clots), or transient ischemic attack (TIA), aspirin should be used at 75 mg daily for several years. There was no evidence that higher doses were more effective (Eccles et al., 1998). The Group did not mention either buffer or enteric coating, both of which seem desirable to this writer. Nor was there convincing evidence for the multi-year use of low-dose aspirin.

Bottom line on primary protection with aspirin

So the answer for *secondary* protection from recurrence of several types of undesirable vascular conditions is: Yes, take aspirin in low doses in order to obtain a moderate (16-22%) reduction in risk for a potentially fatal *second* heart attack. Take the first magnesium-buffered aspirin tablet (325 mg), not enteric-coated, in a hurry; have small sealed packs in your home and car. Switch then to daily enteric-coated tablets (81 mg), and consider stopping in 4-6 weeks if you do not have further heart attacks.

But is aspirin the best protection from MI that there is, considering both effectiveness and freedom from side effects? Probably not, as will be discussed in Part B.

<u>Aspirin in Congestive Heart Failure</u>

The other major lethal heart condition is called congestive heart failure (CHF, often just HF). This is a result of weaker and weaker pumping ability of the heart, not blocked coronary arteries leading to MIs. There is only one recent study, the non-blinded Warfarin/Aspirin Study in Heart failure (WASH). Here 99 CHF patients (28% female) served as controls, 91 (25% female) were given aspirin at 300 mg/day and 89 (24% female) were given warfarin (Coumadin™) at the usual appropriate dosage based on blood tests. Endpoints after 27 months were the combined ones of death, MI and stroke, because of the small size of the groups. There were 26, 32 and 26 events observed in each of the respective groups, thus the poorest results (32 events) were seen with aspirin, but this was not quite significant because of the small size of the groups. For all-cause hospitalization there were 48, 64 and 47 in each of the groups respectively, a significant losing proposition for the aspirin group

(Cleland et al., 2004). The authors' conclusions were that aspirin is neither safe nor effective in the treatment of congestive heart failure.

## Aspirin for Influenza

One of your body's defense mechanisms against bacterial or viral infection includes raising its temperature — running a fever. Overuse of aspirin to "control" fever is thought by many to make infections worse.

According to the Merck Manual, 16th ed., 1992, aspirin use during serious influenza can increase the risk for developing a deadly condition (Reye's syndrome) by as much as 35-fold (RR=35). In children under 18 years old, taking aspirin is considered especially dangerous for this reason. This is one of the reasons that some medical researchers do not think that aspirin would be approved by the FDA if introduced today.

## Summing Up

Not only the medical adviser to Consumers Union (CU), but also many health professionals who recommend aspirin, believe that there is a "high-risk", but not-yet-diagnosed population who should take aspirin for *primary* prevention of heart attack. You may check for yourself in the studies cited — often there is *no* such group. True, males ≥ 50 years old are at higher risk than males or females ≤ 50, but those males ≥ 50 are actually the *low risk* group in most of the large studies on health professionals, because they have had no symptoms.

The study with the most favorable results in terms of reducing heart attacks, PHS 89, used Bufferin, which contains a significant amount of magnesium, not just aspirin. This fact was lost on CU, as well as many others, including the author of a summary in *The Medical Letter* **42** (1072), 21 Feb 00, p18, who cited PHS 89 and failed to cite all the later European studies.

There is no consensus even among cardiologists that use of aspirin in the general population is advisable. For one, Prof. F. Verheught, Dept. of Cardiology, University Hospital, Nijmegen, Netherlands, warned that "...use of aspirin for primary prevention was inadvisable because its use was investigated only in men [before 1998], that the risk of non-fatal heart attacks is < 0.5% per year [and would be cut only by 0.2%], and that there was risk of gastric discomfort and bleeding." (Kmietowicz, 1998).

The studies on low-risk males were carried on for 5-7 years with an insignificant drop in mortality when Bufferin was used, or in an insignificant rise in mortality when plain aspirin was used. Based on life-expectancies, advice to take aspirin beginning at age 50 would mean ≈30 years of exposure to its side-effects, not a great idea.

When women were given aspirin in a large 10-year trial, the number of side-effects far outweighed the reduction in non-fatal clot incidence.

The story is the same for diabetic patients: in primary studies the hazards exceed the benefits.

*****

For *secondary* protection, aspirin has a limited but definite value, and does not have to be taken forever; most of the benefit is obtained from 81 mg per day for 4-5 weeks (see above for details). One may expect 1/4 to 1/6 fewer deaths for about 2 years after the short period of aspirin use; but this amounts to little in absolute terms. Based on available evidence, oral aspirin and intravenous magnesium citrate (see below) are an important part of the preferred treatment for the majority of stroke or myocardial infarction (heart attack) patients at risk of *recurrences.*

However, because of their higher platelet turnover, diabetics who take aspirin for secondary prevention may benefit from higher doses — 300 mg of enteric-coated aspirin daily (Yudkin, 1995).

*****

Aspirin is neither safe nor effective in the treatment of congestive heart failure.

Occasional use of aspirin for headache and arthritis pain should not cause serious side-effects. More than occasional use can hurt you.

## Part B: Alternatives to Aspirin

### What Else Could You Take to Prevent Heart Attacks or Sudden Cardiac Death?

Despite its off-patent status for about 80 years, aspirin is still strongly promoted by some of the same drug companies that invent and promote prescription drugs. As you saw in Part A, aspirin is promoted for secondary protection from heart attacks, which is supported by both actual published evidence and the FDA. However, aspirin is still touted also for primary protection, despite the lack of evidence for any reduction in all-cause death rates. Indeed many people consider their daily aspirin intake to be inviolable! You may be interested to read how safe and effective some common supplements are for both primary and secondary protection from heart attack or congestive heart failure, and you may begin to wonder why aspirin is recommended by so many physicians who almost never recommend any of the following alternatives.

Besides, most of us really have a compulsion to take some kind of daily pill to ward off disease and death. Here are some suggestions.

### Vitamin E for primary protection

Nurses Health Study, 1993

The Nurses Health Study involved 87,245 female nurses aged 34-59 in 1980, who were free from diagnosed cardiovascular disease and cancer, and who completed dietary questionnaires every two years up to eight years. Women who took vitamin E supplements containing, on average, 200 IU (International Units) for more than 2 years had 41% fewer instances of coronary disease of several types, and overall mortality 13% lower than those who did not ($p = 0.05$) (Stampfer et al., 1993). The amount of vitamin E in multivitamin capsules at that time was typically $\leq$ 30 IU, so the larger amount in vitamin E only capsules made a difference.

Health Professionals Follow-up Study, 1993

The Health Professionals Follow-up Study involving about 40,000 males aged 40-75 in 1986 who were free of diagnosed coronary heart disease, diabetes, or "hypercholesteremia" (see Myth 3) completed detailed dietary questionnaires every two years until 1990. Men who took 100-250 IU of vitamin E as supplements for 2-10 years had 37% fewer instances of coronary disease of several types, including fatal events ($p = 0.05$). Higher doses of vitamin E were no more effective. By contrast, the intake of vitamin C and beta-carotene did not lower risk in this study (Rimm et al., 1993).

Health Protection Study, 2004

The Health Protection Study (HPS) on 20,536 adults aged 40-80 at baseline and followed for 5 years had a low-risk group on 600 mg (close to 600 IU) of synthetic vitamin E, 250 mg of vitamin C and 20 mg of beta-carotene daily. Not reported on by the HPSs own directors, this low-risk group had about 1/3 fewer fatal heart attacks and other blood vessel related deaths (Hickey & Roberts, 2004).

These results are far more impressive than the ones for aspirin, especially for women, and also because side-effects were so minimal as not to be mentioned. And vitamin E *could* be bought at almost any grocery store.

## Vitamin E for secondary protection

Cambridge Heart Antioxidant Study, 1996

The Cambridge Heart Antioxidant Study [CHAOS (English humour?)] was a single-center (means one location only), double-blind, placebo-controlled study with 2002 patients who had angiographically proven coronary atherosclerosis (fatty deposits in the arteries supplying blood to the heart muscles). Doses of 400 or 800 IU of natural vitamin E were used in half, and the group was followed for a median of 510 days. Vitamin E gave a significant reduction in non-fatal MI of 77% ($p$ = 0.005); however, there was a non-significant excess (18%, $p$ = 0.61) of cardiovascular deaths in the combined vitamin E groups. The lower dose of vitamin E was better on both counts, including a 13% lower death rate on 400 IU than on placebo, but a 35% higher death rate on 800 IU. The lower dose of vitamin E gave 86% fewer non-fatal MIs and the higher dose 52% fewer. So here, too, vitamin E is far more effective than aspirin, and, again, side effects were negligible at the lower dose (Stephens et al., 1996). These latter data on lower doses do not appear in the abstract, showing the bias of the authors, as did their measurements of total serum cholesterol, rather than of the more meaningful homocysteine (see Myths 2 and 3).

Health Protection Study, 2004

The Health Protection Study mentioned above found no benefit of synthetic vitamin E with vitamin C and beta-carotene in secondary prevention of cardiovascular deaths (Hickey & Roberts, 2004).

GISSI-P trial, 1999

The GISSI-P trial used 300 mg (close to 300 IU) of synthetic vitamin E (GISSI-P, 1999). In the composite endpoint of death and non-fatal MI, vitamin E reduced risk by a barely significant 11% (Brown, 1999). Since the subjects were already eating a "Mediterranean Diet" high in vitamin E, and high in olive oil, which aids in absorption of vitamin E (McCully & McCully, 1999), perhaps this result is not surprising. Again, measurements of total serum cholesterol, HDL, LDL and triglycerides showed no changes at all due to vitamin E intake.

## Natural Vitamin E is a Mixture

So for secondary protection, some recent RCTs have shown good results for Vitamin E at doses of 400 IU per day, which happens to be the most common size of the softgels on the market today. This is usually d-alpha-tocopherol, the predominant form of vitamin E found in plasma and tissues in your body, while gamma-tocopherol is the most common form in USA diets. Yes, the beta and gamma forms also exist, along with the related tocotrienols, alpha, beta, gamma and delta.

Recent research showed that gamma-tocopherol inhibited the growth of prostate cancer cells, but not normal ones. The gamma-tocopherol was also better than alpha at inhibiting colon cancer cell growth. Various tocotrienols cause death in human breast cancer cell lines. Combinations of these isomers had additive or synergistic effects. This finding was patented. Selenium supplements protect against cancer (see Myth 10), but only when gamma-tocopherol concentrations were relatively high (Jiang et al., 2004).

Because of the important differences found between synthetic or natural vitamin E, which is the d-alpha-tocopherol isomer alone, and natural vitamin E with the d-beta, d-gamma and d-delta isomers also present along with the related four tocotrienols, it would be prudent now to select supplements containing the natural mixture, even for primary protection. For example, a recent study on 50 patients with partial blockage of the carotid artery, as found by ultrasound, found that after 18 months, 23 of the 25 given gamma-tocotrienol stabilized or improved, while 12 of the 25 control patients deteriorated and none improved. A Swedish study found that blood levels of gamma-tocopherol, but not alpha, were reduced in patients with heart disease (Hickey & Roberts, 2004).

Therefore, if one wants to maximize the benefits from vitamin E based on recent best data, one should look for a product with mixed isomers of the tocopherols and the tocotrienols, both with the most gamma isomers of each. Such products now exist, not made by the old vitamin E makers, but, for example, by Carotech Associates, USA, Inc., and available from typical supplement suppliers. One brand is Swanson Health Products (www.swanson vitamins.com) and is called Full Spectrum E with Tocotrienols. (I have no financial ties to Swanson.)

### Mainstream medicine reacts to vitamin E

A meta-analysis of vitamin E trials appeared in 2004 that appeared to refute any value of vitamin E for any purpose. Careful examination of the trials used showed selection bias, as described in the Introduction chapter. Thus some of the successful trials discussed above were not included. Not much attention was given to either the form or dose of vitamin E used in each trial. In most of the trials synthetic vitamin E was used, which is considered chemically different and inferior to the natural alpha-tocopherol form, let alone the natural mixture. Most of the trials in this meta-analysis utilized mixtures of supplements, so one could not say whether the vitamin E was responsible alone for any good or bad effect. Many of the trials were on very sick people with a number of specific conditions. The lack of benefit follows what was discussed above under secondary protection, which was not great (Neustadt et al., 2005).

For a recent minor operation I had a preliminary conference with my appointed anesthesiologist, an MD. He asked whether I took supplements (none in particular were specified). When I said I did, he ordered me to stop taking all supplements a week before my scheduled surgery. My reaction was what your reaction should be: "Doctor, are you trying to kill me?" Further discussion revealed that he was concerned that the anticlotting action of vitamin E and gingko biloba might cause excessive bleeding. I agreed to stop these two until after the operation.

### Magnesium for primary protection

Caerphilly Heart Disease Study, 1992

The Caerphilly Heart Disease Study of men aged 45-59 years examined the relation of magnesium in the diet to the incidence of MIs, both fatal and non-fatal. Of the 627 men in the study 38 suffered MIs over a 5-year period. The mean daily intake of magnesium in local water (as the ion Mg++, not the metal) in these was 12% lower than in men who did not have MIs. This is a difference of about 38 mg per day, less than the amount in a Bufferin tablet (Elwood et al., 1992). The inverse relation of magnesium concentrations in drinking water to the rate of heart attacks has been noted many times (Purvis & Mohaved, 1999).

Long-Term Diet Study in India, 1990

In a prospective study of 10-year duration, the 400 "high-risk" subjects were selected about the same way as the Medical Research Council did for cardiovascular disease (see Meade, 1998). Of these, 93.5% were male, living in Moradabad, India. The trial was carried out by assigning half the group to a high-magnesium diet (1,142 mg per day vs. 418 mg in the control group) from fruits, green vegetables, cereals and nuts) and tracking medical events. The high-magnesium group had 35% fewer deaths from all causes ($p < 0.001$), and a 61% reduction of non-fatal cardiovascular events ($p < 0.001$), including a 54% reduction in strokes (Singh, 1990). Unfortunately, this report was marred by a number of arithmetical errors in the table of results. There was also a confounding factor in that the high-magnesium diet was also a high calcium diet (880 vs. 512 mg daily) and a high-potassium diet (3,080 vs. 548 mg daily). This was expected because these three metal ions are present in most plants. Since serum levels of magnesium and potassium were raised, and those of calcium were not, it is most likely that the magnesium and potassium were responsible for the differences in outcomes, which also included significant reductions in serum glucose (see Myth 2) and in total cholesterol (see Myth 3).

Rancho Bernardo, CA, 1987

Healthy men and women from Rancho Bernardo, CA, upper-middle-class and caucasian, were followed for 12 years for fatal stroke. Men with the lowest intake and serum levels of both potassium and magnesium had a RR = 2.6 for fatal stroke; for women, RR = 4.8. Looking at this the other way, a 400 mg increase in daily potassium intake, accompanied by a 230 mg increase in magnesium intake, gave a RR = 0.60 for fatal stroke overall (Khaw & Barrett-Connor, 1987). This report was so focused on potassium intake that the benefits of magnesium intake needed to be dug out of the body of the paper.

Heart arrhythmias in post-menopausal women, 2002

A diet study on 22 post-menopausal women comparing both low- and high-magnesium diets with and without supplements of magnesium gluconate for about 6 months, where the low-intake group had 130 mg/day of magnesium ion, and the high-intake group had ≥320 mg/day, showed about twice the number of heart arrhythmias in the low-intake group (Klevay & Milne, 2002).

How much magnesium and what form to take

The usual recommendations for dietary supplements are to take 300-600 mg of magnesium daily with food (Miller, 1999). The most common form in which to take magnesium is as the compound magnesium oxide, one of the alkalis in Bufferin; but more persuasive is advice to take it as potassium magnesium aspartate for better absorption (Douglass, 1995). This is one of the forms of "chelated magnesium". Women at risk of osteoporosis are advised to take also about half as much magnesium, by mass, as calcium (Lieberman & Bruning, 1990), because calcium intake, as well as vitamin D and phosphates, increase the amount of magnesium needed (Seelig, 1980). Mildred S.

Seelig, MD, also wrote that the typical daily intake of magnesium in American college students was 250 mg, not ≥385 mg as recommended for a 140-lb woman, or ≥500 mg for a 185-lb man.

Unfortunately, I have not found a report on a large clinical study on primary protection using only magnesium supplements in humans, or on a multi-year study that included all-cause death rates. Use of magnesium supplements in many people is probably justified by inference based on their effectiveness on secondary prevention, the clinical experience of a number of physicians, the drinking water studies, and the above diet study by Singh. Singh's diet study would support using potassium magnesium aspartate as the supplement most resembling the high-magnesium diet, and its results were vastly better than those of the aspirin trials, especially so because there were no side-effects, and the ratio of potassium to magnesium is similar to what food provided in the study. Such a supplement has been available from TwinLabs and others for at least 15 years. My experience is that the capsule form is better absorbed than the tablet form.

If you have foot or leg cramps, especially at night, you are likely to benefit from magnesium supplements. The archaic remedy for cramps, quinine sulfate, works less well and for only a few days as well as having more side-effects.

Two excellent and inexpensive books on the value of dietary and supplemental magnesium have just appeared (Dean, 2001; Cohen, 2004). There is more on magnesium in Myth 4.

<u>Magnesium for secondary protection</u>

Intravenous magnesium after hospital admissions for acute MI, 1986

In a double-blind, placebo-controlled study involving 273 patients with suspected acute MI in Hvidovre hospital, Copenhagen, Denmark, 74 received placebo, while 130 received 1.2 g of magnesium as the chloride intravenously during 24 hours, followed by 0.3 g in the next 24 hours. Treatments were begun within 3 hours of hospital admission. During the first 4 weeks after treatment mortality was 7% in the magnesium group and 19% in the placebo group, a mortality reduction of 63%, or RR = 0.37 ($p$ = 0.045). In the magnesium group 21% of the patients had arrhythmias that needed treatment vs. 47% in the placebo group, a reduction of 55% or RR = 0.45 ($p$ = 0.004). No adverse effects of intravenous magnesium were observed (Rasmussen et al., 1986).

Meta-analysis of intravenous magnesium in hospitals, 1991

By 1991 there were 7 placebo-controlled trials in coronary care units in UK hospitals involving 1301 MI patients. Short-term mortality was 3.8% among the treatment groups and 8.2% among the control groups, thus RR = 0.45 for treatment with magnesium based on the most important endpoint (Teo et al., 1991).

Conflicting results from trials in 1990s

Reported in 1992, the second Leicester Intravenous Magnesium Intervention Trial (LIMIT-2) on 2316 patients with suspected acute MI found a 24% reduction or RR = 0.76 ($p$ = 0.05) in 28-day mortality from treatment with intravenous magnesium sulfate (Woods et al., 1992). Reported in 1995, the Fourth International Study of Infarct Survival (ISIS-4) showed <u>no</u> benefit of similar treatment of 29,000 patients (ISIS-4, 1995). How could this be?

By 1996 the discrepancy was explained as follows: LIMIT-2 was double-blinded and placebo controlled, and only 30% of the patients had received treatment for thrombosis (streptokinase) by the time magnesium was begun on average 3 hours after onset of symptoms. ISIS-4 was non-blinded, had no placebo, the alternate treatments being the drugs isosorbide mononitrate or captopril; and 70% of the patients had received treatment (which raises blood magnesium concentrations) for thrombosis (clotting in major blood vessel), and 94% had received aspirin by the time magnesium was begun on average 8 hours (not soon enough) after the onset of symptoms. It is interesting that captopril is a product of Bristol-Myers Squibb, the sponsor of ISIS-4, at a cost for the trial of about $10 million (Baxter et al., 1996; Baxter et al., 1997).

University College Hospitals and Medical School, London, 1996-7

A study appeared simultaneously involving 194 patients considered unsuitable for treatment for thrombosis. In-hospital mortality was 4.2% in the magnesium group and 17.3% in controls, a reduction of 76%; so RR = 0.24 with treatment (Baxter et al., 1996; Baxter et al., 1997).

Where confounding treatments are absent, rapid treatment of patients suffering from MI with intravenous magnesium is of great benefit in secondary prevention, not only of MI, but of arrhythmias. The studies not confounded showed, on average, a greater 4-week benefit than from aspirin, and LIMIT-2 showed that concurrent aspirin did not change the outcome. Side-effects of magnesium were minimal and could be avoided altogether by controlling the rate of administration.

Mainstream medicine accepts magnesium

By 1990 the medical establishment had accepted the role of oral magnesium supplements in countering hypertension, heart attacks, congestive heart failure, and arrhythmias (Lauler, 1989). By 1997 your hospital should have adopted a routine policy of giving intravenous magnesium citrate to incoming heart attack patients. Has it?

## Coenzyme Q10 for primary protection

Coenzyme Q10 is an oily organic compound, like vitamin E, and is found in every cell of the body. It has a number of functions, among which are preventing the oxidation of LDL, and transporting oxygen from hemoglobin into the parts of cells (mitochondria) where ATP, the main source of cellular energy, can be formed. Sharing its status with magnesium, oral coenzyme Q10 supplements for better health in a low-risk population has not been investigated in large-scale controlled experiments (Overvad et al., 1999). Its use for primary protection in older people with some definite symptoms, such as congestive heart failure (CHF or HF), is probably justified by inference based on its effectiveness on secondary prevention, and on the clinical experience of a number of physicians. For details see the website of The International Coenzyme Q10 Association (wwwcsi.unian.it).

The usual doses of coenzyme Q10 as a long-term supplement are from 30-300 mg per day. The orange-red soft-gels are much more effective than the yellow powder in capsules, and are worth the extra expense.

The statin-type drugs used to lower cholesterol, which are of no benefit in lowering mortality rates (see Myth 3), also lower coenzyme Q10 levels (Rundek et al., 2004) by similar amounts. This is a serious side-effect to be avoided at all costs by not taking statin drugs, such as atorvastatin (Lipitor).

## Coenzyme Q10 for secondary protection against CHF

Folkers et al. study, 1985-6

The New York Heart Association (NYHA) has grouped congestive heart failure (CHF) into 4 classes of severity. A cardiac patient in class IV, the most serious, is unable to perform any physical act without discomfort, and symptoms of heart failure, including anginal pain, may be present even at rest. Cardiologists should know that such patients are on a relentless downhill course to death in spite of all conventional therapy. In a study in which all patients in hospitals were in NYHA classes III and IV, all who received conventional therapy (bypass surgery, digitalis, diuretics, vasodilators), about 25% survived for 3 years. The 88 patients treated with Coenzyme Q10 had a 75% survival rate after 3 years; these are absolute percentages. Thus the RR = 0.33 for all-cause mortality with Coenzyme Q10 treatment. (Folkers et al., 1985; Folkers, 1986).

## Morisco et al. study, 1993

Congestive heart failure is always characterized by an energy depletion status correlated with lowered coenzyme Q10 levels. In a 1-year double-blind trial, 641 patients of mean age 67 with chronic congestive heart failure (NYHA classes III and IV) were randomly assigned to receive either 2 mg/kg (≈100 mg) daily of coenzyme Q10 or placebo. The number of patients who required hospitalization for worsening heart failure was 38% lower ($p < 0.001$) in the Q10 group; the incidence of pulmonary edema was cut by 61%, and of cardiac asthma was cut by 51% (both $p < 0.001$) (Morsico et al., 1993). A similar study on 2500 patients showed only 0.5% with side effects thought due to coenzyme Q10.

## Dosage

The main unknown is how much coenzyme Q10 you should take if you are diagnosed with CHF. You should titrate the amount by beginning at 30 mg per day for a week. After that, keep doubling the dose each week until you feel better (more energetic). More than 300 mg per day has not been tested, and is probably a waste; but coenzyme Q10 has no toxicity at all.

## Omega-3 Fatty Acids for Primary Protection

### What are omega-3 fatty acids?

Omega-3 fatty acids include the 18-carbon linolenic acid found in a few vegetable oils, such as canola (7-9%), and the more effective 20- and 22-carbon fatty acids now familiar as EPA and DHA found in fish and fish oil supplements. See Figure 2-2 in Myth 2 for a drawing and an explanation of the omega-x names for fatty acids.

### Chicago Western Electric Study, 1997

The Chicago Western Electric Study used as an example in the Introduction followed the effects of fish consumption in 2,107 men aged 40-55, for 30 years. Those who ate 35 g daily had, for fatal coronary heart disease (CHD) or fatal myocardial infarction (MI) combined, a RR = 0.62 compared with men who consumed none. From the abstract's conclusions: "These data show an inverse association between fish consumption and death from CHD, especially non-sudden death from MI." (Daviglus et al., 1997) In their Table 2, the age-adjusted RRs for all-cause death were: 0g/day, 1.00 (this is the arbitrary reference value); 1-17g/day, 1.00; 18-34g/day, 0.98; 35g/day, 0.90. So the all-cause RR = 0.90 from most to no fish consumption, and was not quite significant. These authors failed to note that the benefits of the highest fish consumption were obtained regardless of any mercury that might have been in the fish.

## Nurses' Health Study, 2002

The Nurses' Health Study, also used as an example in the Introduction, on 84,688 women aged 34-59 years, followed for 16 years for outcomes vs. fish and omega-3 fatty acid intake, had the following conclusions in the abstract: "Among women, higher consumption of fish and omega-3 fatty acids is associated with a lower risk of CHD [same as CVD], particularly CHD deaths." (Hu et al., 2002) In the body of the paper, in text only, for all-cause mortality, the RR = 0.68 for women consuming fish five times weekly vs. once/month; RR = 0.75 for the extreme quintiles of total omega-3 intake; both were significant. These authors also failed to note that the benefits of the highest fish consumption were obtained regardless of any mercury that might have been in the fish.

## Mercury in fish

Because of concerns that mercury in fish might be damaging to health (McLaughlin, 2003), since organic mercury compounds are associated with heart disease and neurological disorders (Geier & Geier, 2003) it is sad that the authors of these 2 long-term studies did not try to allay these fears of eating fish or taking fish oil capsules by addressing the mercury issue directly. Pregnant women have been cautioned to restrict their intake of fish (http://www.cbc.ca/storyview/CBC/2002/10/21/Consumers/mercuryfish_021021) despite evidence that children receive most of their mercury from vaccines (Bradstreet et al, 2003; Geier & Geier, 2003).

## Lemaitre et al. study, 2003

The omega-3 fatty acid content in fish and some vegetable oils (canola, flaxseed, perilla) has been shown in RCTs to be active beneficial components, with long-term protection from *fatal* MIs, unlike aspirin. In healthy patients over 65 years old (42.6% female) and followed for 7 years, based on assays of plasma, the higher EPA and DHA levels were associated with many fewer fatal MIs (RR = 0.30, $p$ = 0.01). Higher levels of linolenic acid from flaxseed, soybean and canola oils were associated with lesser protection (RR = 0.48, $p$ = 0.04). Conversely, higher levels of linoleic acid (an n-6 or omega-6 fatty acid) as in cottonseed, corn, or soybean oils, were associated with a serious increase in fatal heart attacks (RR = 2.42, $p$ = 0.03), (Lemaitre et al., 2003). This and other work described in Myth 2 are at odds with the widely disseminated advice to eat polyunsaturated oils high in linoleic acid, advice whose intensity from the American Heart Association, among others, peaked about 20 years ago.

## Fish oil supplements

The typical amounts of EPA and DHA together in the usual mixture ratio of 3:2 in capsules may be obtained in capsules of 300-500 mg as daily supplements for people who do not eat much oily fish such as salmon, sardines or herring.

## Omega-3 Fatty Acids for Secondary Protection

## High fish diet trial on men, 1989

An RCT on 2033 men who had recovered from an MI had a "fish advice" arm of 847 men who were simply advised repeatedly by dietitians to eat more fatty fish (mackerel, herring, kipper, pilchard, sardine, salmon or trout). Those who would not eat fish (22%) were given fish oil capsules. After 2 years, of those who did eat fish or take fish oil capsules, 90.7% were still alive vs. 87.2% who did neither ($p < 0.05$), (Burr et al., 1989). True, the difference in absolute mortality risk was small, but it was larger than in some of the trials on aspirin and many other drugs to be described in Myths 3, 4 and 10.

## EPA and DHA fish oil supplements, 2002

An RCT on 11,323 survivors of heart attack (14.7% female) had 5679 of them taking just 1 g (1000 mg) of omega-3 supplements per day, apparently EPA and DHA. Of these, after 3.5 years, 91.4% were alive vs. 90.2% of the controls ($p < 0.01$). The protection improved steadily over this time period (Marchioli et al., 2002).

So eating oily fish or taking 1000 mg/day of combined EPA and DHA were of some benefit in secondary protection from heart attack. Some of the benefit is from the effect on cutting down on arrhythmias that lead to sudden heart failure. The benefits are at least as great as those from aspirin, but without the side-effects of aspirin. Fish oils cause some belching in some people as a main side-effect.

## Summing Up

Studies have shown that Vitamin E, magnesium, certain omega-3 fatty acids and coenzyme Q10 each provide much greater long-term benefits than aspirin. All of these supplements have fewer side-effects.

Vitamin E is both more effective and safer than aspirin, and its value in primary protection has been demonstrated in both men and women. The natural mixed isomers of vitamin E are probably better for both primary and secondary protection. More studies are needed.

Magnesium intake is inversely correlated with incidence of cardiovascular problems, the effect being more pronounced in men than in women. Up to at least 1,100 mg daily along with up to 3,000 mg of potassium is strongly protective in the primary sense, and unarguably protective in the secondary sense without the potassium.

Lowering homocysteine levels may be of the greatest value in preventing cardiovascular disease (McCully & McCully, 1999), and both vitamin E and magnesium have roles in lowering those levels, or preventing oxidation of LDL cholesterol (see Myth 2).

The omega-3 fatty acids in fish oils, EPA and DHA, are very protective (much better than aspirin in the long term) against sudden cardiac death, by preventing arrhythmias. About 1-3 g/day of intake of the commercially available 3:2 mixture is usually advised. Linolenic acid, an omega-3 from vegetable oils, is of less value, and the omega-6 loaded oils, such as soybean, are detrimental.

Despite all the evidence for the value of these supplements, your mainstream physician is far more likely to recommend aspirin. Why? It was introduced by a Big Pharma company that is still around — Bayer — and is advertised more than all four supplements together.

### Acknowledgements for Myth #1

The following faculty at The University of the Sciences in Philadelphia provided help: Eric G. Boyce, Donna Gagnier, Daniel A Hussar, Sarah Spinler, Jeannette McVeigh, and William A. Reinsmith, were of great help, but do not necessarily agree with the conclusions. Additional aid was provided by Frances E. H. Pane, MSLS, Charles J. Kelley, PhD, Tom Miller and Mildred S. Seelig, MD.

### Myth 1 References

Anon. (1988). *Consumer Reports* 10/1988, pp616-8.
Anon. (1990). "Meta-Analysis in the Breech", *Science* 249:476-9.

ATC (1994). ATC: Antiplatelet Trialists' Collaboration, *British Medical Journal* 308:81-106.

Baigent C, Collins R, Appleby P, Parish S, Sleight P, Peto R (1998). "ISIS-2: 10-Year Survival Among Patients with Suspected Acute Myocardial Infarction in Randomised Comparison of Intravenous Streptokinase, Oral Aspirin, Both, or Neither", *British Medical Journal* 316:1337-1343.

Baxter GF, Sumeray MS, Walker JM (1996). Infarct Size and Magnesium: Insights into LIMIT-2 and ISIS-4 from Experimental Studies, *The Lancet* 348:1424-6.

Baxter GF, Sumeray MS, Walker JM (1997). reply to letter, *The Lancet* 349:283 .

BMJ 88 (1988): Trialists' Collaboration, *British Medical Journal* 296:320-331.

Bradstreet J, Geier DA, Kartzinel JJ, Adams JB, Geier MR (2003). A case-control study of mercury burden in children with autistic spectrum disorders. *Journal of American Physicians and Surgeons* 8:76-79.

Brown M (1999). "Do Vitamin E and Fish Oil Protect Against Ischaemic Heart Disease? (Commentary), *Lancet* 354:441-2.

Burr ML, Gilbert JF, Holliday RM, Elwood PC, Fehily AM, Rogers S, Sweetnam PM, Deadman NM (1989). Effects of Changes in Fat, Fish, and Fibre Intakes on Death and Myocardial Reinfarction: Diet and Reinfarction Trial (DART). *The Lancet* 8666:758-761.

Cleland JGF (2000a). Preventing atherosclerotic events with aspirin. *British Medical Journal* 324:103-105.

Cleland, JGF (2000b). No reduction in cardiovascular risk with NSAIDS — Including aspirin? *The Lancet* 359:92-93.

Cleland JGF, Findlay I, Jafri S, et al. (2004). The Warfarin/Aspirin Study in Heart failure (WASH); a randomised trial comparing antithrombotic strategies for patients with heart failure. *American Heart Journal,* 148:157-164.

Cohen JS (2004). *The Magnesium Solution for High Blood Pressure,* Garden City, NY: SquareOne Publishers.

Cumming RG, Mitchell P (1998). Medications and Cataract: The Blue Mountains Eye Study, *Ophthalmology* 105:1751-8.

Daviglus ML, Stamler J, Orencia AJ, et al. (1997). Fish consumption and the 30-year risk of fatal myocardial infarction. *New England Journal of Medicine* 336:1046-1053.

Dean C (2001). *The Miracle of Magnesium.*

Derry S, Loke YK. Risk of gastrointestinal haemorrhage with long term use of aspirin: meta-analysis. *BMJ* 2000:321:1183-7.

Douglass WC (1995). A Strong Case for Magnesium, *Second Opinion,* V(7), 1-3 (July).

Douglass WC (1998). Health Breakthroughs, *Second Opinion,* Atlanta GA, Fall, p4.

Eccles M, Fremantle N, Mason J, and the North of England Aspirin Guideline Development Group (1998). North of England based guideline development project: Guideline on the use of aspirin as secondary prophylaxis for vascular disease in primary care. *British Medical Journal* 316:1303-1307.

Eidelman, RS, Hebert PR, Weisman SM, Hennekens CH (2003). An Update on Aspirin in the Primary Prevention od Cardiovascular Disease. *Archives of Internal Medicine 163:2006-2010.*

Elwood PC, Cochrane AL, Burr ML, Sweetman PM, Williams GH, Welsby E (1974). A Randomized Controlled Trial of Acetylsalicylic Acid in the Secondary Prevention of Mortality from Myocardial Infarction. *British Medical Journal,* Part 1:436-440 (9 Mar 74).

Elwood PC, Fehily AM, Sweetnam PM, Yarnell JW (1992). Dietary Magnesium and Prediction of Heart Disease, *Lancet* **340**, 483.

Enstrom E, Kanim LE, Klein MA (1992). Vitamin C intake and mortality among a sample of the United States population. *Epidemiology 3,* 189-91.

Fleming TR, DeMets DL (1996). *Annals of Internal Medicine* 125:605-613.

Feinman SE, Ed., *Beneficial and Toxic Effects of Aspirin,* CRC Press, Boca Raton, FL, 1993, p11.

Folkers K (1986). Contemporary Therapy with Vitamin B6, Vitamin B2, and Coenzyme Q10, *Chemical & Engineering News,* 55-6 (21 Apr 86); Folkers K, Vadhanavikit S, Mortensen SA (1985). Biochemical Rationale and Myocardial Tissue Data on the Effective Therapy of Cardiomyopathy with Coenzyme Q10, *Proceedings of the National Academy of Sciences USA* 82:901-4.

Ford ES (1999). Serum magnesium and ischaemic heart disease: findings from a national sample of US adults. *International Journal of Epidemiology* 28:645-651.

Fored CM, Ejerblad EE, Lindblad P, et al. (2001). Acetaminophen, Aspirin, and Chronic Renal Failure. *New England Journal of Medicine,* 345(25):1801-1808.

Fraser GE, Shavlik DJ (1997). Risk Factors for All-Cause and Coronary Heart Disease Mortality in the Oldest-Old. *Archives of Internal Medicine* 157:2249-2258.

Geier MR, Geier DA. Thimerosal in childhood vaccines, neurodevelopment disorders, and heart disease in the US. *Journal of American Physicians and Surgeons* 2003;8:6-11.

Gent M, Carter CJ (1982) in *Acetylsalicylic Acid: New Uses for an Old Drug.* Barnett H. J. M., et al., Eds., Raven Press, NY, p251-2.

GISSI-P Investigators (1999). Dietary Supplementation with N-3 Polyunsaturated Fatty Acids and Vitamin E after Myocardial Infarction: Results of the GISSI-Prevenzione Trial. *The Lancet* 354:447-55.

Gum PA, Thamilarisan M, Watanabe J, Blackstone EH, Lauer MS (2001). Aspirin use and all-cause mortality among patients being evaluated for known or suspected coronary artery disease. *Journal of the American Medical Association,* 286:1187-1194.

Hickey S, Roberts H (2004). *Ascorbate: The Science of Vitamin C.* Lulu Press, Napa, CA, pp102-105.

Hu FB, Bronner L, Willett WC, et al. (2002). Fish and omega-3 fatty acid intake and risk of coronary heart disease in women. *Journal of the American Medical Association,* 287(14):1815-1821.

ISIS-2 Collaborative Group (1988). Randomised trial of intravenous streptokinase, oral aspirin, both, or neither among 17,187 cases of suspected acute myocardial infarction. *The Lancet,* 349-360 (13 Aug 88).

ISIS-4 Collaborative Group (1995). A Randomised Factorial Trial Assessing Early Oral Captopril, Oral Mononitrate, and Intravenous Magnesium Sulphate in 58,050 Patients with Suspected Acute Myocardial Infarction, *The Lancet* 345:669-82.

Iso H, Hennekens CH, Stampfer MJ, Rexrode KM, Colditz GA, Speizer FE, Willett WC, Manson JE (1999). Prospective study of aspirin use and risk of stroke in women. *Stroke* 30:1764-1771.

Jeffreys D (2004). *Aspirin: The Remarkable Story of a Wonder Drug.* New York, NY: Bloomsbury.

Jiang Q, Wong J, Fyrst H, Saba JD, Ames BN (2004). Gamma-Tocopherol or combinations of vitamin E forms induce cell death in human prostate cancer cells by interrupting sphingolipid synthesis. *Proceedings of the National Academy of Sciences* 2004;101(51):17825-17830.

Kauffman JM (2000). Should you take aspirin to prevent heart attack? *Journal of Scientific Exploration* 14:623-641.

Kauffman JM (2002). "Aspirin Study Flawed", Letter to Editor, *J. Scientific Exploration* 16(2), 247-249 (2002).

Khaw K-T, Barrett-Connor E (1987). Dietary Potassium and Stroke-Associated Mortality. A 12-Year Prospective Population Study. *New England Journal of Medicine* 316:235-240.

Klevay LM, Milne DB (2002). Low dietary magnesium increases supraventricular ectopy. *American Journal of Clinical Nutrition* 75:550-554.

Kmietowicz Z (1998). Aspirin and Warfarin Best for Primary Prevention of Heart Attacks, *British Medical Journal* 316:327.

Knorr J-A (2000). Aspirin, The Multi-Purpose Compound, Not Just for Headaches Anymore. *Life Extension,* 2/2000, pp50-55.

Kronmal A, Hart RG, Manolio TA, Talbert RL, Beauchamp NJ, Newman A (1998). Aspirin use and incident stroke in the cardiovascular health study. *Stroke* 29:887-894.

Lauler DP (1989). A Symposium: Magnesium Deficiency—Pathogenesis, Prevalence, and Strategies for Repletion. *The American Journal of Cardiology* 63(14):1-43G.

Lemaitre RN, King IB, Mozaffarian D, Kuller LH, Tracy, RP, Siscovick DS (2003). n-3 Polyunsaturated fatty acids, fatal ischemic heart disease, and nonfatal myocardial infarction in older adults: the Cardiovascular Health Study. *American Journal of Clinical Nutrition* 77:319-325.

Lieberman S, Bruning N (1990).*The Real Vitamin & Mineral Book,* Avery Publ. Grp., Garden City Park, NY, pp141-2.

Mamdani M, Juurlink DN, Lee DS, et al. (2004). Cyclo-oxygenase-2 inhibitors versus non-selective non-steroidal antiinflammatory drugs and congestive heart failure outcomes in elderly patients: a population-based study. *The Lancet* 363:1751-1756.

Mann CC, Plummer ML (1991).*The Aspirin Wars: Money, Medicine, and 100 Years of Rampant Competition,* Alfred A. Knopf, NY *("Wars").*

Marchioli R, Barzi F, Bomba E et al. (2002). Early protection Against Sudden Death by n-3 Polyunsaturated Fatty Acids After Myocardial Infarction. *Circulation* 105:1897-1903.

McCarty C, Taylor HR. The Genetics of Cataract. Investigative Ophthalmology and Visual Science 2001;42(8):1677-1678.

McCully K, McCully M (1999). *The Heart Revolution. The Extraordinary Discovery that Finally Laid the Cholesterol Myth to Rest,* HarperCollins, New York, NY, and references to peer-reviewed papers therein.

McDonald JWD (1982) in *Acetylsalicylic Acid: New Uses for an Old Drug,* Barnett HJM et al., Eds., Raven Press, NY, p89.

McLaughlin K (2003). Angling for answers: is fish healthy or dangerous? *Wall Street Journal,* Sept. 2, pp D1,D8.

McTaggart L, Ed. (1995). *Medicine: What Works & What Doesn't,* The Wallace Press, no location, pp52-54.

Meade TW with The Medical Research Council's General Practice Research Framework (1998). Thrombosis prevention trial: Randomised trial of low intensity oral anticoagulation with warfarin and low dose aspirin in the primary prevention of ischaemic heart disease in men at increased risk. *The Lancet* 351:233-41.

Miller T, www.execpc.com, last update 23 Jul 99.

Morisco C, Trimarco B, Condorelli M (1993). Effect of Coenzyme Q10 Therapy in Patients with Congestive Heart Failure: A Long-Term Multicenter Randomized Study, *Clinical Investigations* 71(8 Suppl.):S134-6.

Mustard JF (1982) in *Acetylsalicylic Acid: New Uses for an Old Drug,* H. J. M. Barnett et al., Eds., Raven Press, NY, p1.

Nabel EG. Available at: http://www.nih.gov/news/pr/mar2005/nhlbi-07.htm Accessed 13 Apr 05.

Neustadt J, Pizzorno J (2005). Vitamin E and All-Cause Mortality. *Integrative Medicine* 4(1):14-17.

N. I. H., National Eye Institute. Prevalence of Cataract, Age-Related Macular Degeneration, and Open-Angle Glaucoma Among Adults 40 Years and Older in the United States.   http://www.nei.nih.gov/eyedata/pbd_tables.asp Accessed 15 Jun 05.

Overvad K, Diamant B, Holm L, Holmer G, Mortensen SA, Stender S (1999). Coenzyme Q10 in Health and Disease, *European Journal of Clinical Nutrition* 53:764-70.

Pelton R, LaValle JB (2000). *The Nutritional Cost of Prescription Drugs,* Englewood, CO: Perspective/Morton.

PHS 89: Steering Committee of the Physicians Health Study Research Group (1989). *The New England Journal of Medicine* 321:129-135.

Pignone M, Mulrow C (2002).  Aspirin for CHD Prevention in Lower Risk Adults.  *British Medical Journal* Rapid Response, 15 Jan.

Purvis JR, Mohaved A (1999). Magnesium Disorders and Cardiovascular Diseases, *Clinical Cardiology* 5:566-8.

Radin D (1997). *The Conscious Universe,* Harper Edge, San Francisco, CA, pp55-6.

Rasmussen HS, Norregard P, Lindeneg O, McNair P, Backer V, Balslev S (1986). Intravenous Magnesium in Acute Myocardial Infarction, *The Lancet,* 234-5(1 Feb 86).

Ridker PM, Cook NR, Lee I-M, et al. A Randomized Trial of Low-Dose Aspirin in the Primary Prevention of Cardiovascular Disease in Women. New Engl J Med 2005;352(13):1293-1304.

Rimm EB, Stampfer MJ, Ascherio A, Giovannucci E, Colditz GA, Willett WC (1993).  Vitamin E Consumption and the Risk of Coronary Disease in Men, *The New England Journal of Medicine* 328:1450-96.

Rundek T, Naini A, Sacco R, Coates K, DiMauro S (2004). Atorvastatin Decreases the Coenzyme Q10 Level in the Blood of Patients at Risk for Cardiovascular Disease and Stroke. *Archives of Neurology* 61:889-892.

Seelig MS (1980). *Magnesium Deficiency in the Pathogenesis of Disease,* Plenum, New York, NY, pp8,10,169.

Singh RB (1990). Effect of Dietary Magnesium Supplementation in the Prevention of Coronary Heart Disease and Sudden Cardiac Death. *Magnesium & Trace Elements* 9:143-51.

Stampfer MJ, Hennekens CH, Manson JE, Colditz GA, Rosner B, Willett WC (1993).Vitamin E Consumption and the Risk of Coronary Disease in Women, *The New England Journal of Medicine,* **328**, 1444-92.

Stephens NG, Parsons A, Schofield PM, Kelly F, Cheeseman K, Mitchinson MJ, Brown MJ (1996). Randomised controlled trial of vitamin E in patients with coronary disease: Cambridge Heart Antioxidant Study (CHAOS). *The Lancet* 347:781-786.

Teo KK, Yusuf S, Collins R, Held PH, Peto R (1991). Effects of intravenous magnesium in suspected acute myocardial infarction: overview of randomised trials. *British Medical Journal* 303:1499-1503.

Vane JR, Botting RM, Eds. (1992). *Aspirin and Other Salicylates,* Chapman & Hall Medical, London, p10.

Weil J, Colin-Jones D, Langman M, Lawson D, Logan R, Murphy R, Rawlins M, Vessey M, Wainwright P (1995). Prophylactic aspirin and the risk of peptic ulcer bleeding. *British Medical Journal* 310:827-829.

Whitaker J (1996). *Health & Healing* **6** (8), 8/96, pp1-3. (Dr. Whitaker is one of the most courageous advocates of new or alternate treatments for many conditions.  He has risked life, liberty, and financial ruin in trying to protect other practitioners from the FDA and in campaigning for easy availability of supplements.)

Windholz M, Ed. (1976). *The Merck Index,* 9th ed., Merck & Co., Inc., Rahway, NJ, p114.

Wolfe SM, Sasich LD (2002). *Worst Pills, Best Pills 2002 Companion,* Washington, DC: Public Citizen Health Research Group, pp35-36, 39-41.

Woods KL, Fletcher S, Roffe C, Haider Y (1992). Intravenous Magnesium Sulphate in Suspected Acute Myocardial Infarction: Results of the Second Leicester Intravenous Magnesium Interventional Trial (LIMIT-2). *The Lancet* 339:1553-8.

Yudkin J (1995). Editorial, Which Diabetic Patients Should be Taking Aspirin?, *British Medical Journal* 311:641-2.

# Myth 2: Low-Carbohydrate Diets are Unsafe and Ineffective for Losing Weight

*"There is no nonsense so arrant that it cannot be made the creed of the vast majority by adequate governmental action."* Bertrand Russell, *An Outline of Intellectual Rubbish*, 1950 (Ottoboni & Ottoboni, 2002, p173).

An Analysis of Diet Nonsense by Spacedoc

Because so many of us in the USA adopted the recommended high carbohydrate/low fat diet in the past fifty years, we now are faced with a massive ongoing epidemic of obesity and type-2 diabetes. Yet those agencies and foundations responsible for this incredible nutritional *faux pas* are still denying their role. Instead of admitting they have made a gross error in judgment these past many decades, they have become the principal perpetrators of the myth that carbohydrate restriction is harmful. They have also taken the position of sniping at every attempt being made by *responsible* advocates to get this country's diet back on track.

On the one hand, we doctors were taught in biochemistry courses that consumption of fat and protein placed minimal demands on the pancreas for insulin production, yet at the same time and in the very same educational institutions, we were instructed to use the standard diabetic diet with its emphasis on ample carbohydrates in the form of bread, potatoes, pasta and rice. All of these carbohydrates placed heavy demands on insulin secretion. Even today, some fifty years later, I can vividly recall my surprise at these conflicting lectures; but as a fledgling doctor I could not even conceive the thought of challenging traditional medical concepts. Now we find a growing trend among diabetes specialists to restrict carbohydrates in their patients' diet because it works. Not only does it work but it works far better than fifty years of traditional diabetes treatment.

When I read of the accomplishments of such medical scientists as Richard K. Bernstein, MD, himself a juvenile diabetic, who as a young engineer had to take his diabetes treatment into his own hands to save his life, I am filled with shame at how inadequate have been our treatment standards. Bernstein later went to medical school in mid-life primarily so that having an MD degree, his studies could be published in medical journals so he could better inform other doctors. This is a sad commentary of the reality of challenging orthodoxy.

As you review these low-carb high-fat diets you will observe how very basic they are, even primitive, for to eat in this manner is to regress, nutritionally speaking, 10,000 years to the time before our encounter with agriculture and the preponderance of carbohydrate in our diet. We humans think of ourselves as highly evolved - the epitome of the evolutionary process, yet our metabolic system is unchanged from that of our primitive ancestors. A carbohydrate-restricted diet is natural for [many of] us, the one to which we are best adapted physiologically.

Our present USDA Food Pyramid is wrong and this chapter is an excellent review of the reasons why. No more than 40-50% of our daily caloric intake should be from carbohydrates, even if we are not carb-sensitive or diabetic. For fats we must return to the natural fats that were the foundation of the American diet ten decades ago. We also should remember that our strongest antagonists in our what I chose to call "back to basics" diet will be our food industry, for there is relatively little profit in basic foods. I fondly remember the words of Paul Dudley White, MD, cardiologist to the President back in the mid-fifties. When pressed to support the politically motivated "prudent" diet of fat and cholesterol restriction, he replied, "See here, I began my practice as a cardiologist in 1921 and never saw a myocardial infarction patient until 1928. Back in the MI-free days before 1920, the fats were butter, whole milk and lard, and I think we would all benefit from the kind of diet that we had when no one had ever heard of corn oil." Today most people have forgotten all about Dr. Dudley White and his prophetic words of advice, but he was right and all the other experts were wrong. If Dudley White had been in control of our dietary destiny then, cardiovascular disease would not be the immense problem it is today.

    ----Duane Graveline, MD, MPH, astronaut, flight surgeon, family physician

## Diet Dogma

For the last 50 years government agencies in many countries and non-governmental associations have recommended high-carbohydrate diets. Recently this has come to mean lots of starch, often in the form of unrefined or "whole" grains. This also meant that we were to restrict our intake of fats, especially animal fats, because of their content of cholesterol and saturated fatty acids. Doing so necessarily meant eliminating most meats and eggs. Then about 25 years ago, plant oils high in saturated fatty acids joined the list of "harmful" foods, with coconut and palm oils departing from grocery shelves. And anything containing polyunsaturated oils was touted for better health, namely corn, cottonseed, safflower, soybean, and sunflower oils. The partially hydrogenated versions of these oils, the source of the ubiquitous *trans* fatty acids, the ones found in Crisco™, Oreo™ cookies, Triscuit™ crackers, pie crust, cake icing, and a zillion other products, became as common as classic Coca Cola™, a high-carbohydrate drink. This campaign was intensified in the last 20 years, coinciding with a massive increase in the proportion of people in the USA and UK who are overweight, obese, and/or diagnosed with adult-onset diabetes. The simple rationales and supposedly scientific evidence for the "eat carbs" advice is shown in this chapter to be flawed.

At no time in the last 50 years have diet experts had a consensus, as is so often claimed. Reasoned objections to high-carb low-fat diets co-existed for the entire period; but these were overwhelmed by the financial power of the high-carbohydrate advocates, and the prestige of the medical and government spokespeople they controlled.

## Opposition to Dogma

Conversely, other writings from the medical and nutritional literature, based on studies and trials, show real benefits of low-carbohydrate diets, both in weight loss and in improved values in conventional tests on blood for hypertension (high blood pressure, see Myth 4), inflammation, and "hyperlipidemia". This last term means "high" serum total cholesterol (TC) and triglyceride (TG) levels. A lipid is a general term for both cholesterol and fats or oils. The latter pair are also called triglycerides.

These benefits of low-carbohydrate diets are often found in the actual data in journal articles on studies designed and claimed to provide evidence of the opposite! These are articles in which conclusions in the abstracts are used to promote high-carb diets, but these conclusions often do not match their actual data. Many studies also show that adherence to low-carbohydrate diets is better than for other types of diet, despite claims of "experts" that no diets work for long.

The authors of the books reviewed in Appendix B have recommended low-carbohydrate diets, some with no restrictions on intakes of fat and/or protein. Not only do all of the books have a plausible biochemical rationale for their advice, but they present histories of extremely long adherence to low-carbohydrate diets by individuals, many with medical degrees, with good health being the result. Examples are given later in this chapter. Clinical observations by 9 of the authors who have extensive experience treating obese and diabetic patients support the value of low-carbohydrate diets. Many other advantages of low-carbohydrate diets are shown by improvements in a diverse area of afflictions, from Crohn's and celiac diseases, to cancer, multiple sclerosis and arthritis. Even the performance of athletes who believed they were better served by high-carbohydrate diets was improved with low-carbohydrate diets. However, many other aspects of diet advice in these books are not in agreement with each other, and a majority of them contain diet advice based on unproven assumptions or contain some technical errors.

This chapter also shows that the energy content of specific foods listed on food labels, as determined by burning samples of them in a laboratory, often has little relation to their varied levels of digestibility and actual energy content as foods. The misguided diet stances of agencies and foundations is shown to have led to misleading food labels in both the USA and UK.

Low-carbohydrate diets, even if maintained for decades, have been demonstrated to be safe and effective for weight loss and preventing diabetes. Nevertheless, they are still considered to be alternative, and thus targets of attack by certain associations and governmental agencies. One of the most insidious attacks is calling low-carbohydrate diets a fad or craze. Another is the pernicious misrepresentation of low-carb diets as high-protein diets. Even the BBC erroneously supported this misconception (http://news.bbc.co.uk/2/hi/health/3545850.stm). Evidence will be given that effective low-carb diets contain about the same amount of protein as low-fat diets do, while the fat content remains the same or must increase. This is the chief bone in the throat of critics of low-carb diets, making it psychologically difficult for low-carb dieters to persist and succeed when bombarded with messages that eating fat is bad.

## Diet Wars

One of the fiercest battles in medicine and nutrition concerns nutritional advice about which diets will best preserve health and prolong life, especially to curb obesity and related conditions. Now we are living in an advice war on how much carbohydrate (carb) should be in our diets. Seemingly every government agency and private association recommends high-carb diets (more than 50% of metabolic energy from carbs, the rest from fat and protein), while every book reviewed in Appendix B recommends the opposite! For the last half-century high-carb diets have been recommended in order to limit intakes of fat and cholesterol in the simplistic belief that eating fat makes one fat, and that eating cholesterol leads to atherosclerosis (also referred to as cardiovascular disease, CVD). Also, these agencies and associations, along with processed food producers, control the mass media, the editorial policies of major journals, and the major sources of research funding. Some results of such control will be discussed below. True, there are many books, articles, pamphlets, websites and broadcasts that adhere to the mainstream view; this will be shown to be due to fear of job loss or to confirmation bias (copycats).

So whom should you believe? This chapter is an attempt to resolve the controversy by examining the rationales and the results obtained in books authored by those recommending low-carb diets, as well as the results of controlled trials in the medical literature. This is bolstered by reviews of 12 individual books in Appendix B, leading off with Dr. Robert C. Atkins' last book. These books were chosen because all contain recommendations for low-carb diets, and because all of them were written for educated readers such as you. The detailed reviews of these books point out differences in diet recommendations that are surprisingly at odds with one another. You ought to be able, after going over those reviews, to decide which diet advice to follow (if any). These books also have recipes and menus, which are not included here.

In order to limit the number of citations to individual research papers, a citation without a date of publication, but with a page number, will refer to one of the books reviewed in Appendix B. Example: Atkins, p100. In most cases, the book will have cited the original peer-reviewed articles.

47

Some Basic Food Chemistry

A century and a half ago the starch in certain foods and the sugars then known were found to have 1 carbon atom for each 2 hydrogen atoms and each oxygen atom, so the most simplified formula for many of these starches and sugars was $CH_2O$, making them appear to be "hydrates of carbon" — carbohydrates. This is also called an "empirical" formula, and it tells only which elements are present and their simplest whole-number ratio. The simplest common sugars were determined to have actual molecular formulas of $C_6H_{12}O_6$. Glucose is one of these, and chemistry students are all supposed to learn that there are many other sugars with this formula, but with slightly different arrangements of atoms. Common table sugar called sucrose looks like two of these fused together with loss of a water molecule, so its molecular formula is $C_{12}H_{22}O_{11}$. In sucrose, one of the two halves is from glucose, while the other half is derived from fructose.

For definitions, composition of, and physical and chemical changes in food, an excellent reference book exists (deMan, 1999), which is without bias or judgment or recommendations. For example, it explains that the technical term for "complex carbohydrates" is polysaccharides (pp183-206). Most are polymers (repeating units) of glucose, which is a monosaccharide. Glucose is also called dextrose, blood sugar, grape sugar, and corn sugar (not to be confused with corn syrup). Glucose is a distinct entity different from fructose (fruit sugar) or sucrose (common table sugar or cane sugar). The word "sugar" means sucrose in this book. "Sugars" means any kind of sugar.

One of the most common polymers of glucose is cellulose, which can be written $(C_6H_{10}O_5)_n$, and humans cannot digest it. It is the usual form of what is called fiber. Starches are also polymers of glucose with the same molecular formulas, but their slightly geometrically different hook-ups and branches make starches digestible by humans. Starch, called amylose by biochemists, is what we call flour when it is ground up. Starch is a complex carbohydrate that is converted to glucose in your body. A great many promoters of diets do not know this, and glorify complex carbohydrates, blithely ignorant of the fact that most starches have more calories than simple sugars, and raise blood glucose levels more. The starch in potato and corn is almost totally digestible, first being converted to glucose. Some starchy foods are not totally digestible, so they must contain some form of what is called "soluble fiber". Examples are durum wheat, bulgur, rye and oat flours, which are not totally digested.

The quantities of carbohydrates in food, as shown on food labels, are not assayed directly, as are fat, protein, ash or water, but are calculated by difference, so these carb quantities are not so accurate (Atkins, p173). All carbohydrates are not alike, either in digestibility or in their effects on blood glucose and insulin levels.

*Some* indigestible polysaccharide amounts in foods are listed on US and UK labels as fiber, or fibre, or dietary fiber, for which no calories are counted. This is what is also called "crude dietary fiber" and was determined by an older simple assay. This method missed soluble fiber, which is usually present in 2-16 times greater amounts (deMan, 1999, pp203-206), thus the caloric content for carbs on US food labels tends to be too high, because the quantity of soluble fiber is not listed, and because the fiber is only partially digested. The caloric values of the main food groups were originally determined by oxidizing (burning) foods in a bomb calorimeter under pressurized oxygen to form nitric acid, water and carbon dioxide, thus the honest older designation for the caloric values was "fuel values" (Atwater & Snell, 1903). These simple end-products are not nearly all of what is really formed in our bodies. The heat generated by burning was measured by how much it raised the temperature in the water surrounding the calorimeter.

A calorie is the unit of heat used in the USA. It is the heat energy needed to raise the temperature of 1 g of water by 1°C. Food energy values (the fuel values) are actually in kilocalories (kcal), which equal 1000 calories. Sloppily, the "k" has been left out on USA food labels, but will be

48

used accurately in this book. The older caloric values of food were: carb, 4.0 kcal/g; fat, 9.3; and protein, 5.25 or 5.6 (Wiley & Bigelow, 1898).*

Now it is understood that the net metabolizable energy (NME) from carbs in humans ranges from 0-2 kcal/g from fiber (Livesy, 2001) through 3.9 for sucrose to 4.2 for starches (Ottoboni & Ottoboni, p79). For example, the FDA food label on celery stalks gives 15 "calories" (should be kilocalories or kcal, but being off by 1,000x is good enough for government work) per 65 g serving based on the old fuel values, while the Geigy Tables on Food Composition give 11 kcal (Lentner, 1981, p246), which is 38% lower and correctly represents the digestible portion. Natural fats have different digestibilities, so their NME ranges from 5.5-8.5 kcal/g (see Appendix C). Proteins have been recognized to have an NME of 4.1 kcal/g (Kekwick & Pawan, 1969). So for clarity and consistency with most other authors, most of the discussion below is based on the conventional values of: carb, 4 kcal/g; fat, 9; and protein 4, despite the knowledge that 2 of 3 are usually wrong.

Compounding the problem of counting calories is the fact that meat contains hidden fat. A serving of lean beef brisket, for example, with no visible fat, still contains 44% of its total calories as fat, because the cell membranes of the meat are composed of fat (Enig & Fallon, 2005, p44-45). So the energy contents of diets given by conventional "experts" really contain much more fat, less carb and less protein than they calculate from the fuel values.


## Diabetes and the Glycemic Index

The glycemic index (GI) is the effect of a food on serum glucose level compared with the effect of an equal weight of glucose as a standard with a value of 100. If eating 75 g of glucose raised your serum glucose by 30 mg/dL, and eating 75 g of some food raised your serum glucose by 15 mg/dL, the food would have a GI of 50. The GI values of food range from 0 (fat) to 115 for tofu non-dairy frozen dessert. Old-fashioned ice cream has a GI of about 65. The glycemic load (GL) equals the GI times the dietary carbohydrate content in grams. Both GI and GL are important. A list of GI values may be seen at: http://wave.prohosting.com/rmendosa/gi.htm

Non-insulin-dependent diabetes mellitus (NIDDM) is a result of excessive carbohydrate consumption, which leads to excessive insulin production in people genetically so disposed. NIDDM is also called adult-onset or Type-II or Type-2 diabetes. Milder cases are called insulin resistance or Syndrome X. "Several prospective observational studies have shown that the chronic consumption of a diet with a high glycemic load is independently associated with an increased risk of developing type 2 diabetes, cardiovascular disease, and certain cancers." (Foster-Powell, et al., 2002). This is a very important concept, since it has been shown that NIDDM leads to so many other medical problems.

IDDM, also called juvenile onset or Type-I or Type-1 diabetes, is a result of destruction of most of the insulin-producing beta cells of the pancreas, and injected insulin is an essential component of successful treatment. According to Richard K. Bernstein, MD, "Prior to the availability of insulin...[in 1925]...people with Type I diabetes usually died within a few months of diagnosis. Their lives could be prolonged somewhat with a diet that was very low in carbohydrate and usually high in fat. Sufferers from...Type II diabetes frequently survived on this type of diet... When I became diabetic [with IDDM in 1947]...many people were still following very low carbohydrate, high-fat diets" (Bernstein, p310). About this time it was noted that the artificial induction of "atherosclerosis" in vegetarian animals force-fed with animal fats led to the assumption that some of the complications

---

*The rest of the civilized world uses the joule (J), 4.18 of which equal 1 calorie, so if you see "kJ" on a non-USA food label, you will know what it means.

of diabetes (atherosclerosis, CVD) were caused by high fat diets. "Therefore, I and many other diabetics...[were] treated with a high-carbohydrate, low-fat diet...as adopted by the American Diabetes Association (here ADbA), the American Heart Association (AHA) and other groups around the world. On the new diet many of us had even higher serum cholesterol levels, and still developed the grave complications of diabetes. Seemingly unaware of the importance of blood sugar control, the ADbA raised the recommended carbohydrate content to 40% of calories, and then more recently to 60%" (Bernstein, p310).

A rogues gallery of low-fat diet guidelines in the following section will seem very familiar to any of you who watch, read or listen to the mass media.

## Official Recommendations *Against* Low-Carb Diets

American Dietetic Association, 2003

"With nearly 70,000 members, the American Dietetic Association (ADA, here ADtA) is the nation's largest organization of food and nutrition professionals. The ADtA serves the public by promoting optimal nutrition, health and well-being." The AdtA endorses the Food Guide Pyramid of the United States Department of Agriculture (USDA) unequivocally, thus recommending high-carb diets with 75% carb, 10% fat and 15% protein. None of the books under review in Appendix B appear on the ADtA reading list. (http://www.eatright.org/Public/NutritionInformation/92_fgp.cfm)

United States Department of Agriculture, 1907 and 2004

USDA Bulletin No. 42 of 1907 says that "...as the chief function of the fats and carbohydrates is to serve as fuel, it is of more importance that they should be in sufficient amount than that they should be in definite relative proportions to each other" (Williams, 1907). How times change! The latest Food Guide Pyramid now has carbs in 5 different places, and seemingly recommends 20 servings of them to just 1 of fats (http://www.nal.usda.gov.8001/py/pymap.htm).

American Diabetes Association, 2003

The American Diabetes Association (ADbA) recommends 60% high-GI carbs in the diet without reservation: "The message today: Eat more starches! It is healthiest for everyone to eat more whole grains, beans, and starchy vegetables such as peas, corn, potatoes and winter squash. Starches are good for you because they have very little fat, saturated fat, or cholesterol. They are packed with vitamins, minerals, and fiber. Yes, foods with carbohydrate -- starches, vegetables, fruits, and dairy products -- will raise your blood glucose more quickly than meats and fats, but they are the healthiest foods for you. Your doctor may need to adjust your medications when you eat more carbohydrates. You may need to increase your activity level or try spacing carbohydrates throughout the day. On average Americans eat around 40-45% of our calories as carbohydrate. This is a moderate amount of carbohydrate, not high. Currently some controversy about carbohydrates is raging due to a number new diet books. These books encourage a low carbohydrate, high protein and moderate fat intake. These diets are not in synch with the American Diabetes Association nutrition recommendations, which are based on years of research and clinical experience. In addition, these trendy diets are hard to follow year after year."
(http://www.diabetes.org/nutrition-and-recipes/nutrition/starches.jsp)

US Food and Drug Administration, 2003

The US Food and Drug Administration (FDA) recommends high-carb diets with caloric content of 55% carb, 30% fat (1/3 each saturated, monounsaturated, polyunsaturated) and 15% protein. The % daily value (DV) of each on US food labels reflects this and utilizes the conventional caloric values of foods (http://www.cfsan.fda.gov/~dms/foodlab.html). Crude fiber is sometimes counted at 4 kcal/g instead of 0, and soluble fiber is not listed separately, or counted at 0-2 kcal/g, as it should be (Livesy, 2001).

National Cholesterol Education Program, 2003

The National Cholesterol Education Program (NCEP), seemingly sponsored by the National Heart, Lung and Blood Institute (NHLBI) of the National Institutes of Health (NIH), recommends high-carb diets with caloric content the same as those of the FDA. Many high GI foods are recommended as well as margarine, mayonnaise and vegetable oils, including for diabetics (www.nhlbisupport.com).

American Heart Association, 2003

The American Heart Association (AHA) recommends the use of a food pyramid with about the same caloric content from each of the food groups as in the USDA pyramid. Differences are that the AHA recommends no egg yolks at all, and otherwise to avoid saturated fat and cholesterol intake at all costs; also the positions of some foods are changed. The AHA favors small amounts of soft margarine, and large amounts of milk and low-fat milk and other dairy products, with no exceptions for diabetics that are apparent on the website. On their new web pages for diabetics: "Type 2 diabetes is a progressive disease that develops *when the body does not produce enough insulin* and does not efficiently use the insulin it does produce (a phenomenon known as insulin resistance)..." (Italics added.) The AHA notes that the World Health Organization Study (WHO) Group recommends that 15% of total calories be derived from fat, and is concerned that certain key nutrient levels will not be met in certain population groups at this level. The AHA still quotes the work of Ancel Keys stating that the consumption of saturated fat is the best predictor in the diet of heart disease (www.americanheart.org). The overall diet recommendations of the AHA, the ADtA and other groups were published in 1999 as the result of a conference (Deckelbaum et al., 1999).

American Medical Association, 2003

The American Medical Association clearly recommends a low-fat diet (http://www.ama-assn.org/ama/pub/article/4197-6132.html). By implication this means a high-carb diet.

Health Canada, 2003

Health Canada recommends very high-carb diets with caloric content of 78% carb, 9% fat and 13% protein. The Food Rainbow (instead of a pyramid) favors grains, then fruits and vegetables without regard to GI or exceptions for diabetics, followed distantly by "Other Foods" such as milk products, meats, and meat substitutes such as beans and peanut butter!
(http://www.hc-sc.gc.ca/hpfb-dgpsa/onpp-bppn/food_guide_rainbow_e.html)

National Advisory Committee, UK, 2003

In 1983-4, two UK committees, the National Advisory Committee for Nutrition Education and the Committee on the Medical Aspects of Food Policy recommended that the intake of fats be reduced "to prevent heart disease" (Groves, p25). Based on the information on the food label from Walkers Ready Salted Crisps the anonymous nutrition professionals of the United Kingdom recommend for average adults a daily fat-calorie energy consumption of 3.5% of total energy intake for women and 3.8% for men.

## Evidence Presented *Against* Low-Carb Diets

Dr. Felix Niemeyer, 1860s

As early as the 1860s, in reaction to the success story of William Banting's low-carb diet (see below), Dr. Felix Niemeyer of Stuttgart, on thermodynamic grounds later shown to be fallacious, recommended a high protein diet with both carb and fat restricted, which is still the basis of some slimming diets to this day (Groves, p19).

Sir William Osler, 1920s

Sir William Osler, an immensely influential professor of medicine in both the USA and UK, "recognized" about 100 years ago that atherosclerosis and angina pectoris were "afflictions of the better classes, not of the working classes", and ascribed the afflictions to consumption of eggs and milk rather than cereals, vegetables, fruit, fish and meat. Atherosclerosis was not found in wild animals, but in vegetarian lab animals fed cholesterol around 1911-4. Later study indicated that the cholesterol was oxidized, making it dangerous.

William Dock, MD, 1953

The writer of that bit of history on Osler, William Dock, MD, was positive that a diet with eggs, butter and cream killed 1/3 of all physicians (Dock, 1953). Of course, these observations influence nutrition to this day, but none has stood the test of time. For example, Osler's observations did not discern whether "the better classes" manifested their afflictions at greater ages than those of "the working classes". Even now, despite the leveling effects of national health services, the life expectancy of professional people in both the UK and Finland is 7.2 years longer than that of unskilled laborers (Cohen, 2003), making both Osler's and Dock's observations useless or worse as diet advice.

Diet-Heart Theory, 1950

The Diet-Heart Theory (DHT) was the notion that eating saturated fat and cholesterol made people fat and caused atherosclerosis leading to cardiovascular disease (CVD). The DHT was said to have begun in earnest in 1950 when Gofman et al. described a method for isolating the lipoproteins of blood by ultracentrifugation, and made 2 proposals: (1) that the concentration of serum low-density lipoprotein (LDL) was a useful index of atherogenesis, and (2) that the concentration could be influenced meaningfully by diet (Mann, 1977). Even though low-carb diets for diabetes were found beneficial at least since 1800 (Allan & Lutz, p7), the American Diabetes Association abandoned them around 1950 without a single trial (Atkins, p282). By 1977 it was already known that the DHT was false, that LDL was no better a predictor than total cholesterol (TC), and that high-density lipoprotein (HDL) concentration was supposedly inversely related to the incidence of cardiovascular disease, (Mann, 1977).

## Dr. Ancel Keys, 1953-1970

The DHT was inflated by Prof. Ancel Keys in 1953, who eventually published a graph showing that cardiovascular disease (CVD, blocked coronary arteries leading to heart attacks) was correlated with available food fat in 6 (later 7) countries, while ignoring data then available from the WHO on 16 other countries that did not fall nicely on the line of his graph. This was scientific misconduct at best, or outright fraud, and was used a an example of phony evidence in the Introduction. Moreover, the variation in CVD rates of 5-fold by location within 2 of the countries was not mentioned or resolved (Allen & Lutz, pp76-82; Groves, pp60-61; Mann, 1977; Ravnskov, pp15-19).

Sparked by Keys' earlier reports, in the mid-1950s, the AHA contracted with a team of investigators to evaluate evidence that the fat content of North American or European diets caused CVD. The report was submitted in 1957 with the conclusions that there was nothing to support the DHT. The AHA could have changed its direction or clung to the DHT with greater fervor; it did the latter after 4 years, beginning in 1961, recommending that *all* Americans reduce their consumption of fat and cholesterol (Smith, 1991, p8). The Special Communication of the AHA on these topics in *JAMA* also strongly recommended switching to polyunsaturated oils, the ones with linoleic acid, an omega-6 fatty acid, in particular. Perhaps it is revealing that none of the members of the Central Committee for Medical and Community Program put his name on this paper (Anon., 1961).

## Ernst Wynder, MD, 1965-1979

Animal fats have been associated with colon cancer by certain "authorities", beginning in 1965 when Ernst Wynder, MD, gave a presentation at a meeting. He projected a slide with a supposed correlation of animal fat consumption in many countries with the incidence of colon cancer. His figures were erroneous in that most of the fat consumed in most of the countries was vegetable fat (or oil). For the US he misrepresented as animal fat what was actually 89% processed vegetable fats, which would have encompassed *trans* fats as well. In 1973 his hypothesis was said to have been confirmed by examination of the diets of Japanese Hawaiians by staff of the NIH, yet their own findings implicated macaroni, beans, peas and soy, not beef. In 1979 Wynder's hypothesis received yet more support in a review in the American Journal of Epidemiology based on his false data (Enig, 2000, pp84-85).

## Nurses' Health Study II, 2003

Evidence supposedly correlating the intake of animal fat with breast cancer appeared recently. A prospective analysis of the relation between dietary fat intake and breast cancer risk among 90,655 premenopausal women in the Nurses' Health Study II, in which the subjects were followed for eight years, showed, according to the results in the abstract of the paper in the *Journal of the National Cancer Institute*: "...Relative to women in the lowest quintile of fat intake, women in the highest quintile of intake had a slight increased risk of breast cancer (RR = 1.25, 95% CI = 0.98 to 1.59; $p$ trend = 0.06). The increase was associated with intake of animal fat but not vegetable fat; the [multi-variables adjusted] relative risks for the increasing quintiles of animal fat intake were 1.00 (referent), 1.28, 1.37, 1.54, and 1.33 (95% CI = 1.02 to 1.73; P trend = 0.002)..." The conclusions in the abstract of this paper are: "Intake of animal fat, mainly from red meat and high-fat dairy foods during premenopausal years, is associated with an increased risk of breast cancer." (Cho et al., 2003)

First off, note that the arbitrarily adjusted risk in the fourth quintile of animal fat intake is larger than the fifth quintile. This is very suspicious, since the fifth and highest quintile of intake should have had the highest risk for breast cancer if there were any real trend. In fact the fifth quintile had only the third highest risk after the arbitrary adjustments.

The absence of absolute risk levels is misleading. The Tables 1 and 2 in the paper allow us to calculate what the *unadjusted* chances *not* to get breast cancer are. Here are the median energy percentage intake as animal fat/percentage who did *not* get breast cancer for each quintile: 12% energy intake from animal fat / 99.3% who did *not* get breast cancer, 15%/99.2, 17%/99.2, 20%/99.1, 23%/99.3. Many of the adjustments used were of doubtful soundness, such as for body-mass index and alcohol intake, and there was *no* trend in the *unadjusted* data. See that the percent of nurses who did *not* get breast cancer hardly changes from the lowest to highest intake. It runs from 99.1 to 99.3%, not enough difference to be a concern. Thus the drumbeat that animal fat consumption causes cancer continues to this day, while the actual data in this paper make a mockery of its conclusions (Kauffman, 2004a).

Framingham Study, 1948-2000

By 1970 the Framingham Study, begun in 1948, had examined about 1000 people by dietary recall; it was reported that there was *no* correlation between dietary saturated fat or cholesterol intake and measured serum cholesterol (Groves, pp61-2; Mann, 1977). After 30 years of follow-up the AHA and the National Heart, Lung and Blood Institute of the NIH (NHLBI) reported in 1990 in *The Cholesterol Facts* that: "The results of the Framingham Study indicate that a 1% reduction...of cholesterol [corresponds to a] 2% reduction in CHD risk". But in their *JAMA* paper based on the same data the authors wrote that those [subjects] whose cholesterol had *decreased* by itself during those 30 years ran a greater risk of dying than those whose cholesterol had *increased*. And: "For each 1 % *drop* of cholesterol there was an 11% *increase* in coronary and total mortality." (Anderson et al., 1987; Ravnskov, pp57-8). You read that correctly: the result reported for the public was the opposite of what was reported from the same data in *JAMA*, formerly the *Journal of the American Medical Association*.

Multiple Risk Factor Intervention Trial, 1982

Beginning in 1972 the Multiple Risk Factor Intervention Trial (MRFIT), sponsored by the NHLBI, was a randomized clinical trial (RCT), potentially the most scientific sort of comparative study, as described in both the Introduction and in Myth 1. Of the approximately 361,662 men who were screened, a group of 12,866 men aged 35-57 said to be at high risk of CVD were selected. Those at *very* high risk, namely men who had a previous heart attack, angina, diabetes, TC >350 mg/dL, diastolic blood pressure over 115 mm Hg, high BMI or in treatment with most common drugs, were actually excluded as well! Subjects in the intervention group were asked to eat much less animal fat (high-carb diet) and to smoke less, and they were reported to have a non-significantly lower death rate from CVD after a mean follow-up of 7 years compared with the control group (MRFIT Res. Grp., 1982). However the *overall* mortality rate in the intervention group was slightly *higher* due to more cancer. Since smoking does increase cancer rates, one must conclude that eating animal fat protected against cancer (Allan & Lutz, pp84-5).

NHLBI/AHA Consensus Development Conference,1984

These and other trials moved the NHLBI and the AHA to hold a Consensus Development Conference in December of 1984. A 14-member panel and 600 attendees showed considerable disagreement on the effect of diet on TC levels and on the frequency of CVD, which was supposedly associated with high levels of TC or LDL. Written *before* the meeting (Enig, 2003) a statement, quickly incorporated into a press release, and claimed to be a result of *consensus*, proclaimed that: "The blood cholesterol of most Americans is undesirably high [>200 mg/dL], in a large part because of our high intake of calories, saturated fat, and cholesterol". This became the genesis of the National

Cholesterol Education Program (NCEP), which was quickly supported by the AMA, Kellogg (breakfast cereal producer), Merck (producer of cholesterol-lowering drugs even then) and American Home Products (which had an agricultural division at the time that promoted soybeans), (Moore, 1989, pp56-81).

New Cholesterol Guidelines, 2001

The New Cholesterol Guidelines were approved by the NCEP, and released to the public on 15 May 2001. The Guidelines ignore the adverse effects of excess dietary carbohydrates as well as the imbalance of essential fatty acids created by their recommendation of vegetable oils instead of animal fat. Despite the acknowledgement that the low-fat diets recommended and used by many for 40 years exacerbated obesity and NIDDM, the new recommendation was to intensify the use of the failed diets! (Ottoboni, pp177-182). This was supposed to be supported by a meta-analysis of 9 RCTs on low-fat (high-carb) diets; but both CVD and total mortality were unchanged in 7 trials, up in 1 and down in another. Another meta-analysis supported "...a central role of dietary fat intake in the causation of CVD...", but to reach this conclusion the authors included a trial with more heavy smokers in the control group, and excluded the trial with the most contradictive result. This folderol was reported by Uffe Ravnskov, MD, PhD, a world-famous cholesterol expert. (Ravnskov, 2002a).

Scott R. Grundy, MD, 2002

Evidence *for* the value of low-carb diets has been attacked at least twice by Scott R. Grundy, MD, in publications. As a spokesman for the AHA, he cited 10 studies in support of the AHA's diet recommendations of 1982. On close examination of this first attack, 6 of the 10 studies used inappropriate liquid formula diets, 1 failed to report the effect of its diet on TC, 2 by Ancel Keys reported almost no effect of dietary cholesterol on serum cholesterol levels, and the final study indicated a *decrease* in serum cholesterol with the *addition* of dietary cholesterol (Smith, 1991, pp188-9).

More recently, an article by Gary Taubes in *Science* critical of the NCEP's low-fat recommendation was attacked by Grundy, who wrote that many studies showed that saturated fatty acids as a class, compared with unsaturated fatty acids and *carbohydrate,* raise serum LDL and thus cause CVD. Grundy cited two reviews in support. In one there are no references. In the other, of which Grundy is a co-author, there are 12 references used as support. On close examination, none of the 12 were really supportive, and some did not even directly address his issue (Ravnskov et al., 2002). Dr. Grundy has received honoraria from Merck, Pfizer, Sankyo, Bayer, and Bristol-Myers Squibb (ATPIII, 2001).

Dena M. Bravata et al., Stanford CA Medical, 2003

In a study partially funded by the *American Medical Association* (AMA), a prodigious literature review on articles in English on low-carb diets was performed by use of MEDLINE and other searches for articles published between 1 Jan 1966 and 15 Feb 2003. All 2609 potentially relevant articles were perused. Bravata et al. excluded all but 107 articles on 94 studies on 3268 subjects receiving 0-901 g/day of carbohydrates for 4-365 days, but the reasons for exclusion of so many of the trials were obscure. Only 5 studies (non-randomized and no control groups) lasted more than 90 days.

The Conclusions of the paper in the *Journal of the American Medical Association* on this review included the following: "...these [low-carb] diets have not been adequately evaluated for use longer than 90 days, or for individuals aged 53 years or older, or for use by participants with hyperlipidemia, hypertension, or diabetes". Only books by Atkins, Sears and Heller were cited, and incorrectly said to recommend more protein and less carb, where, in fact, more fat was recommended. The Abstract's Conclusions verbatim are: "There is insufficient evidence to make recommendations for or against the use of low-carbohydrate diets, particularly among participants older than age 50 years, for use longer than 90 days, or for diets of 20 g/d or less of carbohydrates. Among the published studies that were reviewed, participant weight loss while using low-carbohydrate diets was principally associated with decreased caloric intake and increased diet duration but not with reduced carbohydrate content." (Bravata et al., 2003).

Of the 2 main "low-carb" groups into which the trials were divided by Bravata et al., the under 60 g/d group's mean intake of carb was 29 g/d, and the total energy intake all foods was 1446 kcal/day (fuel values). In the over 60 g/d group the mean intake of carb was 236 g/d, and total intake of all foods was 1913 kcal/day (from their Table 3). But in the books reviewed in Appendix B, any intake over about 150-200 g/d of total carb would not be considered low-carb. In the true low-carb group (under 60 g/d) the mean weight loss in trials was 17 kg (37 lbs), while in the higher-carb group it was only 2 kg (4 lbs) as found in Table 5 of Bravata et al., who do not consider this significant and attribute the result to the lower total caloric intake as quoted above. Low-carb diets were said to have no adverse effects on serum lipid, fasting serum glucose, fasting insulin levels, or blood pressure, according to Bravata et al. This clever wording is different from writing that there was a beneficial effect of low-carb diets on these measured parameters, which studies in the next section do show.

The caloric intake view (all calories are the same) has been falsified in several studies. For example, controlled trials in a hospital have shown that a diet of just 1,000 kcal/day, which was 90% carbohydrate, led to weight gain, and intakes of 1,000 to 2,600 kcal/day with a very low carbohydrate content led to weight loss (Groves, pp21-2). A female "dieter" lost a little weight on a diet of 5,000 kcal/day which contained only 30-40 g (2.4-3.2% of energy intake) of digestible carb (Eades & Eades, pp50-1). Thus the trick used by Bravata et al. to trash low-carb diets was to combine trials on them with other trials which were actually on medium-to-high-carb diets.

*****

Thus you can see that most of the evidence supposedly invalidating the use of low-carb diets is misleading at best, and may be outright fraud at worst. Therefore, there is no solid evidence behind the numberless advertisements for low-fat or low-cholesterol foods.

### Recommendations and Evidence *Favoring* Low-Carb Diets

*Individual Observations*

So what is the evidence for the safety and efficacy of low-carb diets? The examples following are all of multi-year observations that support the thesis that low-carb diets are safe and effective for long periods, as well as promoting quality-of-life. Granted these are anecdotes, but of a number and duration to make the overall weight of evidence persuasive.

These are followed by the results of short-term randomized clinical trials (RCTs). While the RCT is supposed to be the ultimate for making medical decisions, it is not the only source of acceptable data. The differences in outcomes observed between study centers in a number of multi-center drug RCTs is so extreme as to question their lack of bias (O'Shea et al., 2001). It is true that RCTs on low-carb diets of durations longer than a few months are scarce, and that none have been carried beyond 1 year as of this time. It is true that clinical experience as in some of the examples given may be biased, but there is support for the possibility that clinical data may be less biased than some RCTs (O'Brien, 2003).

## William Banting, 1860s

Undertaker to the rich and famous, William Banting became obese in his thirties. An eminent surgeon and friend recommended extreme exercise, which Banting carried out, only to increase his appetite, so he stopped it. Baths, cathartics and low-calorie starvation diets did no better. At the age of 64, in 1862, Banting weighed 91 kg (200 lbs) and was 1.65 m (5 ft, 5 in) tall, and had failing eyesight and deafness. William Harvey, MD, advised Banting to give up bread, butter, milk, sugar, beer and potatoes. After 38 weeks on a fairly low-carb diet, Banting had lost 21 kg (46 lbs), felt better, and no longer had any other ailments. Delighted, he published the details at his own expense and gave away 1000 copies of his now famous *Letter on Corpulence*. He remained a normal weight until his death at age 81 after 17 years on his low-carb diet (Groves, 15-19; Allan & Lutz, 12-13).

## Vilhjalmur Stefansson, MD, 1920s-1960s

Vilhjalmur Stefansson, MD, and Anthropology Instructor at Harvard University (Braly & Hoggan, p204), beginning at age 27 in 1906, spent a total of 15 years with the Canadian Eskimos, including eating their obviously healthful high-fat no-carb diet, which he grew to prefer. There are reports of many Eskimos living into their 90s in the 18th century (Michener, 1988). In 1928 Stefansson and a former companion, Karsten Anderson, MD, entered Bellevue Hospital in New York for a 1-year trial of Eskimo diets. Anderson did well with an all-meat diet, but Stefansson required considerable fat to feel his best, finally settling on 80% fat and 20% protein, with a total caloric intake of 2000-3100 kcal/day. His TC went *down* about 10 mg/dL. All kinds of other tests were done, but no bad effects of his diet were seen (Lieb, 1929; McClellan & Du Bois, 1930). In the last 6 years of his life, Stefansson returned to his Arctic diet until his death at age 83, spending a total of 22 years on such a diet (Allan & Lutz, 14-17; Groves, 20-21).

## Jan Kwasniewski, MD, and colleagues, 1970s to present

Jan Kwasniewski, MD, who ran a clinic in Poland (see review of his book in Appendix B), has used a low-carb diet for 30 years, and is still practicing medicine at age 66. His colleague, Marek Chylinski, has used one for about 14 years, according to their book translator, Bogdan Sikorski, who has used one for 6 years and looks like a football player at age 45.

## Michael R. Eades, MD and Mary Dan Eades, MD, 1980s to present

Michael R. Eades, MD and Mary Dan Eades, MD have consumed a low-carb diet themselves for about 19 years, as well as recommending such for thousands of their patients (see review of their book in Appendix B).

## Richard K. Bernstein, MD, 1960s to present

Richard K. Bernstein, was diagnosed with insulin-dependent diabetes mellitus (IDDM) at the age of 12 in 1946. Following the advice of the AHA and ADbA to eat a high-carb (40%, then 60% carb) diet, his condition worsened and most of the complications of IDDM began to appear. He found that he could not normalize his blood sugars with any insulin regimen, and that exercise in his condition did not help. By doing a literature search himself, he realized the potential benefits of normal blood sugars. By using himself as the test animal he found that about 30 g/day of slow-acting carbohydrate (essentially fiber with no simple sugars or high GI starches at all) was necessary to normalize his blood glucose levels, the rest of his diet being fat and protein. He obtained an MD degree at about age 45 partly to have his observations published in medical journals, because the papers were rejected when he did not have the MD degree. He has continued the diet for 35 years so far, which includes on many days, 3 eggs for breakfast and no fruit. His TC dropped from 300 mg/dL to 179, of which LDL = 63 and HDL = 116 (that is not a misprint). His TG dropped from 250 to 45. His lipoprotein(a) level, a marker of inflammation, became undetectable. In 1983 he began his own medical practice for diabetics. At age 72 he still works 12-14-hour days in his medical practice on diabetics (Bernstein, pp xii-xx, 127).

## Robert C. Atkins, MD, 1960s-2003

Robert C. Atkins, MD, as a young cardiologist in 1963, gained weight rapidly and needed a hunger-free way to deal with it. Finding that a low-carb diet worked, he remained on it until his death from trauma 39 years later at age 71 (Atkins, p306).

## Barry Groves, PhD, 1960s to present

Barry Groves, PhD, e-mailed that he has eaten a low-carb diet for 41 years and enjoys excellent health at age 67 exemplified by his status as a British and World Champion Archer.

## Wolfgang Lutz, MD, 1950s to present

Wolfgang Lutz, MD, who has been operating a clinic for internal medicine in Vienna, has used a low-carb diet (72 g/day) for 50 years, and is still active at age 90. His colleague Christian Allan, PhD, age 42, and his wife Jenny Allan, have each used low-carb diets for 7 years, and are healthy (all from a recent e-mail from C. Allan).

### Clinical Observations

Lutz followed many of his patients on low-carb diets for many years. The most desirable level for serum glucose after 12 hours of fasting is 90 mg/dL; under 125 is usually not treated in any way. The mean baseline fasting serum glucose levels for 15 of Lutz's patients with slight non-insulin-dependent diabetes mellitus (NIDDM) was 167 mg/dL; a low-carb diet reduced the level to 125 after 6 months. (These are almost identical with the glucose level changes in myself after 6 months of low-carb diet.)

The glucose tolerance test shows how rapidly a person can lower her serum glucose levels after eating or drinking about 75 g of glucose. The glucose tolerance curves of 7 patients before and after they adopted a low-carb diet for several months showed how much hyperinsulinemia was brought down (Allan & Lutz, pp37-49). Since too much insulin in the blood is thought to cause some of the damage to many organs, one does not want any higher insulin level than is needed to knock down glucose levels.

Both too little or too much hemoglobin in the blood is unhealthful; the latter is called polycythemia, with which condition the blood of the patient is more likely to clot, leading to heart attacks and strokes. Levels of 14-16 g/dL are normal. Before beginning a low-carb diet the mean hemoglobin level of 130 patients was 17.3 g/dL. After 10 months on the diet the 40 patients still available were down to 15.8, and after 30 months the 12 patients still available were down to 15.6 (Allan & Lutz, pp94-95).

Before beginning a low-carb diet the mean systolic blood pressure in 38 patients was 194 mm Hg (see Myth 4). After 1 week and up to 5 years on a low-carb diet this varied between 160-172 for the 2-27 patients available.

One of the longest-lasting fears expressed about low-carb diets is that too much protein will cause gout or kidney stones due to increased levels of uric acid in the blood. Before beginning a low-carb diet the mean level of uric acid in 193 patients was 7.3 mg/dL; this plunged to 5.8 after 4 months on a low-carb diet for the 38 patients available, and did not go above 6.9 during 46 months. True, the sickest patients might have been the ones to disappear, skewing the results.

It is normal for total cholesterol (TC) levels in serum to rise with age, and people over 60 with the highest TC levels live the longest (see Myth 3). In patients over 60 years old, mean TC was 307 mg/dL before the low-carb diet began, and 310 25 months afterwards; among those 40-60 years old, TC was 297 before and 280 25 months afterwards; among those under 40 years old, mean TC was 285 before and 230 8 months afterwords. The downward direction of the changes in TC from very high levels in those under 60 years old may be considered beneficial, since the drops were not caused by severe infection, inflammation or cancer.

Electrocardiograms (EKGs) from 7 patients were presented and said to be improved after a low-carb diet was adopted (Allan & Lutz, pp94-108). Of course, one must trust that these were not selective data.

*Epidemiological Studies*

Using data from the Nurses Health Study on 65,173 women aged 40-65 years and free from CVD, cancer and diabetes at the start, who completed a detailed dietary questionnaire and were followed for 6 years, and after adjustment for age, BMI, smoking and many other factors, those eating a diet of the highest quintile in glycemic index (GI, high-carb diet) had a RR of 1.37 for the 915 cases of diabetes observed. Using glycemic load (GL), those in the highest quintile had RR of 1.47. When high GL was combined with low cereal fiber intake the RR became 2.5; all RRs were highly significant because of the huge numbers of subjects involved (Bernstein, p444; Salmeron et al., 1997).

Another study, this one done by a team at the Department of Nutrition at the Harvard School of Public Health, Boston, MA, on 75,521 nurses followed for 10 years, found that high GL predicted CVD better than high GI, which was still a better predictor than whether the carb content of the diet was simple or complex (Liu et al., 2000). Thus for CVD the RR = 1.57 for the highest quintile of GL vs. the lowest. When adjusted only for age and smoking, $p$ was < 0.0001, meaning that there was only a 1/10,000 probability of the difference being due to chance. This is one of many confirmations that eating complex carbs (starches) is no panacea for disease; the GI and GL are what counts, and starches are usually high in both. This invalidates the claims of many writers, including Arthur Agatston, MD, in *The South Beach Diet,* 2003, that switching to complex carbs will make you healthy.

Contrarily, a prospective (see footnote in Myth 1) study on 2286 men and 2030 women aged 40-69 and initially free of NIDDM, with a 10-year follow-up, was reported to show an inverse relation of NIDDM with whole-grain consumption (RR = 0.65) and much more so with cereal fiber intake (RR = 0.39), (Montonen et al., 2003). Many adjustments to other variables were made to obtain these figures. The authors did not remark on the notably inverse relation of magnesium intake with diabetes which they found, which should have been highlighted. Others have emphasized the connection (Dean, 2003, p113-116). Magnesium is important to carb metabolism by its influence on the release and activity of insulin (Cohen, 2004, p42-45).

*Controlled Trials*

More evidence is now provided to show that the common contentions of health authorities — that all calories are alike, and that only caloric restriction will suffice for weight loss — is wrong. For this purpose, studies of shorter duration will have to serve. Water loss of 2-4 kg is generally completed within a week (Atkins, p84-5), and is not an explanation for the success of low-carb diets.

In 1956 Prof. Alan Kekwick and Gaston Pawan, MD, at Middlesex Hospital, London, England, conducted tests of 4 varieties of 1,000 kcal/day diets: 90% fat (by fuel values), 90% protein, 90% carbohydrate, and a normal mixed diet. Subjects on the high-fat diet lost much more weight than any of the others. Several subjects on the high-carb diet actually gained weight, even at only 1000 kcal/day! Even at 2,600 kcal/day of very low-carb diet, subjects lost weight (Groves, p21-2). A patient of Eades & Eades (pp50-1) lost a little weight on a diet of 5,000 kcal/day which contained only 30-40 g (2.4-3.2%) of digestible carb. Thus the dogma that a "balanced" diet is best for almost everyone had been falsified a half century ago.

Reported in 1988, a small study (n = 7) measured serum TC, HDL, TG, and fasting serum glucose after adult subjects with high baseline TC levels ate a diet of fatty beef, fruit and vegetables (and no sucrose, milk, or grains) for 3-18 months (mean 8 months). Mean TC dropped from 263 to 189 mg/dL; HDL rose from 57 to 63 mg/dL (n = 6); TG dropped from 113 to 73 mg/dL; and fasting glucose from 167 to 96 mg/dL (n = 2). Patients became ill if they ate beef *without* bulk fat (Newbold, 1988).

Numerous other studies confirm these findings (Atkins, pp282-4; Groves, 21-2; Kauffman, 2002; Mann, 1977) so, not to abuse your patience, just 6 very recent trials will be cited to demonstrate that not all calories are equal in effects on obesity, and further falsify the notion that either a "balanced diet" or low-fat diet is optimal.

(1) A recent one-year diet trial supposedly designed to evaluate the Atkins (low-carb) diet examined 63 subjects, of whom the 33 assigned to the Atkins diet were given a copy of Atkins' book (reviewed in Appendix B) and were instructed to follow it, including no restriction on the amount of fat and protein that could be eaten. The 30 assigned to the low-fat diet (60% carb, 25% fat, 15% protein by fuel values) were restricted to 1200-1500 kcal/day for women and 1500-1800 kcal/day for men, definitely slimming diets by conventional standards. All subjects met with a registered dietitian 4 times. Since registered dietitians are indoctrinated by the ADtA to promote high-carb diets, this variable was not properly controlled, since the controls would have had reinforcement (placebo effect) and low-carb subjects would not (nocebo effect, O'Mathúna, 2003). In addition, subjects were excluded if they were ill, had NIDDM, were taking lipid-lowering medications or ones that affect body weight (see Atkins book review in Appendix B), or were pregnant or lactating. *In other words, most of the potential subjects who would have benefited the most from the Atkins diet were excluded.* Nevertheless, there was more weight loss among subjects on the Atkins diet, highly significant at 3 and 6 months, but claimed not to be significant at 12 months by using data from all participants, including those who did not complete the study, but whose values were extrapolated! The absolute difference in weight loss as % body weight was actually 3% between groups at 12 months among those actually completing the study, favoring the low-carb group. Low-carb dieters had increased HDL and decreased TG. Adherence was poor and attrition high in both groups, but adherence was better in the low-carb group. More trials were recommended, and all the usual unfounded dreads about low-carb diets were resurrected, probably to preserve the researchers' status as low-fat flunkies and grant-getters (Foster et al., 2003).

(2) The subjects of a 12-week RCT on adolescents were 13-17 years old, and had an initial mean weight of 92.1 kg (203 pounds) in the low-carb group and 99.5 kg (219 pounds) in the low-fat group. The low-carb group used an Atkins diet, with very appropriate increases of carb over time, and consumed 1830 kcal/day. The low-fat group at under 40 g/day of fat and 75 g of whole-grain carb, consumed 1100 kcal/day. The low-carb group lost 9.9 kg (22 pounds) vs 4.1 kg (9 pounds), ($p < 0.05$)

for the low-fat group (Sondike et al., 2003), despite both the lower initial weight of the low-carb group and the disparity in calories— much more in the low-carb group. Chalk up another win for Atkins.

(3) A 10-week RCT on obese women (ages 45-56 years) carried out at the University of Illinois Urbana-Champaign, followed the USDA Food Guide Pyramid for the high-carb group, consuming 55% carb, 30% fat and 15% protein in energy content using the fuel values. In the "low-carb" group, which actually ate a moderate-carb diet comprised of 41% carb, 30% fat and 29% protein, very close to Barry Sears' Zone Diet. Both ate 1700 kcal.day, both had 30% energy as fat and equal fiber. Several weeks involved all food being served in the laboratory, and the diets otherwise were strictly controlled. Slightly more weight was lost in the lower-carb, high-protein group, which had a significantly higher fat loss (as in Sears, pp40-53), significantly lower TG and TG/HDL, and these subjects were less hungry (Layman et al., 2003).

(4) Another assault on the Atkins diet claims that it "...restricts carb to less than 10% of daily caloric intake, causes ketosis, and promises fat loss, weight loss, and satiety, which have not [sic] been established as outcomes." Brehm and his team at the University of Cincinnati and Children's Hospital Medical Center aired the usual shibboleths that the increased fat, especially saturated fat, will lead to CVD, and used selective citations "linking" high fat to increased triglycerides (TG), insulin resistance, glucose intolerance and obesity (Brehm et al., 2003). So an RCT of 6 months duration was performed on 53 healthy obese women, BMI 33.6, who were randomized to either an Atkins low-carb diet or a 55% carb diet said to be recommended by the AHA (which actually recommends 75%). Exclusion criteria included CVD, hypertension and diabetes, so again, subjects who might have benefited the most were absent. Both groups were subjected to registered dietitians, so the caveats above apply.

Both groups were free-living *and had reduced calorie consumption by similar amounts* at 3 and 6 months. Adherence was good and there were only 3 dropouts in each group. The low-carb group lost 8.5 kg vs 3.9 kg ($p = < 0.001$) in the high-carb group, including more body fat: 4.8 kg vs 2.0 kg ($p < 0.01$, only 1/100 the probability that this result was due to chance). Both groups had "improved" blood lipid concentrations (see Myth 3) and no changes in EKGs.

The authors were so honest as to write: "This study provides a surprising challenge to prevailing dietary practice". Moreover, gleaned from one of their figures but not stated, indicated that the weight loss in the high-carb group was leveling out, while the loss in the low-carb group was continuing down.

(5) The target of an RCT, also of 6 months duration, at the Philadelphia Veterans Affairs Medical Center was *The Protein Power Lifeplan* (see review of Eades & Eades book in Appendix B). Stratified randomization of 132 severely obese subjects (mean BMI =43) ensured that the low-carb and low-fat groups would have equal numbers of diabetics and women. The exclusion criteria were thus reasonable, including inability to monitor one's own glucose, participation in another weight loss program, use of weight-loss drugs, or severe, life-limiting conditions. The low-fat group was to follow the NHLBI guidelines (55% carb, 30% fat, 15% protein) with calorie restriction to create an energy deficit of 500 kcal/day. The low-carb group was instructed to use 30 g of carb per day, which was incorrectly imputed to Eades, who actually recommend less than 40 g of total carb/day, even to start, and by the 6-month phase, in Maintenance mode, less than 120 g digestible carb per day (Eades & Eades, p335).

Both free-living groups were given an exceptional number of contacts with "experts in nutritional counseling", so the placebo and nocebo effects postulated by this reviewer for the study of Foster et al. would be even more intense here. No wonder then, that adherence was poor and dropout rates were high. But the dropout rate at the 3-month mark was 47% in the low-fat group and 33% in the low-carb group ($p$ = 0.03). The difference between the two groups in consumption of energy from carbs was quite narrow: 51% in the low-fat group, and 37% in the low-carb group, pretty close to the 40% carb energy recommended by Sears. Total energy intake at the 6-month mark was 1576 kcal/day in the low-fat group and 1630 kcal/day in the low-carb group. Nevertheless, the low-carb group lost 5.8 kg (and was still losing weight at 6 months) vs 1.9 kg (and leveled off) in the low-fat group ($p$ = 0.002). TG dropped 20% in the low-carb group. vs 4% in the low-fat group ($p$ = 0.001). The low-carb group became more insulin-sensitive ($p$ = 0.01). Yet the authors want these results to be interpreted with caution "given the known benefits of fat restriction" (Samaha et al., 2003).

(6) Besides being best for weight loss in carb-sensitive people, a low-carb diet can slow the progression of cardiovascular disease (CVD), as found by researchers at 5 universities in Boston, MA, Winston-Salem, NC and Seattle, WA. A prospective (defined in a footnote in Myth 1) study was carried out on 235 postmenopausal women whose normal diets, whatever they were, were compared with the narrowing of openings of their coronary arteries, as determined by angiography, before and after a 3.1-year trial period. Here a "dye" that shows up on Xray is injected and the pictures obtained can show differences in the diameter of the opening of 0.02 mm. Greater carbohydrate intake by quartile was strongly associated with more narrowing of the arteries ($p$ for trend = 0.001), and even more so when the GI was high. (Mozaffarian et al., 2004) The carbohydrate included the whole grains in typical diets.

One of the study's sponsors was the NHLBI. One must wonder how much longer the NHLBI's and NCEP's diet recommendations for high-carb diets as given above will remain unchanged Or why this type of trial, which could have been done 30 years ago, was delayed so long.

All these controlled trials confirm the findings of an observational study called "The Spanish Paradox". After 1975 the Spanish became more prosperous, ate more meat and saturated fat as well as much less cereal and pasta. Their CVD mortality dropped by about 35% from 1975 to 1990 (Serre-Majem et al., 1995).

*****

All these recent studies confirm what had already been known: calorie content is not as predictive of weight loss as reduced carb consumption. Low-carb diets have other demonstrable benefits besides better adherence, and no deleterious effects whatever in people of the appropriate metabolic type, that is, people who tend to convert too much of their carbohydrate intake to fat — the "carb-sensitive types". Several of the journal articles discussed above indicate bias and attempts to make trial results conform to diet dogma which is negative to low-carb diets.

Starting a Low-Carb Diet

Whether persons adopting a low-carb diet should plunge in at once to the very low carb levels, or approach them gradually is not yet clear. In the practice of Herbert H. Nehrlich, MD, a gradual approach cut down the problems with gallbladder overreaction to the required high fat content.

## Allergies to Grain, Wheat, Soy or Milk Proteins

Recommendations to eat lots of grains, from government and non-government agencies, and some popular diet books, rarely include warnings on common allergies to grain. Grain proponents are so focused on the mystique of the "complex carbohydrates" of grains that they ignore the consequences of grain allergies. The symptoms can range from frequent stomach aches to diarrhea alternating with constipation. Another manifestation is chronic fatigue syndrome. More serious cases may be called celiac disease, or the even more debilitating Crohn's disease. This leads to emaciation due to malnourishment caused by a compromised ability of the gastrointestinal system to digest food. Multiple sclerosis, IDDM, infertility, brain disorders, chronic pain or problematic pregnancies are typical signs of grain allergies that lead to autoimmune reactions. Breast cancer, in the families of celiac disease patients, is twice as common as in the general population. Other cancers of the digestive tract are 10-12 times as frequent in celiac sufferers (Braly & Hoggan, p113). Some forms of cancer of the gastrointestinal system may be the ultimate result (see Myth 10). Grain allergies, sometimes to wheat specifically, are among the most under diagnosed conditions in much of the developed world.

Grain allergies are strongly associated with thyroid gland problems, which may be over- or underproduction of thyroid hormones (Braly & Hoggan, pp81,123). Mild thyroid failure is found in 10% of the USA population and in up to 20% of older women. Another reason for the increasing incidence of thyroid failure is water fluoridation (see Myth 11). (Shames & Shames, 2001, pp4,12)

Grains are a recent addition to human diets, only being added beginning about 10,000 years ago for some populations, and much more recently for others. Whole grain proteins, including lectins, glutens, and gliadins are not healthful for 10-40% of typical populations. People who have grain allergies, but who are not carb-sensitive, may be better off with refined grains than whole grains. Ubiquitous recommendations for whole grains for everyone are not based on real evidence, and dangerous for people who are allergic. Blanket recommendations for unrefined grains over the corresponding refined ones, as is supported by at least one study (Liu et al., 2003) must be tempered by the fact that their sometimes lower GI is not accompanied by a lower GL (Foster-Powell, 2002), and more gluten and other allergens are found in the proteins of unrefined grains (Braly & Hoggan, p101).

To find out about having a grain allergy, you can be tested. Some of the best non-invasive tests on blood serum are described in Smith's book (see Appendix B). Allergies to soy or milk proteins are common enough to be considered. Elimination of these from the diet may be tried for a month instead of testing. This is not as simple as we might like, since "textured vegetable protein", a soybean product, is used in many packaged products whose labels do not necessarily show the word "soy". Worse, the stuff is often used as a meat extender in fast foods which do not have labels with ingredients (Daniel, 2005). Milk chocolate may contain enough milk protein to be allergenic.

Usually the range of allergenic foods in limited, and the diet restrictions are much less than those for very low-carb dieters. Sometimes a low-carb diet that eliminates grains, soy products or milk will make the dieter feel much better by accident, because an allergen has been eliminated. Testing and finding a specific allergy may allow many foods to return to an over-restricted diet.

The books by Braly and Hoggan and by Smith (both reviewed in Appendix B) are focused on grain allergies. Eades & Eades (reviewed in Appendix B) has a entire chapter on such allergies.

<u>Food Fights over Fat, Fructose, Fiber, etc.</u>

Limiting Fat and Protein Intake

Whether the amounts of protein and fat should be limited is disputed, and probably depends on the individual. Since protein does have a glycemic response, it seems as though the amount should be limited to what is needed to maintain lean body mass. Sears fixes the calories from fat as equal to the calories from protein. Bernstein and Eades & Eades advise that, if weight loss is still desired after a period of very low-carb diet, the fat intake will have to be cut, whatever it was. All four of these authors show how to work out how much protein is ideal for maintenance of lean body mass (Appendix B).

Best and Worst Fats for Health

Since an effective low-carb diet must be both medium-protein and medium-to-high-fat, the nature of the fat is important, and the most healthful mix of fats is still disputed. One of the main disagreements among the authors is on the healthful level of saturated fat (Figure 2-0) in the diet, ranging from none to unlimited, with some authors espousing 1/3 of all fat, as recommended by the FDA and NHLBI. Based on a review of diet studies most trusted by this reviewer, done by Uffe Ravnskov, MD, PhD, saturated fat does *not* increase the risk of CVD (Ravnskov, 1998), and animal fat may well be protective against cancer (Allan & Lutz, pp84-5). The medium-chain-length saturated fats in butter and coconut and palm kernel oils have both antiinflammatory and antimicrobial effects (Enig, 2000, p87ff).

The benefits of canola oil are greatly disputed among our authors based on its perceived content of desirable omega-3 fats (actually fatty acids) and undesirable *trans* fats. Canola is an acronym for Canadian Oil Association. The Canadian, Eddie Vos, a materials engineer, and author of a dozen peer-reviewed publications on diet, is certain that there is very little *trans* fatty acid in canola oil (www.health-heart.org). Certainly the partially hydrogenated canola oil used to make hard margarine is loaded with *trans* fats; this should be avoided altogether. Of the non-hydrogenated types, deodorized, or otherwise finished canola oil from Belgium, France, Germany and the UK retained most of their desirable omega-3 linolenic acid (8-10%), and contained only 1-3% *trans* fatty acids. They contained only 2-3 times as much omega-6 as omega-3 fatty acids, all determined by gas chromatography of the methyl esters obtained from the fatty acids in the oil samples, an excellent method (Wolff, 1992; Wolff, 1993; Hénon et al., 1999). A sample of commercial deodorized canola oil obtained from the Cereol refinery in France contained 0.4% total *trans* 18:2* and 1.26% total *trans* 18:3 (Hénon et al., 1999). The latest type of deodorizers, *SoftColumn™*, can be operated to give canola oils with as little as 0.02% total *trans* 18:2 and 0.08% total *trans* 18:3 (Ahrens, 1999). But according to e-mails from Fred and Alice Ottoboni, processed canola oil in the USA contains more *trans* fat and very little omega-3.

Some self-styled diet experts still confuse canola oil with rapeseed oil, which contained a large fraction (50%) of a peculiar fatty acid, erucic acid, a 22:1 type, never shown harmful to humans, but some old tests on rodents cast suspicion on it. So selective breeding produced canola oil with well under 1% erucic acid content.

Randomized clinical trials (RCTs) have shown that there is no health benefit in using olive oil or, worse still, corn oil, compared with animal fats (Rose et al., 1965), or in using unhydrogenated polyunsaturated oils in general (Morris et al., 1968; Pearce et al., 1971), despite reductions in serum total cholesterol (TC) with the polyunsaturated oils. Therefore, consuming more than the minimal requirements of such oils, the ones with too much omega-6 fatty acid present, is a serious contributor to chronic health conditions. This is contrary to advice in many diet books and from the AHA. The exceptions, of course, have been noted: the polyunsaturated EPA and DHA of fish oils (see Myth 1), and the alpha-linolenic acid based vegetable oils, such as canola and flaxseed oils. These all contain the desirable omega-3 linolenic acids which are very widely recommended by those giving advice on health foods. However, a recent review of studies on how omega-3 oils from plants, whose main

---

*This ultra-compact way of describing the fatty acids in fats is very easy to understand. "18:2" simply means that the fatty acid has 18 carbon atoms and 2 carbon-carbon double bonds. Double bonds are what makes the fatty acid or fat "unsaturated" or "polyunsaturated" in the case of 18:2. A formula of an 18:0 fatty acid is shown in Figure 2-0, and a formula of a typical 18:2 is shown in Fig. 2-1.

# Figure 2-0. General Structure of a Saturated Fat

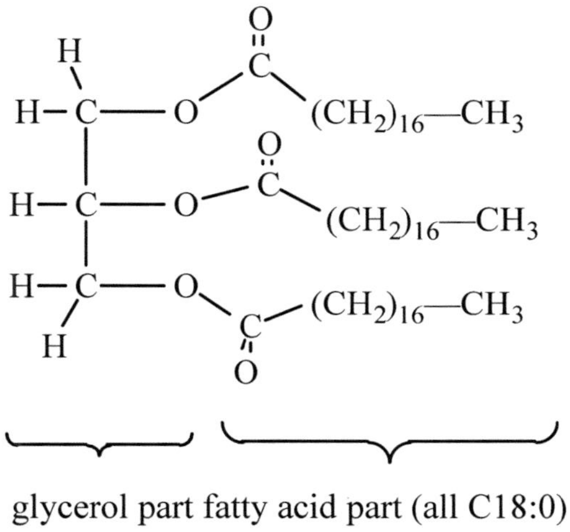

glycerol part    fatty acid part (all C18:0)

## Figure 2-1. The Structural Formula of the Linoleic Acid Isomer 18:2,n-6,t-10,c-12

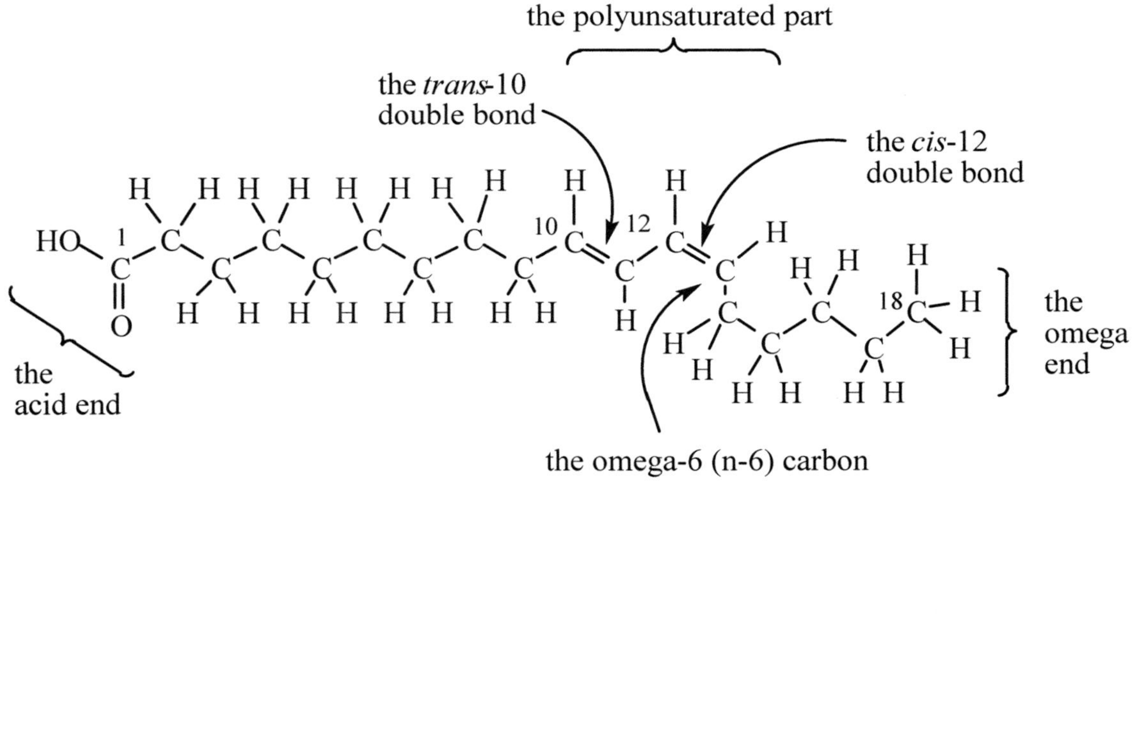

the polyunsaturated part

the *trans*-10 double bond

the *cis*-12 double bond

the acid end

the omega-6 (n-6) carbon

the omega end

omega-3 component is alpha-linolenic acid, showed, based on 9 research studies utilizing stable isotopes, that alpha-linolenic acid is converted to only small amounts of the very desirable EPA and DHA (Burdge, 2004). So eating fish or taking supplemental fish oils to get EPA and DHA is better.

Further on fat, Barry Sears was among the first to popularize the findings that omega-6 fatty acids are converted to arachidonic acid, a 20-carbon polyunsaturated fatty acid (20:4). This is metabolized to thromboxane $A_2$, which raises blood pressure and increases clotting. Several other undesirable substances are formed as well (Ottoboni & Ottoboni, p49; Enig, 2000, p28). Since the main omega-6 fatty acid is linoleic, found in corn, cottonseed, grapeseed, safflower, soybean, and sunflower oils, the recommendation of diet "authorities" to consume such oils was misguided from the beginning, and continues unabashed to this day. The reduction in serum total cholesterol, which had been the unsound basis for these recommendations, was mostly a reduction in the supposedly more desirable HDL, not in LDL (see Myth 3).

This result was also found in a diet study at Texas A & M University which also confirmed the unhealthful nature of *trans* fatty acids and omega-6 fatty acids, and the benign nature of butter and palm oil (Wood et al., 1993). In this carefully controlled study, foods prepared with particular fats and oils were served to the subjects in a cafeteria at Texas A & M University for months. Blood tests for lipids were done several times. Palm oil growers supported the study, but the researchers "swore" that the results were honest, and that the agreement was to publish no matter what the findings.

A 7-year multi-center study of 5201 men and women aged ≥65 years correlated types of dietary oils with their concentrations in plasma. Higher intakes of omega-6 oils were strongly correlated with higher incidence of fatal CVD. This finding did not appear in either the abstract or conclusions of this paper (Lemaitre et al., 2003).

Still further confirmation came from a 3.1-year study on 235 postmenopausal women whose normal diets were compared with the narrowing of openings their coronary arteries, as determined by angiography. Here a "dye" that shows up on Xray is injected and the pictures obtained can show differences in the diameter of the opening of 0.02 mm. Differences in total fat intake had little effect, but higher intake of saturated fat was very beneficial, monounsaturated fat less so, and higher intake of polyunsaturated fats narrowed the coronary arteries (Mozaffarian et al., 2004).

A 5-year study on Swedish women showed that those eating mostly corn and safflower oils had 3 times the breast cancer rate of those eating mostly canola and olive oils (Wolk et al., 1998; Ottoboni & Ottoboni, p37).

*****

Conjugated is the word used by Organic Chemists to indicate that there are 2 carbon-carbon double bonds separated by a single bond (C=C—C=C). The n-6 means omega-6: that means that the carbon-carbon double bond furthest from the acid end is between the 6th and 7th carbons from the other end. The t stands for *trans* and the c for *cis*. Figure 2-1 shows the structural formula for this toxic isomer of linoleic acid, including the geometries of the *trans* and *cis* double bonds. See Enig, 2000.

Recent work on *trans* fats, actually *trans* fatty acids as components of fats and oils, has uncovered a common very bad one. One particular form (isomer) of conjugated linoleic acid (18:2,n-6,t-10,c-12) formed by partial exposure to hydrogenation of the natural linoleic acid (18:2,n-6,c-9,c-12) in vegetable oils, soybean in particular, has been found to increase insulin resistance (Risérus et al., 2002) and oxidative stress (Risérus et al., 2002a) in humans. Thus there is evidence that not only a high carb intake can cause insulin resistance, but also fats containing the particular *trans* fatty acid shown in Figure 2-1, justifying the recommendations to avoid *trans* fats. Here one picture really is worth 1000 words. Please look at the structural formula in Figure 2-1. The various chemical bits you have read about are clearly identified and easy to understand.

How could the diet research giants have made such a staggering error in recommending against saturated fats and in ignoring *trans* fats? Among other diet researchers, David Kritchevsky, Wistar Institute, University of Pennsylvania, beginning in the 1950s, used partially hydrogenated vegetable fats in feeding studies, but counted the *trans* fat content as saturated fat!

When Walter Willett, Harvard School of Public Health, Boston, Massachusetts, realized that *trans* fats were lumped in with saturated fats in early reports, and that their amounts were underestimated in foods, his papers began to recognize some of the ill effects of *trans* fats, in 1993 (Willett et al., 1993). Beginning then, Willett began to use the accurate assays for *trans* fat of Mary Enig (Enig, 1995). What was reported in the abstract and press releases was that the 85,000 women in the Nurses Health Study who ate the most *trans* fat (highest quintile compared with lowest quintile) were 1.5 times (RR = 1.5) as likely to have CVD, fatal or non-fatal, or an MI. What was not mentioned in the abstract or press releases was that the RR = 1.78 when the *trans* fats were from vegetable oils, and 0.59 when the *trans* fats were from animal fats! This buried treasure received little attention. Imagine that their risk of CVD including MI, after just 8 years, was tripled, *tripled,* in women eating the most partially hydrogenated vegetable oil compared with those eating the most animal fat! And the reaction of both corporate executives, government agency hacks, and spokespersons for non-government organizations, such as the American Heart Association, damning animal fat? Defend the *status quo* no matter what!

Mary G. Enig, PhD, pointed out that manufacturers of food containing *trans* fats nearly always said that these fats were perfectly healthful, yet they always tried to conceal or underestimate the *trans* fat content (Enig, 1995). When you see news releases that "low fat diets reduced cancer", etc., that usually means *trans* fats were lower in the test group, not just animal fats. Combining the two out of ignorance might have been forgivable in the 1940s-1950s, but was carried on far beyond the time when alarms about *trans* fat were raised (Fallon, 2001, p15).

Much nonsense has been written on the Okinawan diet, which has changed radically since 1945. Stephen C. Byrnes, who lived in Honolulu, HI, has friends raised in Okinawa. They ate fish, rice and vegetables, but pork and lard "...have always been the mainstay of this people's diet". At least before the USA occupation of Okinawa, that is; afterwards the consumption of vegetable oil skyrocketed, and, since 1986, Okinawan longevity is no longer the highest in the world. By 1990 it had dropped to fifth among Japanese prefectures. The youngest have more violent death now, and the middle generations have more CVD. Only the oldest generations still live quite long, and they usually die of respiratory diseases. A major change in diet among younger Japanese consists of a 3.5-fold increase in the intake of vegetable oils containing omega-6 fatty acids. This is believed to have increased rates of western-type cancers as well as CVD and allergies (Okuyama et al., 1997). Conversely, higher intakes of animal fat and cholesterol since 1955 reduced the incidence of fatal hemorrhagic stroke very significantly among Japanese (Sauvaget et al., 2004).

Fats and Gallstones

Opponents of low-carb high-fat diets warn that such diets cause gallstones. A typical daily fat intake is about 125 g (4.5 oz). This has been addressed by Robert C. Atkins, MD: "There is now overwhelming scientific evidence that gallstones (responsible for over 90% of gallbladder disease) are formed when fat intake is *low.* In a study that examined the effect of a diet that provided 27 g of fat per day, gallstones developed in 13% of the participants. The reason is that the gallbladder will not contract unless fat is taken in, and if it doesn't contract, a condition called biliary stasis develops, and the bile salts crystallize into stones. Our gall bladders need to be kept active to prevent stone formation. It is not uncommon to find gallstones in people who are obese, although the gallstones may not be causing discomfort. People with existing gallstones may, however, have trouble with high fat meals. If you are one of these people you may have to slowly increase the level of fat you eat according to your own tolerance, meaning how you feel. Remember, gallstones are not formed overnight. So anyone who tells you they started doing Atkins and two weeks later developed gallstones doesn't fully understand the medical situation." (Atkins, 2002, p87).

## Virtues and Vices of Fructose

Fructose is another conundrum, because its low GI (Foster-Powell et al., 2002) does not account for the delayed hyperglycemia it causes, observed by Bernstein (p124-5) and Mercola (p106), but not by Smith (p27). It does raise TG levels, worsening one of the best indicators of ill-health — the TG/HDL ratio (Eades & Eades, pp95-6), which should be as low as possible. Eating fruit, in which the main sugar is fructose, is encouraged by some low-carb authors, limited by most, and banned by two of them. Contrast this caution with the zeal with which high fruit consumption is ballyhooed by diet "authorities". Sugary fruit is not healthful for the carb-sensitive among us. We must abstain from dates and most melons in favor of berries, cherries, and some citrus.

Recent studies show that fructose, besides raising TG levels, causes insulin resistance (Thresher et al, 2000), and that men are more sensitive to fructose than women (Bantle et al, 2000). Most fructose is converted slowly to glucose in the human liver; but it is first metabolized to the 3-carbon pyruvate (Berg et al., 2002). It seems, then, that the high GL of fructose counts more in causing health problems than its low GI. This means that modest amounts of fructose may be OK, but large amounts, perhaps in the form of high-fructose corn syrup, are not.

## Low-Carb Sweeteners

There is no agreement on which, or any, low- or non-caloric sweeteners are most healthful. Trials have shown mixed results, but a recent trial pitting sucrose against aspartame, acesulfame-K, cyclamate and saccharin showed that the non-caloric sweeteners led to weight and fat loss, as well as lower blood pressures, compared with unwanted gains in the sucrose group (Raben et al., 2002). Atkins prefers sucralose (Splenda™) and avoidance of aspartame. Bernstein (pp 137-139) advises avoiding artificial sweeteners in packets, as even the gram of lactose or other sugar they contain counts for diabetics. He advises tablet or liquid forms. He is not concerned about aspartame. Eades & Eades (pp 151-172) are, and prefer sucralose and stevia. Mercola (pp 118-119, 237) bans them all, especially aspartame and stevia. The sugar alcohols, such as sorbitol, mannitol, lactitol or xylitol, will not raise blood glucose levels and are non-caloric, but may cause gas and diarrhea, and are not well-tolerated by many people. Eades & Eades advise using only small amounts.

Without presenting results from actual trials on low-carb sweeteners, my sense from reading the complaints about aspartame (Equal™) is that 5% or fewer people in the USA are badly affected by it, at least when it is not heated. Some of the alarms about sucralose, which seems safe for now, claim that it is as dangerous as a chlorinated hydrocarbon, such DDT, PCBs, chloroform, etc. While there are 3 chloro groups in the sucralose molecule, replacing 3 of the 8 hydroxyl groups in sucrose, sucralose is very soluble in water, like sucrose, and unlike the fat-soluble chlorinated hydrocarbons.

## Fiber is No Panacea

One study found benefits of eating fiber for prevention of NIDDM (Montonen et al., 2003) and another study found no benefit in cancer prevention (Fuchs et al., 1999). Since some long-term followers of low-carb diets and some ethnic groups ate no fiber at all, and remained in good health, the benefits of fiber are probably moderate at best, and possibly might be due to an associated nutrient such as magnesium.

## Nuts to Nut Allergies

For the majority of us who are not allergic to nuts, restrictions on consumption of nuts (except walnuts) (Mercola & Levy, p111) is at odds with the findings of epidemiological studies (Fraser et al., 1997), in which the benefits promoting longevity are usually attributed to the high omega-3 content of nuts (Lee et al., 2003); but there is an equally good argument for the benefits being due to the copper content of nuts (Klevay, 1993). The magnesium and selenium found in nuts does not hurt, either. If you are not allergic to them, most kinds of nuts make a great snack food as part of a low-carb diet.

## Soybean Products Overpromoted

Soy products are both promoted and disparaged. Soy protein may be acceptable for vegetarians, according to Richard K. Bernstein (Bernstein, p132). According to Kilmer S. McCully in his e-mail of 24 Jun 03, "...soy products are undesirable in the diet in any quantity. The exception would be fermented soy foods in small quantities, as eaten by Asian populations. Soy contains multiple toxic proteins that are anti-thyroid and phytoestrogens that have antifertility and other toxic effects." The usual cautions about soy products relates to their phytate content <http://www.westonaprice.org/soy/soy_alert.html> which inhibits absorption of many minerals. However, actual assays of flours shows the phytate content of soy to be the same as that of rye and refined wheat, with whole wheat being 2.5 times higher (Lentner, 1981, p265). Kaayla T. Daniel, PhD, wrote a passionate and well-referenced article and book about the dangers of soy products (http://www.mothering.com/10-0-0/html/10-6-0/soy-story.shtml), (Daniel, 2005).

## Many Alcoholic Drinks Contain Carbs

Recommendations for alcohol consumption vary from nearly none to several glasses daily of red wine only, to 1.5 drinks daily of any variety (40 mL of ethanol daily in any form), all based on the long-known protection from CVD (see Myth #5). In fact, there is no *significant* difference in *all-cause* death rates between non- and moderate drinkers (Theobald et al, 2001; Malyutina et al., 2002). No alcohol is proper for those with the "leaky gut" syndrome (Braly et al., p150; Smith, p148-9). For the carb-sensitive the carb content matters most, so ales and stouts with up to 18 g/355 mL (12 fl oz) should be avoided in favor of diet beers with ≤ 5 g/355 mL. Low-sugar red wine such as pinot noir at ≤ 150 mL per day is equivalent, but most wines contain serious levels of sugars. Those of you interested in the antioxidants in wine can obtain them by eating grapes (watch high GI) and berries (Smith, p149), but see Myth 5.

## Water Can Kill

Recommendations for water consumption range from whatever one drinks because of natural thirst (*ad libitum*) to 12 glasses per day! The Ottobonis saw no evidence for drinking more than what is governed by thirst (Ottoboni & Ottoboni, p168). There are 3 reports in journals of deaths from drinking excess water. Drinking fluoridated water should be avoided. Some very serious researchers have amassed hard evidence that the benefits for teeth are quite minimal, and that the health problems are serious (Kauffman, 2005), (see Myth 11).

## Nutritional Supplements: None, Some or Many?

Recommendations for supplements range from a multivitamin only, to a half dozen known 50 years ago that are to be taken only when needed, to a dozen recent ones, to a dozen or so with good clinical studies. This reviewer believes that the definitive work on the actions of supplements, along with the symptoms they relieve (Atkins, 1998), does not really indicate who should take which; but like other books on the topic, Atkins' may lead one to believe that dozens should be taken by almost everyone. It is true that there are almost universal deficiencies in the intake levels of vitamin C and magnesium, for example (Eades & Eades., pp129-30, 205-26), that cannot be reached by food choices alone, especially when high GL foods such as sweet fruits are to be limited.

What do you do? If you have some health complaint, see whether it is due to a deficiency of something that can be treated by taking a supplement. Watch out for over promotion of many supplements. Often the evidence given is that test animals or even humans taking the supplement for a few weeks had some substance change in concentration in some body fluid. This is not good enough. Longer term trials with all-cause mortality rates are needed, such as the ones given for coenzyme Q10 in Myth 1.

## Exercise Can Kill

As nearly all the low-carb authors provide total lifeplans including exercise, not just diet advice on the contents of meals, it is hard to determine what fraction of the benefits of their interventions are due to each factor. The benefits of exercise are very dependent on its intensity and the condition of the individual (Dorn et al., 1996), and see Myth 6.

## Kilocalorie Kounts Konfused

There is no simple laboratory method of analysis at present to account for the fact that the net metabolizable energies (NMEs) for carb and fat are not 4 and 9 kcal/g. Insoluble fiber has no NME, soluble fiber provides 0-2 kcal/g (Livesy, 2001), partially digestible starches run 2-4 kcal/g, and the mean energy content of common fats is nearer 8 kcal/g than 9 (Appendix C). Counting a mean NME of 2.5 kcal/g for the low GI, low GL carbs usually recommended, and 8 kcal/g for fat, the 40:30:30 diet of Sears and others is really nearer to 30:33:37 carb:fat:protein in energy content. Thus the calorie counts on US food labels are barely to be trusted. It is better to look up the GI and GL of each ingredient. However, Dr. Robert C. Atkins showed how to partially translate US FDA food labels into some useful information (Atkins, pp108-112).

## FDA Food Labels Foolish

But FDA labels list saturated fat and cholesterol as undesirable. They fail to list *trans* fat or linoleic acid contents of foods, ignoring that these are really undesirable. The "%DV" (daily value) on FDA food labels is supposed to indicate what % of the recommended allowance per day is supposed to be of a few components in a serving of the food, such as sodium in salt. As has been shown, this is sheer nonsense and can be ignored, because the %DV numbers are based on high-carb, low cholesterol, low saturated fat diets, and make no allowance for anybody's metabolic type. Some of the nonsense is based on the outmoded notion that we need only enough of most micronutrients to prevent deficiency diseases. Linus Pauling's insight that there is an optimum higher amount of each micronutrient for optimum health continues to be ignored.

## Major Findings

• The symptoms of carb sensitivity are a 12-hour fasting blood glucose level over 125 mg/dL, sleepiness or fainting from hypoglycemia, which is a rebound effect of hyperglycemia from high-carb foods, or simply by noticing a big belly.

- About 3/4 of us would benefit from reducing the carb content of our diets to 40% of energy intake or less based on the combustion values of 4 kcal/g for carb or protein and 9 kcal/g for fat.
- About 1/4 of us who are obese, carb-sensitive, have hypoglycemic episodes, or are diabetic should reduce the digestible carb content of diet to ≤15% of energy, or whatever is needed to normalize blood glucose levels, or to reverse obesity.
- At least 1/3 of those carbs should be fiber, as in low-GI vegetables and fruit, such as string beans and berries, in order to obtain the other nutrients in these foods. These nutrients include potassium, calcium and magnesium, which may be more important than the fiber or the antioxidants.
- Fish, meat, eggs and most cheeses are very healthful foods, and do not lead to obesity or cancer or CVD (Hu et al., 1999; Hu et al., 2002; Malhotra, 1967). Most of these foods have such low concentrations of toxins that they are safe for most people to eat frequently. According to Richard K. Bernstein, MD, and others, a reasonable amount of protein to eat at each meal is a volume equal to that of one's own palm, or about the size of a deck of cards. Or see Eades & Eades, p310-317.
- Saturated, monounsaturated, and smaller amounts of omega-3 fats and oils, whether animal or vegetable, are healthful, and do not lead to obesity or cancer. Saturated fats are low-calorie fats (5.5-8 kcal/g).
- Vegetable oils with high omega-6 content cause CVD and cancer, so should be avoided, even if they are not partially hydrogenated. Examples are soybean, corn, cottonseed and safflower oils. These are also high-calorie oils (9.3 kcal/g).
- All products containing *trans* fat should be avoided. Since it is lawful for US food labels to omit small amounts of *trans* fat, one must look for the words "partially hydrogenated" among the ingredients, and avoid all such products.
- Those who have grain allergies should avoid grains.
- Those who have protein allergies to soybean protein, milk protein, or other types should avoid them.
- A "balanced" diet has no meaning; it is a propaganda term. There is no requirement for carbohydrate in the diets of humans at all. People who are are grain-sensitive, carb-sensitive or diabetic are harmed by "balanced" diets.
- So much diet advice is contradictory or fails because people react so differently to foods.
- "Calories in equals calories out" is another propaganda term not based on actual trials in humans. Many constituents of foods, such as fiber, are not digested. Long-chain saturated fatty acids, especially 18:0, are not fully digested, for example. The digestible carb content of foods is what leads to fat bellies, not the size of the total calorie count, as shown by actual trials.
- Restaurants in civilized areas are now very cooperative about replacing starches with vegetables, salad or cole slaw. Ask nicely. Bring your own rye crispbread.

### A Day's Fare Containing about 100g (4 oz) of Digestible Carb or 15% Energy from Carb

Breakfast: Omelette from 2 jumbo eggs, 25g (1 oz) ham, 25 g celery, coffee with light cream, 2 pieces of rye crispbread with sesame seeds (Ryvita™) with butter and 10 g total jelly sweetened with grape juice.

Lunch: Sliced cheese on 2 pieces of rye crispbread (or German pumpernickel), coffee with light cream, salad with tomato, olive, cucumber, lettuce, mushroom, radish, olive oil and vinegar. Dessert: 25 g of 70+% chocolate.

Dinner: Risotto, 50g, undercooked, with a bouillon cube, bok choy, broccoli, garlic, bell pepper, and 100g of kielbasa (Polish pork sausage). Dessert: blueberries and whipped cream.

Snack: 25 g of 70+% chocolate or 50g of nuts.

*****

Several of the books reviewed in Appendix B have much more extensive low-carb menus, which are very nice to avoid diet boredom.

<u>Countering the Delusions of Diet "Experts"</u>

• Cutting out simple sugars and substituting "complex carbohydrates" (starches) is worse for carb-sensitive people, since the glycemic load may be higher and the glycemic index may not be any lower. Starches are converted to glucose with its glycemic index of 100. One must look up the glycemic indexes and loads of foods, either in one of the low-carb diet books reviewed in Appendix B, or in the original literature (http://wave.prohosting.com/rmendosa/gi.htm; Foster-Powell et al., 2002).

• Using "whole grains" instead of refined grains may well sicken people who have grain, gluten or wheat allergies, leading to autoimmune diseases from celiac disease to cancer (see reviews of books by Braly & Hoggan and Smith in Appendix B). Such people who are not generally carb-sensitive may only have to cut out grains, but not potato, rice, or ice cream.

• Many people who are justly cynical about all diet advice try to follow both the low-fat and low-carb advice-givers by eating only protein and high-fiber vegetables. This does not work because fat gives the greatest feeling of fullness from eating, delays stomach emptying, and because some saturated and omega-3 and omega-6 fats are essential for health. Protein does have a glycemic index of about 22, while fat has a glycemic index of zero.

• Many new food products claiming low-carb status have appeared which may contain allergenic proteins from grains, gluten, wheat, soybean, or milk . Most of these products are also low in fat, so they do not satisfy, and the undersized portion sizes on the package are quickly exceeded. Few of these products have had long-term diet trials to prove their merits.

• Many foods that never contained any carbs are suddenly sporting labels saying "low-carb" just as many foods that never contained any fat sported labels saying "low-fat". Ignore such labeling, and check the ingredients.

• The selected types of carbohydrates, fats, oils and certain minerals found on USA and UK food labels, along with their supposed caloric values, were based mostly on disproven diet dogma and outmoded methods of measurement. Serving sizes are usually unrealistically too small. This allows the manufacturer to omit listing anything undesirable, such as *trans* fat, if less than 0.5 g per serving is present.

• Low-carb diet critics have collaborated in using the pejorative term "fad" for low-carb or Atkins diets. Such diets have been in use for 200 years (Allan & Lutz, p7). The low-fat diets advised for 50 years might better be called fad diets, since there is no accurate evidence supporting their use.

<u>Individual Book Reviews</u>

All of the authors of the books reviewed individually in Appendix B recommend low-carb diets for all diabetics, most people who are obese, and people suffering from certain other conditions including hypoglycemia, hyperlipidemia, NIDDM, polycythemia, hypertension, stroke, CVD, cancers, GI problems such as Crohn's disease, as well as multiple sclerosis, rheumatoid arthritis, osteoporosis and others. The length of this list of afflictions may strain your credulity, but for each condition evidence for a cause by excess carb of some type is given, often from the author's own clinical experience. Most authors advise on exercise, water, alcohol, coffee, tea and supplement consumption as well, so these topics are addressed. There is a great difference of opinion among these authors in

72

many of the other topics, which are best examined in these individual book reviews, which will also help you decide which of these books to use in your own program.

Each of the books individually reviewed in Appendix B describes aspects of low-carb diets that are both unique and useful. At least 1 or 2 should be read for proper implementation of a low-carb or low-grain diet. All of the authors of these books who are also practicing physicians must be considered courageous for using effective treatments in their practices that are not recommended by mainstream authorities.

## Conclusions

Based on the long-term effects of low-carb diets in a number of individuals, mostly MDs; the long-term results in their patients; the favorable results in all controlled trials, allowing for bias, and using the actual data and not necessarily the trial directors' conclusions, the safety of low-carb diets is established, and their efficacy for weight-loss and prevention of the complications of diabetes is indisputable.

Barry Sears showed that young athletes, who were supposedly not insulin-resistant, at the peak of their training on high-carb diets, improved their performance on a medium-carb diet. He and others estimate that 3/4 of all people of European descent are insulin resistant to some degree, so at least this fraction would benefit from eating a low-carb diet. A study from the Centers for Disease Control and Prevention (the US CDC), using indirect methods, estimated that 1/4 of all Americans over age 20 have the metabolic syndrome, and that >42% of those over 60 do (Ford et al., 2002); these groups would obtain the greatest advantages from a low-carb diet.

Overlapping any of these populations are people who suffer from gluten or grain sensitivity; those people should use low-grain diets as their form of low-carb diet, and some may have to limit all carb intakes as well. Since at least 10% of all Americans have grain, gluten or wheat allergies, caused by the proteins in whole grains, any increase in whole grain consumption must be felt to be free from digestive problems. Blood tests are necessary if you think you have a grain allergy. Blanket recommendations for whole grains are irresponsible and ignorant.

Obesity and diabetes are strongly associated with CVD (Liu et al., 2000). Even though the absolute values of TC and LDL in serum are not predictive for identifying specific individuals in a given age group who will suffer from CVD soonest (Stehbens, 2001), several authors of the books reviewed have noted how a low TG level, and more so a low TG/HDL ratio, a strong predictor of CVD (Gaziano et al., 1997), both drop in people using low-carb diets, as do homocysteine levels. Insulin produced to deal with glucose activates production of the enzyme HMG-CoA reductase, one of the catalysts for cholesterol synthesis.

For diabetics, reversal of complications in IDDM has been noted when blood glucose levels are normalized, and adopting a low-carb diet is an essential factor (van Dam et al., 2002), regardless of the insulin regimen or use of antidiabetes drugs. A surprising number of other afflictions are stabilized or reversed with a low-carb diet. Since diabetes is the major risk factor for CVD, blindness, and circulatory problems leading to infections that lead to amputations, avoiding NIDDM by using a low-carb diet prevents all the other problems.

Much of the evidence for low-fat (high-carb) diets is a result of poorly designed studies, misinterpretation, exaggeration and outright fraud. Remember, the original reason for the recommendations for low-fat (high-carb) diets was to limit the intake of cholesterol and saturated fats, especially animal fats, tropical fats and eggs, and to substitute omega-6 and *trans* fats. "An almost endless number of observations and experiments have effectively falsified the hypothesis that dietary cholesterol and [saturated] fats, and a high [serum] cholesterol level play a role in the causation of atherosclerosis and CVD" (Kauffman, 2001; Ravnskov, 2002b).

A quandary with all the books reviewed in Appendix B is that one is not told how much longer one might live when following the low-carb diet program, or what the cause of death might become. For example, the lower incidence of heart deaths in France and Japan are accompanied by a higher incidence of cancer deaths.

The extent of the evidence for the benefits of low-carb diets in both time and volume is so great as to invite questioning of the the motives among all the government agencies and private foundations still recommending high-carb diets and presently coordinating a world-wide attack on low-carb diets, despite the obvious result of weight loss among at least 40,000,000 Americans alone (based on book sales) who use low-carb diets. Could the vast difference in interpretation of studies be an honest scientific controversy? More likely it is simply resistance in defense of an entrenched organizational position that should not have been adopted originally, an attitude all too familiar to those of you who observe the interpersonal relationships in bureaucracies. Could it also be seen as negligence (or worse) that has led to lower quality of life and premature death for millions of dieters, for which compensation in the courts might be sought?

*"Men occasionally stumble over the truth, but most pick themselves up and hurry off as if nothing had happened."* Winston Churchill (in McGee, 2001, p82).

## Acknowledgment

Expert online searches and editorial aid were provided by Leslie Ann Bowman, AMLS, and other faculty at the University of the Sciences in Philadelphia, including a complete critical reading of the manuscript by William Reinsmith, DA, and Frances E. H. Pane, MSLS, and Duane Graveline, MD, MPH. The searching skills of Wendy H. Kramer, MLS, at the Eastern Regional Research Center of the USDA, Wyndmoor, PA, were extremely valuable. Many members of The International Cholesterol Skeptics Group provided information and/or editorial aid <www.THINCS.org>. Thanks to Henry H. Bauer, PhD, Editor of the *Journal for Scientific Exploration* for suggesting the original format (published as Kauffman, 2004).

## Myth #2 References

Ahrens D (1999). Industrial thin-film deodorization of seed oils with SoftColumn™ technology. *Fett/Lipid 101*, 230-234.

Anderson KM, Castelli WP, Levy D (1987). Cholesterol and Mortality. 30 years of follow-up from the Framingham Study. *Journal of the American Medical Association* 257:2176-2180.

Anon. (1961). Dietary Fat and Its Relation to Heart Attacks and Strokes. *Journal of the American Medical Association* 175:389-391.

Atkins RC (1998). *Dr Atkins Vita-Nutrient Solution*, London, England: Pocket Books, Simon & Schuster.

ATPIII ( 2001). *Journal of the American Medical Association* 285(19):2536.

Atwater WO, Snell JF (1903). Description of a Bomb Calorimeter and Method of Its Use. *Journal of the American Chemical Society* 25(7):659-699.

Bantle JP, Raatz SK, Thomas W, Georgopoulos A (2000). Effects of dietary fructose on plasma lipids in healthy subjects. *American Journal of Clinical Nutrition* 72:1128-1134.

Berg JM, Tymoczko JL, Stryer L (2002). *Biochemistry,* 5th ed., New York, NY: W. H. Freeman, pp440-441.

Bravata DM, Sanders L, Huang J, Krumholz HM, Olkin I, Gardner CD, Bravata DM (2003). Efficacy and Safety of Low-Carbohydrate Diets: A Systematic Review. *Journal of the American Medical Association* 289(14):1837-1850.

Brehm BJ, Seeley RJ, Daniels SR, D'Alessio DA (2003). A Randomized Trial Comparing a Very Low Carbohydrate Diet and a Calorie-Restricted Low Fat Diet on Body Weight and Cardiovascular Risk Factors in Healthy Women. *The Journal of Clinical Endocrinology & Metabolism* 88(4):1617-1623.

Burdge G (2004). alpha-Linolenic acid metabolism in men and women: nutritional and biological implications. *Current Opinions in Clinical, Nutrition and Metabolic Care* 7:137-144.

Cho E, Spiegelman D, Hunter DJ, et al. (2003). Premenopausal fat intake and risk of breast cancer. *Journal of the National Cancer Institute* 95:1079-1085.

Cohen BL (2003). Risks in Perspective. *Journal of American Physicians and Surgeons* 8(2), 50-53.

Cohen JS (2004). *The Magnesium Solution for High Blood Pressure,* New Garden City, NY: Square One Publishers.

van Dam RM, Rimm EB, Willett WC, Stampfer MJ, Hu FB (2002). Dietary Patterns and Risk for Type 2 Diabetes Mellitus in U. S. Men. *Annals of Internal Medicine* 136:201-209.

Daniel KT (2005). *The Whole Soy Story,* Washington, DC: New Trends Press.

Dean C (2003). *The Miracle of Magnesium,* New York, NY: Ballantine Books.

Deckelbaum RJ, Fisher EA, Winston M, Kumanyika S, Lauer RM, Pi-Sunyer FX, Jeor SSt, Schaefer EJ, Weinstein IB (1999). Summary of a Scientific Conference on Preventive Nutrition: Pediatrics to Geriatrics. *Circulation 100,* 450-456.

Dock W (1953). The Reluctance of Physicians to Admit That Chronic Disease May Be Due to Faulty Diet. *The Journal of Clinical Nutrition* 5:1345-1347.

Dorn J, Naughton J, Imamura D, Trevisan M (1999). Results of a Multicenter Randomized Clinical Trial of Exercise and Long-Term Survival in Myocardial Infarction Patients. *Circulation* 100:1764-1769.

Enig MG (1995). *Trans* Fatty Acids in the Food Supply: A Comprehensive Report Covering 60 Years of Research, 2nd ed. Silver Spring, MD: Enig Associates, 11120 New Hampshire Ave., Suite 500.

Enig MG (2000). *Know Your Fats,* Silver Spring, MD: Bethesda Press.

Enig MG (2003). NHLBI Consensus. Personal e-mail of 9 Aug.

Enig MG, Fallon, S (2005). *Eat Fat, Lose Fat,* New York, NY: Hudson Street Press.

Fallon S (2001). *Nourishing Traditions,* 2nd ed., Washington, DC: New Trends Publishing.

Ford ES, Giles WH, Dietz WH (2002). Prevalence of the Metabolic Syndrome Among US Adults. *Journal of the American Medical Association* 287(3):356-359.

Foster GD, Wyatt HR, Hill JO, McGuckin BG, Brill C, Mohammed BS, Szapary PO, Rader DJ, Edman JS, Klein S (2003). A Randomized Trial of a Low-Carbohydrate Diet for Obesity. *New England Journal of Medicine* 348(21):2082-2090.

Foster-Powell K, Holt SHA, Brand-Miller JC (2002). International table of glycemic index and glycemic load values: 2002. *American Journal of Clinical Nutrition* 76:5-56.

Fraser GE, Shavlik DJ (1997). Risk factors for all-cause and coronary heart disease mortality in the oldest-old. The Adventist Health Study. *Archives of Internal Medicine* 157:2249-2258.

Fuchs CS, Giovannucci EL, Colditz GA, Hunter DJ, Stampfer MJ, Rosner B, Speizer FE, Willett WC (1999). Dietary Fiber and the Risk of Colorectal Cancer and Adenoma in Women. *New England Journal of Medicine* 348(3):169-176.

Gaziano JM, Hennekens CH, O'Donnell CJ, Breslow JL, Buring JE (1997). Fasting Triglycerides, High-Density Lipoprotein, and Risk of Myocardial Infarction. *Circulation* 96:2520-2525.

Hénon G, Kemény Z, Recseg K, Zwobada F. Kovari K (1999). Deodorization of Vegetable Oils. Part I.: Modeling the Geometrical Isomerization of Polyunsaturated Fatty Acids. *Journal of the American Oil Chemists Society* 76:73-81.

Hu FB, Stampfer MJ, Rimm EB, Manson JE, Ascherio A, Colditz GA, Rosner BA, Spiegelman D, Speizer FE, Sacks FM, Hennekens CH, Willett WC (1999). A Prospective Study of Egg Consumption and Risk of Cardiovascular Disease in Men and Women. *Journal of the American Medical Association* 281(15):1387-1394.

Hu FB, Bronner L, Willett WC, Stampfer MJ, Rexrode KM, Albert CN, Hunter D, Manson J-AE ( 2002). Fish and Omega-3 Fatty Acid Intake and Risk of Coronary Heart Disease in Women. *Journal of the American Medical Association* 287(14):1815-1821.

Kauffman, J. M. (2001). Book Review of "The Cholesterol Myths" by Uffe Ravnskov (2000), *Journal of Scientific Exploration* 15(4):531-540.

Kauffman JM (2002). Alternative Medicine: Watching the Watchdogs at Quackwatch. Website Review. *Journal of Scientific Exploration* 16(2):312-337 (2002).

Kauffman JM (2004). Low-Carbohydrate Diets, *Journal of Scientific Exploration* 18(1):83-134 .

Kauffman JM (2004a). Bias in Recent Papers on Diets and Drugs in Peer-Reviewed Medical Journals, *Journal of American Physicians & Surgeons* 9(1):11-14.

Kauffman JM (2005). Water Fluoridation: A Review of Recent Research and Actions, *Journal of American Physicians & Surgeons* 10(2):38-44.

Kekwick A, Pawan GLS (1969). Body-Weight, Food, and Energy. *The Lancet* 19 Jun:822-825.

Klevay LM (1993). Copper in Nuts May Lower Heart Disease Risk. *Archives of Internal Medicine* 153:401-402.

Layman DK, Boileau RA, Erickson DJ, Painter JE, Shiue H, Sather C, Christou DD (2003). A Reduced Ratio of Dietary Carbohydrate to Protein Improves Body Composition and Blood Lipid Profiles during Weight Loss in Adult Women. *Journal of Nutrition* 133:411-417.

Lee KW, Lip GYH (2003). The role of omega-3 fatty acids in the secondary prevention of cardiovascular disease. *Quarterly Journal of Medicine* 96:465-480.

Lemaitre RN, King IB, Mozaffarian D, Luller LH, Tracy RP, Siscovick DS (2003). n-3 Polyunsaturated fatty acids, fatal ischemic heart disease, and nonfatal myocardial infarction in older adults: the Cardiovascular Health Study. *American Journal of Clinical Nutrition* 77:319-325.

Lentner C, Ed. (1981). *Geigy Scientific Tables,* Excerpts, 8th ed., West Caldwell, NJ: CIBA-Geigy.

Lieb, C. W. (1929). The Effects on Human Beings of a Twelve Months' Exclusive Meat Diet. *Journal of the American Medical Association* 93(1):20-22.

Liu S, Willett WC, Stampfer MJ, Hu FB, Franz M, Sampson L, Hennekens CH, Manson JE (2000). A prospective study of dietary glycemic load, carbohydrate intake, and risk of coronary heart disease in US women. *American Journal of Clinical Nutrition* 71:1455-1461.

Liu S, Sesso HD, Manson JE, Willett WC, Bering JE (2003). Is intake of breakfast cereals related to total and cause-specific mortality in men? *American Journal of Clinical Nutrition* 77:594-599.

Livesy G (2001). A perspective on food energy standards for nutrition labeling. *British Journal of Nutrition* 85:271-287.

Malhotra SL (1967). Serum lipids, dietary factors and ischemic heart disease. *American Journal of Clinical Nutrition* 20:462-474.

Malyutina S, Bobak M, Kurilovitch S, Gafarov V, Simonova G, Nikitin Y, Marmot M (2002). Relation between heavy and binge drinking and all-cause and cardiovascular mortality in Novosibirsk, Russia: a prospective cohort study. *The Lancet* 360:1448-1454.

deMan JM (1999). *Principles of Food Chemistry,* 3rd ed., Gaithersburg, MD: Aspen.

Mann GV (1977). Diet-Heart: End of an Era. *New England Journal of Medicine* 297(12):644-650.

McClellan WS, Du Bois EF (1930). Prolonged meat diets with a study of kidney function and ketosis. *The Journal of Biological Chemistry* 87:651-668.

McCully KS (2003). E-mail of 17 Dec 03.

McGee CT (2001). *Heart Frauds: Uncovering the Biggest Health Scam in History,* Colorado Springs, CO: HealthWise Pubs.

Michener JA (1988). *Alaska,* New York, NY: Random House, p179.

Montonen J, Knekt P, Järvinen R, Aromaa A, Reunanen A (2003). Whole-grain and fiber intake and the incidence of type 2 diabetes. *American Journal of Clinical Nutrition* 77:622-629.

Moore TJ (1989). *Prescription for Disaster. The Hidden Dangers in Your Medicine Cabinet,* New York, NY: Simon & Schuster.

Morris JN et al. for the MRC Social Medicine Research Unit (1968). Controlled Trial of Soya-Bean Oil in Myocardial Infarction. *The Lancet* 28 Sep:693-699.

Mozaffarian D, Rimm EB, Herrington DM (2004). Dietary fats, carbohydrate, and progression of coronary atherosclerosis in postmenopausal women. *American Journal of Clinical Nutrition* 80:1175-84.

MRFIT Research Group (1982). Multiple Risk Factor Intervention Trial. Risk Factor Changes and Mortality Results. *Journal of the American Medical Association* 248(12):1465-1477.

Newbold HL (1988). Reducing the Serum Cholesterol Level with a Diet High in Animal Fat. *Southern Medical Journal* 81(1):61-63.

O'Brien LJ (2003). Misplaced notions of simplicity, denial of complexity (i. e., value of randomized controlled clinical trials). *British Medical Journal Electronic, 11 July.*

Okuyama H, Kobayashi T, Watanabe S. (1997) Dietary Fatty Acids — The N-6/N-3 Balance and Chronic Elderly Diseases. Excess Linoleic Acid and Relative N-3 Deficiency Syndrome Seen in Japan. *Progress in Lipid Research* 35(4):409-457.

O'Mathúna DP (2003). The Placebo Effect and Alternative Therapies. *Alternative Medicine Alert* 6(6):61-69.

O'Shea JC, DeMets DL (2001). Statistical issues relating to international difference in clinical trials. *American Heart Journal* 142:21-28.

Ottoboni A, Ottoboni, F (2002). *The Modern Nutritional Diseases: heart disease, stroke, type-2 diabetes, obesity, cancer, and how to prevent them.* Sparks, NV: Vincente Books.

Pearce ML, Dayton S (1971). Incidence of Cancer in Men on a Diet High In Polyunsaturated Fat. *The Lancet* 6 Mar:464-467.

Raben A, Vasilaras TH, Møller AC, Astrup A (2002). Sucrose compared with artificial sweeteners: different effects on *ad libitum* food intake and body weight after 10 wk of supplementation in overweight subjects. *American Journal of Clinical Nutrition* 76:721-729.

Ravnskov U (1998). The Questionable Role of Saturated and Polyunsaturated Fatty Acids in Cardiovascular Disease. *Journal of Clinical Epidemiology* 51:443-60.

Ravnskov U (2000).*The Cholesterol Myths: Exposing the Fallacy that Saturated Fat and Cholesterol Cause Heart Disease,* Washington, DC: New Trends Publishing.

Ravnskov U, Allen C, Atrens D, Enig MG, Groves BM, Kauffman JM, Kronfeld R, Rosch PJ, Rosenman R, Werkö L, Vesti-Nielsen J, Wilske J, Worm N (2002). Studies of Dietary Fat and Heart Disease. *Science* 292:1464-1465.

Ravnskov U (2002a). Is atherosclerosis caused by high cholesterol? *Quarterly Journal of Medicine* 95:397-403.

Ravnskov U (2002b). A hypothesis out-of-date: The diet-heart idea. *Journal of Clinical Epidemiology* 55:1057-1063.

Risérus U, Abner P, Brismar K, Vessby B (2002a). Treatment with Dietary *trans*10*cis*12 Conjugated Linoleic Acid Causes Isomer-Specific Insulin Resistance in Obese Men with the Metabolic Syndrome. *Diabetes Care* 25(9):1516-1521.

Risérus U, Basu S, Jovinge S, Fredrikson GN, Årnlov J, Vessby B (2002b). Supplementation with Conjugated Linoleic Acid Causes Isomer-Dependent Oxidative Stress and Elevated C-Reactive Protein. A Potential Link to Fatty Acid-Induced Insulin Resistance. *Circulation* 106:1825-1929.

Rose GA, Thomson WB, Williams RT (1965). Corn Oil in Treatment of Ischaemic Heart Disease. *British Medical Journal* 12 Jun:1531-1533.

Salmeron J, Manson JE, Stampfer MJ, Colditz GA, Wing AL, Willett WC (1997). Dietary fiber, glycemic load and risk of non-insulin-dependent diabetes mellitus in women. *Journal of the American Medical Association* 277(6):472-477.

Samaha FF, Iqbal N, Seshadri P, Chicano KL, Daily DA, McGrory J, Williams T, Williams M, Gracely EJ, Stern L ( 2003). A Low-Carbohydrate as Compared with a Low-Fat Diet in Severe Obesity. *The New England Journal of Medicine* 346:476-483.

Sauvaget C, Nagano J, Hayashi M, Yamada M (2004). Animal Protein, Animal Fat, and Cholesterol Intakes and Risk of Cerebral Infarction Mortality in the Adult Health Study. *Stroke* 35(7):1531-7.

Serre-Majem J, Ribas L, Tresseras R, et al. (1995). How could changes in diet explain changes in coronary heart disease mortality in Spain? The Spanish Paradox. *American Journal of Clinical Nutrition* 61(suppl):1351S-1359S.

Shames RL, Shames KH (2001). *Thyroid Power,* New York, NY: HarperCollins.

Smith RE, Pinckney ER (1991). *The Cholesterol Conspiracy.* St. Louis, MO: Warren H. Green, Inc.

Sondike SB, Copperman N, Jacobson MS (2003). Effects of a Low-Carbohydrate Diet on Weight Loss and Cardiovascular Risk Factors in Overweight Adolescents. *The Journal of Pediatrics* 142:253-258.

Stehbens WE (2001). Coronary Heart Disease, Hypercholesterolemia, and Atherosclerosis II. Misrepresented Data. *Experimental and Molecular Pathology* 70:120-139.

Theobald H, Johansson S, Bygren L, Engfeldt P (2001). The Effects of Alcohol Consumption on Mortality and Morbidity: A 26-Year Follow-Up Study. *The Journal of Studies on Alcohol* 62(6):783-789.

Thresher JS, Podolin DA, Wei Y, Mazzeo RS, Pagliasotti MJ (2000). Comparison of the effects of sucrose and fructose on insulin action and glucose tolerance. *American Journal of Physiology, Regulatory Integrative and Comparative Physiology* 279:R1334-R1340.

Wiley HW, Bigelow WD (1898). Calories of Combustion in Oxygen of Cereals and Cereal Products, Calculated from Analytical Data. *Journal of the American Chemical Society* 20:304-316.

Willett WC, Stampfer MJ, Manson JE, et al. (1993). Intake of *trans* fatty acids and risk of coronary heart disease among women. *Lancet* 341:581-585.

Williams KI (1907). The Chemical Composition of Cooked Vegetable Spreads. *Journal of the American Chemical Society* 29:574-582.

Wolff RL (1992). *trans*-Polyunsaturated Fatty Acids in French Edible Rapeseed and Soybean Oils. *Journal of the American Oil Chemists Society* 69(2):106-110.

Wolff RL (1993). Further Studies on Artificial Geometrical Isomers of a-linolenic Acid in Edible Linolenic Acid-Containing Oils. *Journal of the American Oil Chemists Society* 70(3):219-224.

Wolk A, et al. (1998). Various fats may have specific opposite effects. *Archives of Internal Medicine* 147(4):342-352.

Wood R, Kubena K, Tseng S, Martin G, Crook R (1993). Effect of palm oil, margarine, butter, and sunflower oil on the serum lipids and lipoproteins of normocholesterolemic middle-aged men. *Journal of Nutritional Biochemistry* 4:286-297.

# Myth 3: Using Cholesterol Lowering Drugs, Especially The Statins, Would Benefit Nearly Everyone

*"Reported to the FDA: A forty-year-old nurse with mild hypertension and a total cholesterol of 276 (LDL-C 150) was started on 40 mg [daily] of Zocor. After seven days, she began having difficulty breathing. The Zocor was stopped, but she died three months later from a rare lung disease... that was attributed to the Zocor by her doctor and an independent medical examiner."*   ----*Jay S. Cohen, MD, 2005*

### Spacedoc Disillusioned

As a former astronaut, medical research scientist, flight surgeon and family doctor, Duane Graveline, MD, was appalled by the lack of information in his own medical community on the true side effects of the statin drugs.

In the past several years he learned: 1) that statin drugs work their cardiovascular effect not by cholesterol manipulation but by their now well-established anti-inflammatory role and: 2) cholesterol, which the pharmaceutical industry would have us believe is our major adversary is not only vital to our general health, but is mandatory for proper brain function. The pharmaceutical industry would rather you did not know this. Their shameful profits from statin drug sales alone depend a great deal upon your continuing ignorance and compliance with your physician, who may have been paid up to $2,000 to start you on some statin drug such as Crestor™, Lipitor™, or Zocor™.

When Spacedoc first experienced Lipitor-associated amnesia, his reaction was surprise, for in his clinical use of the earlier cholesterol lowering drugs in his family practice, he had never knowingly encountered cognitive dysfunction in a patient. Patients, even less aware of this relationship, are reluctant to report amnesia, confusion and altered memory coming on months or even years after statin drugs are started, thinking it is just old age, an inevitable touch of senility or possibly early Alzheimer's disease. When such patients are brought to the doctor's office with these complaints, all too frequently the doctor fails to consider the very real possibility that such side effects might be due to their statin drug, the very drug he had placed them on for health maintenance purposes, the very drugs purported to do so much good for public health.

Statin drugs, while lowering serum cholesterol levels, must inevitably inhibit the production of other vital intermediary products that originate further along the metabolic pathway, beyond the statin blockade. As a result, the side effects we are seeing from the statin class of drugs are extraordinarily diverse, reflecting a multiplicity of causes. From lack of sufficient bio-availability of cholesterol to excessive inhibition of the Coenzyme Q10 (see Myth 1) and dolichols, both sharing the same biochemical pathway as cholesterol, to the consequences of the newly recognized anti-inflammatory action of statins, the opportunity for serious side effects are legion.

Physicians such as Spacedoc are led to believe that such side effects are so uncommon as to be disregarded. Tens of thousands of patient case reports, slowly accumulated, document how self-serving and untrue is the denial of these side-effects by Big Pharma. Patient case reports are anecdotal, they say, implying they can comfortably be disregarded. This is patently untrue. Spacedoc recalls the words of Dr. Ellsworth Amidon of Vermont College of Medicine to his medical students. "Listen carefully to the words of the patient, my young doctors, for they are telling you the diagnosis." One thing Spacedoc learned in his 25 years of family practice was the truth of Doctor Amidon's wise counsel. Just listen to the patient, he emphasized. I shake my head in memory of this fine doctor as I review the hundreds of case reports I receive each month where distraught patients complain that their doctors don't listen to them and their complaints about statins are ignored.

"One must ask if the ever-increasing use of statin drugs is cost-effective? It is true that we doctors can reduce cardiovascular risk with statin use very slightly, but not enough to affect all-cause mortality much. Having learned that atherosclerosis is an inflammatory disease, our focus should be on presence of inflammation, not on cholesterol level. Doctors need to be far better informed of the true legacy of statin drug side effects. They should be seeking out better ways of identifying those at risk for cardiovascular disease. They should keep in mind that many safe and readily available supplements have been shown to have very substantial anti-inflammatory benefits…" (Spacedoc)

A few alert and courageous MDs like Spacedoc are discovering that our 40-year war on cholesterol through the use of drugs and the now infamous low fat/low cholesterol diet has been grossly misdirected. We have become a nation of fattened sheep, prone to Type 2 diabetes and with unchanged proneness to atherosclerosis. Despite the mounting evidence for cholesterol's irrelevance and our growing awareness of inflammation as one of the bases of atherosclerosis, our public still remains desperately focused on cholesterol, as planned by Big Pharma by multi-billion-dollar promotions. Statin drugs have never been more aggressively marketed.

The only thing we can be absolutely certain of is that lowering everyone's cholesterol produces the incredible profits realized by the pharmaceutical industry. Money absolutely wasted because of the harm done. Read on.


## The Scam

In the previous chapter, Myth 2, ample evidence was given that low-carb diets would tend to normalize lipid levels, especially to lower the triglycerides/high-density-lipoprotein (TG/HDL) ratio with no ill effects. Even CRP levels (C-reactive protein, an inflammation indicator) can be brought down by low-carb diets and certain supplements. Normalizing lipid levels by such an indirect approach that eliminates infection or inflammation is desirable. Doing it by stopping biosynthesis of cholesterol in the liver by using drugs will be shown to be undesirable, since there is so much collateral damage.

The National Cholesterol Education Program (NCEP) sponsored by the National Heart, Lung and Blood Institute (NHLBI) of the National Institutes of Health (NIH), recommends high-carb diets with caloric content the same as those of the FDA as the initial treatment for lowering total cholesterol (TC) and low-density-lipoprotein (LDL). Many high glycemic index foods are recommended, even for those with diabetes. The fats endorsed are margarine, mayonnaise and vegetable oils, as noted in Myth 2 (see www.nhlbisupport.com). These high-carb, high omega-6 and high *trans* fat diets raise TC, LDL, TG (triglycerides) and CRP levels. This is the opposite of what the promoters say high-carb diets are supposed to do. High-carb diets, accompanied by omega-6 and *trans* fats, the very diet recommendations of the NCEP, are bound to fail, and do fail (Ottoboni & Ottoboni, 2002, pp120-122). They are atherogenic and carcinogenic.

The Center for Science in the Public Interest with 35 physicians and other health professionals sent a petition to the NCEP, NHLBI and the Director of the NIH asking for an independent review panel to reevaluate the cholesterol guidelines. A month later the NHLBI responded, refusing, of course, and repeating the dogma. (Hecht, 2004-2005).

*Then every person "who failed to lower her cholesterol on the diet" to ≤200 mg/dL TC is prescribed a cholesterol lowering drug.* The implication is that those who take these drugs will have fewer heart attacks and live longer, *as a result of lowered TC or LDL levels.* There are assurances that side-effects will be minimal, or are a worthwhile trade for the benefits of these drugs. You may have seen beautifully prepared "medical articles" handed out to MDs and patients both to explain how cardiovascular disease (CVD) develops, how it is related to abdominal obesity, and finally how only a statin-type anti-cholesterol drug will be a wonderful solution to "high LDL" (Grundy, 1997).

What is certain is that the total revenues to their manufacturers of anti-cholesterol drugs in the statin class, such as Zocor™ and Lipitor™, were about $15 billion per year, even back in 2002 (Figure 3-1). The retail value of the prescriptions is much higher. One would think that the benefits of drastically lowered levels of TC, often down to 140 mg/dL, have proven value. One would be wrong.

Even before the first statin drug appeared in 1987, there were other cholesterol-lowering drugs, such as colestipol from Upjohn. In the early 1970s a major clinical trial was carried out with such poor randomization of patients (no double or even single blinding) that the favorable results reported with colestipol were neither real or repeatable (Ravnskov, 2000, pp150-151).

Wyeth's clofibrate (Atromid-S™) was touted as a great success in a trial in which the number of non-fatal heart attacks in the treatment group was 25% lower. (Note from Myth 1 that this is a much poorer result than men can obtain from Bufferin!) This "25%" was a relative risk, thus it means nothing without an absolute risk, as explained in the Introduction. However, the number of fatal heart attacks was the same in both groups in this trial, and the all-cause death rate was 47% higher in the clofibrate group, along with more cases of gallstones. And this drug is still prescribed! (Ravnskov, 2000, p151. Moore, 1989, pp51-53) At least it had a Black Box warning (the most serious — see Introduction) in the 1996 Physicians Desk Reference (PDR).

Cholestyramine (Bristol-Myers Squibb's Questran™) was no better, and the major trial quoted to promote this drug had serious manipulation of data (Ravnskov, 2000, pp165, 167-168).

The infamous NHLBI/AHA Consensus Development Conference in December of 1984 exposed in Myth 2 actually claimed a consensus with a press release saying that: "...the entire U. S. population should lower its cholesterol..." (Kolata, 1985); but there was no evidence, even then, from clinical trials, that lowering cholesterol saves lives.

A 1990 conference of the NHLBI quietly published graphs and data showing hardly any difference in all-cause death rates vs. TC for men or women. Fewer CVD deaths with lower TC levels were counterweighted by deaths from cancer, trauma, or digestive causes (Jacobs et al., 1992).

The following year John Allred of Ohio State University published a paper with a clear pair of graphs (Figure 3-2) for the relation of all-cause death rates to TC levels in serum for men and women of all ages based on the data from that same 1990 NHLBI conference (Allred, 1993). It is obvious that women live longer (lower all-cause mortality) with higher cholesterol levels, so they should never be

Figure 3-1. Total Revenues to Drug Manufacturers from Sale of Statings - $ Millions

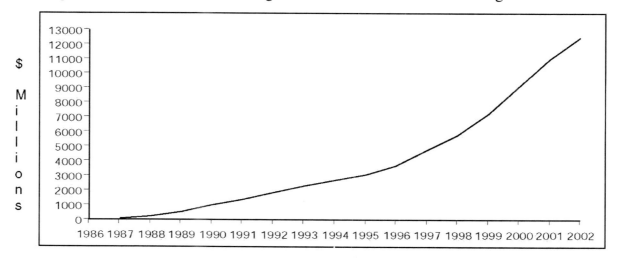

Mevacor & Zocor, 1987-1992, Graham Bell, Director of Investor Relations, Merck & Co., telecon 29 Aug 03. Total Statins, 1998-2002, *Business Week,* 21 Jul 03, p28, *via* IMS Health.

treated to lower TC, and the difference in men is so slight as not to be worth treating. The high TC right-hand side of Figure 3-2 does not end at 239 mg/dL; the fourth data point is for ≥239 mg/dL on up to and including the highest levels of TC. Allred's graphs do not really reveal what the effects are of extremely high or low TC, since Allred's graphs bunch together all TC levels below 160 or above 239. People who die with TC levels of 300-400 tend to do so at advanced ages, say 80-100 years old. As you can see, levels below 200 are progressively less desirable for adult humans. This old data was available to Big Pharma for at least 30 years (Mann, 1977).

In the Quebec Cardiovascular Study on 4576 men aged 35-64 years to start, serum TC levels were not associated with CVD or all-cause mortality (Dagenais et al., 1990).

Even in dialysis patients, all-cause mortality was highest at the lowest TC levels, being 30% lower when TC was ≥240 mg/dL compared with TC <160. Also, mortality was 17% lower at LDL ≥190 mg/dL compared with LDL <130 (Liu et al., 2004).

Among the elderly the effects of *low* serum total cholesterol (TC) and low low-density-lipoprotein (LDL) were found to be deadly. In a study on residents of northern Manhattan, NY, 2,277 subjects were followed for 10 years. Two-thirds were female and 1/3 of the total were Hispanic, Afro-American and white. Subjects were 65-98 years old at baseline, mean age 76. The chance of dying was twice as great in the lowest quartile of TC or LDL levels, while HDL and triglyceride levels were not related to all-cause mortality in this age group (Figure 3-3). Women had higher baseline TC and LDL levels (206 and 124) than men (191 and 117), yet the women lived longer. Men with the same TC and LDL levels as women lived as long. Of the subjects, 1/5 were taking statin drugs to lower TC and LDL, which would have pushed them into the lowest quartile (Schupf et al., 2005). This is an excellent confirmation that *high* TC and LDL levels are beneficial, certainly in the elderly who are most likely to be prescribed a statin drug. The emphasis on the value of lowering LDL, rather than lowering TC, taken by Big Pharma in the last few years, is invalidated by this study.

Figure 3-2. Relative risk of all-cause mortality in males (left graph) and females (right graph) as a function of serum cholesterol (TC) concentration. The Figure was drawn with data from Jacobs et al. (1992). Relative risk estimates for males were recalculated using a weighted average of subjects in the Multiple Risk Factor Intervention Trial (MRFIT) and non-MRFIT trials, based upon the relative numbers of participants. From Allred, 1993.

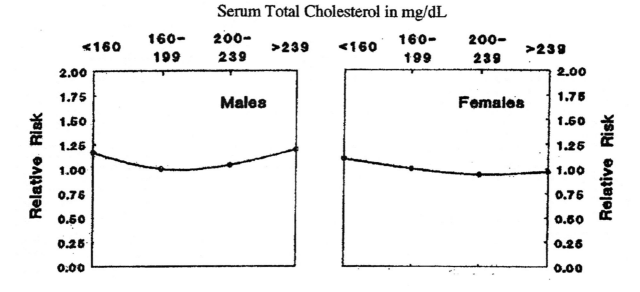

Serum Total Cholesterol in mg/dL

# Figure 3-3. Plasma Lipids vs. Mortality in 2,277Non-Demented Elderly

Ages 65-98 (mean 76), 66% female, followed 10 years in Manhattan, NY
Hispanic 38%, Afro-Am 31%, white 31%, other 1%
Baseline TC (mean): men 191, women 206
Baseline HDL-C (mean): men 117, women 124

| Total Cholesterol | No. Subjects at Risk | Deaths, (%) | Rate Ratio |
|---|---|---|---|
| ≤ 175 mg/dL | 580 | 97 (16.7) | 1.8 |
| 176-199 | 574 | 78 (13.6) | 1.2 |
| 220-226 | 556 | 57 (10.3) | 0.9 |
| > 226 | 567 | 59 (10.4) | 1.0 |
| **LDL Cholesterol** | | | |
| ≤ 97.8 | 572 | 90 (15.7) | 2.0 |
| 97.9-120.6 | 568 | 83 (14.6) | 1.6 |
| 120.7-144.0 | 571 | 65 (11.4) | 1.2 |
| > 144.0 | 566 | 53 ( 9.4) | 1.0 |

HDL Cholesterol - no difference          Triglycerides - no difference

Adapted from Schupf N, et al., 2005

 

Serum TC rises naturally with age from a mean level of 178 mg/dL in 18-24 year-olds to a maximum mean level of 230 mg/dL in 55-64 year-olds (Mann, 1977). Men over 55 and women of all ages who have the highest cholesterol levels live the longest, since high TC protects against cardiovascular disease (CVD) and infections (Ravnskov, 2003), as well as the afflictions listed previously — cancer, trauma, or digestive system ailments. The rise in TC with age is accompanied by the greater likelihood of dying at greater age from any cause. As an example of a similar effect, people develop more skin wrinkles as they age, but no one thinks that the greater number of wrinkles causes death, or that removing the wrinkles will put off death.

Dr. Bernard Forette and a team of French researchers from Paris found that women of mean age 82 with high cholesterol and followed for 5 years lived the longest. When the data of Forette are graphed, the age-adjusted data show a minimal risk of dying out to TC = 320 mg/dL for elderly women (Figure 3-4). The minimum death rate occurred with a TC level of 272 mg/dL, far higher than

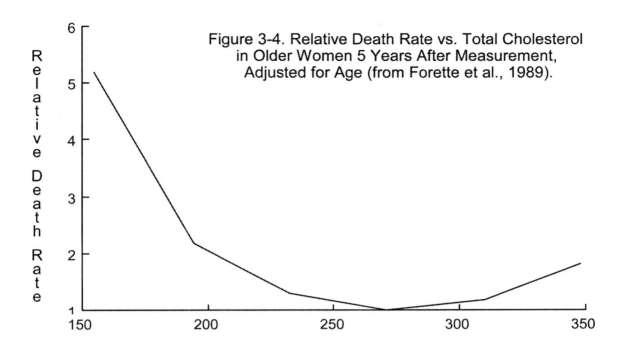

Figure 3-4. Relative Death Rate vs. Total Cholesterol in Older Women 5 Years After Measurement, Adjusted for Age (from Forette et al., 1989).

Total serum cholesterol at baseline in mg/dL

the current NCEP recommendations of ≤200 mg/dL for everyone. The death rate was 5.2 times higher for women who had very low cholesterol, specifically, 155 mg/dL. The death rate was 1.8 times higher for women who had very high cholesterol, specifically, 348 mg/dL, and also 1.8 times higher at 200 mg/dL (Forette et al., 1989). What possible basis could there be for the NCEP recommendations? In their report, the French doctors warned against lowering cholesterol in elderly women.

For people of a narrow age range, even in a 13-year span, say ages 50-62 years, a graph of TC levels of men who did and did not have CVD has been published recently (Figure 3-5), (Stehbens, 2001). Note that there is so much overlap between the men with or without CVD that there is no likelihood that the slightly greater chance for CVD at the higher TC levels could be used for prediction in any one individual, even in this group spanning 13 years in age. This is the reason that drug advertising claims that higher TC means quicker death from CVD are false — in large groups of people, the older ones will have higher TC and LDL, and older people die sooner than younger ones, not necessarily from CVD.

An observational study from the University of Innsbruck, Austria, on 150,000 subjects showed that low cholesterol levels predict premature death in men of all ages, and in women over the age of 50 (Ulmer et al., 2004).

Therefore, the TV ads for Lipitor™ showing one man of a pair of the same age, the one with "high" cholesterol, running into a door, or a woman with "high" TC collapsing in the street, or a body in a morgue to symbolize death from "high" TC, have no basis in fact. In my opinion, the Federal Trade Commission and the FDA are derelict in allowing these ads to run anywhere.

Figure 3-5. Serum cholesterol (TC) levels in Framingham
Study males of age 50-62 years with (- - - -) and without
(———) CVD. Some levels below 140 mg/dL were deleted.
From Stehbens, 2001.

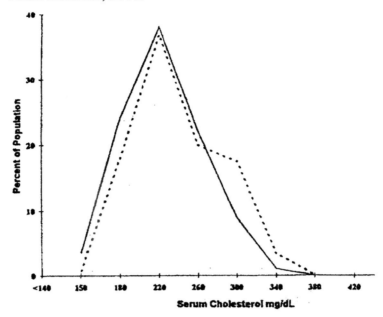

The National Cholesterol Education Program (NCEP) guidelines on "desirable" TC levels were of no value in predicting the existence of calcified plaques in coronary arteries as shown by two separate studies utilizing electron beam tomography to visualize the plaques (Raggi et al., 2001; Hecht et al., 2001). There was simply no correlation of serum TC with the existence or extent of late-stage (calcium-containing) arterial deposits in either of these two completely independent studies. This merely confirmed a study from 1936 in which a pathologist and a biochemist from the Department of Forensic Medicine at New York University found no correlation between the degree of atherosclerosis and serum TC in a number of individuals who had died a violent death. Their work was independently confirmed and an unfounded criticism of it was falsified 26 years later by a researcher who measured TC at intervals for up to 16 hours after death (Ravnskov, 2000, p118; Ravnskov, 2002a).

Patients with baseline LDL levels of 84, 117 and 158 mg/dL were given large doses of statin drugs to lower LDL levels to 76, 74 and 85 mg/dL. After about 1.2 years electron beam tomography showed no difference between the groups in the amount of plaque progression (Hecht et al, 2003). Thus LDL levels both pre- and post-treatment with statin drugs in 176 patients with moderate atherosclerosis were equally as useless as TC as predictors of atherosclerotic plaque progression.

In the huge INTERHEART study on 30,000 subjects in 52 countries, the effect of many modifiable risk factors on heart attacks (MIs) was studied. Smoking led the list, but total cholesterol (TC) and LDL were not even listed, perhaps because the outcomes were not the ones desired by some of the sponsors of the study, which included AstraZeneca, Novartis, Aventis, Abbott Labs, Bristol-Myers Squibb, King Pharma and Sanofi-Synthelabo (Yusuf et al., 2004).

Cholesterol is always present in our blood, and is necessary for life as an essential component of membranes, of nerve junctions, and of brain function (Mauch et al., 2001), and as a source of hormones. The common and true observation that LDL is the form of cholesterol delivered to the cells does not make it "bad cholesterol", since all cells need it to function, especially in the brain. Raised blood TC and LDL levels fail all tests as a necessary cause of atherosclerosis or its CVD form (Sutter, 1994).

Since high TC is beneficial, except in the 0.5% of people with an inherited condition called familial hypercholesterolemia where TC >400 mg/dL, there was never a valid reason to lower it. The famous comedian Bill Cosby's TC level of 700 mg/dL does not slow him down much at age 71. Even screening for cholesterol is not worthwhile, and is said to be a waste of resources of the UK's National Health Service, since it is such a poor predictor of who will have CVD (Kmietowicz, 1998). The opposite stance, a steady drumbeat of "bad cholesterol" bashing supporting the NCEP, can always be found for a quotation in the media, including promotion of high-carb diets (LaRosa, 1996). Advertising cholesterol-lowering drugs never lets up.

*There was never satisfactory evidence that lowering TC or LDL in most people would be of the slightest benefit. While a correlation does not necessarily prove a cause, a lack of correlation necessarily proves a lack of cause. Pretending otherwise is the scam.*

### Dangers of Low Cholesterol Levels

The previous section showed that lower TC and LDL levels have no benefit. This section shows that very low levels are a serious danger.

When TC levels decrease (yes, decrease) on their own, death is imminent. The Institut National de la Santé et de la Recherche Médicale, Unit 258, Hopital Broussais, Paris, France, studied 6230 working men, age 43-52 years at baseline, whose TC was measured 3-5 times annually. There was a weak *inverse* association between baseline TC and cancer mortality. After 17 years of follow-up, those whose TC dropped the most, the bottom quartile, were 30% more likely to die from cancer when allowance was made for age, baseline TC level, TG, BMI, smoking, and systolic blood pressure. When the adjustment of the raw data was made for age alone, those whose TC dropped the most from a mean baseline level of 222 mg/dL were about 25% more likely to die from cancer. Those men whose TC dropped below 180 mg/dL were in this bottom quartile (Zureik et al., 1997).

Published simultaneously in the same journal, *Epidemiology,* a study from the Medical Statistics Unit, London School of Hygiene and Tropical Medicine, England, used data from the Framingham Study on 5209 men and women. The odds of cancer death were up to twice as great (RR = 2) if a large prior fall in TC occurred over any 4- to 6-year period. This was a ≥38 mg/dL drop from the mean level of 230 mg/dL in men or women when they were 46-50 years old who were about to die of cancer. Here, too, the degree of drop in TC was more predictive than the baseline level of TC (Sharp & Pocock, 1997).

From the Leiden University Medical Center, Netherlands, a report appeared on people older than 85 initially and followed for 5 years (38% male). Those people with TC ≥252 mg/dL were half as likely to die as those with TC ≤194. Between those levels of TC, the subjects were 2/3 as likely to die (Weverling-Rijnsberger et al., 1997).

Patients with advanced congestive heart failure (CHF), about 1/4 female, admitted to the Ahmanson-UCLA Cardiomyopathy Center, Los Angeles, CA, were checked for TC, which was proportional to HDL, LDL, TG, and left ventricular ejection fraction (higher is better), and total cardiac output. Those who survived 1 year had mean TC = 185 mg/dL; non-survivors had mean TC = 165. Patients in the *lowest* quintile of TC, <129 mg/dL, were twice as likely to die as those with the *highest* TC. Those in the second quintile (129-160) were 1.4 times as likely to die. All results were very significant. Using deciles of TC, survival was better even at the highest TC levels measured, >250 (Horwich et al., 2002).

In several locations in Europe a group of 303 patients with CHF were followed for 3 years. Of those with TC >201 mg/dL, 72% were alive; of those with TC <201 mg/dL, just 50% were alive. The chance of survival *increased* 25% with each 40 mg/dL *increase* in TC (Rauchhaus et al., 2003).

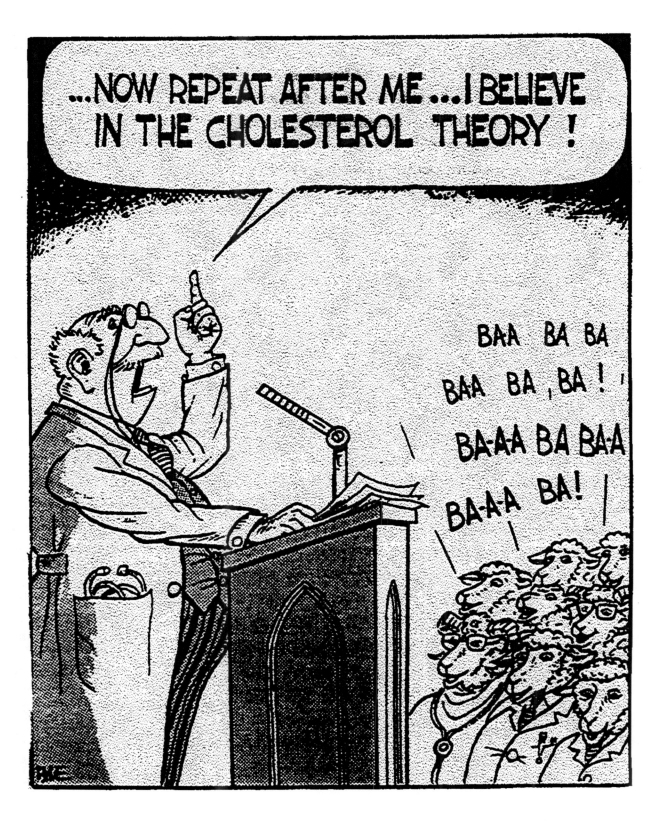

With permission from Charles T. McGee, MD, *Heart Frauds, HealthWise, Colorado Springs, CO, 2001.*

A large number of clinical studies showed that TC levels <180 were associated with depression, accidents, suicide, homicide, antisocial personality disorder in criminals and army veterans, cocaine and heroin addiction, and high relapse rates after detoxification (Buydens-Branchey & Branchey, 2003). To be fair, no increase in the death rate from accidents was seen with lower serum TC by other researchers (Pekkanen et al., 1989); but, on the other hand, a recent review on 32 studies found a strong association of low TC (especially below 200 mg/dL) with violent behaviors and violent death (Golomb, 1998).

At this point it is important to note that patients in a 16-week study who took 80 mg per day of Lipitor™, the best-selling statin drug, had their TC cut down to 140 mg/dL in 6 weeks (Schwartz et al., 2001). Not only was there no evidence in the study that this was beneficial, but plenty of the evidence given above shows that such low levels of TC are quite harmful.

The American Heart Association (AHA), in July of 2002, recommended that children should have their blood TC and LDL levels tested at about the age of five. No evidence was presented by the AHA, which one might suspect was trying to help sell statin drugs to children. An actual comparison of TC levels was made for boys aged 7-9 in six countries vs. mortality rate of children under five in these same countries (Table 3-1). You can see that lower TC means higher mortality. Incidentally, *lower* saturated fat calories in the diet were also correlated fairly well with *higher mortality.*

## What are the Statin Drugs?

HMG-CoA reductase is an enzyme (a catalyst) that is essential for the synthesis of cholesterol in your body. Most of your cholesterol is synthesized; vegetarians would die quickly if it were not. An enzyme inhibitor normally works by binding to the active site of the enzyme tightly enough so that the enzyme cannot do its normal job because it cannot bind to its normal target. When the statin drugs inhibit this enzyme, which helps turn 2-carbon units that could come from almost any food into larger molecules, not only the synthesis of cholesterol is inhibited, but also the synthesis of a number of other biomolecules. These are as essential as cholesterol and all the hormones made from it, as well as

Table 3-1. Mortality Rate of Children Under Five per 1,000 Newborns vs. Serum Cholesterol (TC) in Boys Aged 7-9 in the Same Countries

| Country | Serum TC | Mortality |
|---|---|---|
| Ghana | 128 | 145 |
| Philippines | 147 | 72 |
| Italy | 159 | 12 |
| United States | 167 | 12 |
| Netherlands | 174 | 9 |
| Finland | 190 | 7 |

Adapted from Deutsch M, Ravnskov U, Poster at the 18th International Conference of Clinical Chemistry and Laboratory Medicine, Kyoto, Japan, 20-25 Oct 2002.

dolichols and coenzyme Q10, the latter being essential for using the oxygen you breathe to make the cellular energy source ATP (adenosine triphosphate). So ubiquitous was the presence of Q10 in cells that the original name for it was ubiquinone. All this was known before 1990 (Folkers et al., 1990).

The statin drugs are essentially the HMG-CoA reductase inhibitors: atorvastatin (Lipitor™), cerivastatin (Baycol™, withdrawn 8/01), fluvastatin (Lescol™), lovastatin (Mevacor™), pravastatin (Pravachol™), simvastatin (Zocor™), pitavastatin and rosuvastatin (Crestor™), which were introduced to lower total cholesterol TC levels, and especially LDL-cholesterol (LDL) levels, ostensibly to prevent CVD. The shorthand structural formulas are shown in Appendix D.

Lovastatin was the first, introduced in the USA in 1987. It is a molecule identical to one in a red yeast which grows on a type of rice that has been used in China for more than 1200 years, and had been available in the USA since 1950. Rather than refusing to allow Merck to patent lovastatin, since it is a natural product, the reason vitamin E and coenzyme Q10 could never be patented, the FDA allowed the patent and banned the sale of some forms of red rice yeast (Ottoboni & Ottoboni, 2002, p157-168). The other statin drugs are "me, too" products of slightly different structures that can cause different levels of TC lowering and different types and levels of side-effects.

## Do Statin Drugs Lengthen Lives?

In this book no assertions are made without evidence. Despite the caveats given about the problems in medical papers on randomized clinical trials (RCTs), some important facts can be extracted with difficulty from the data in the body of such papers even when such facts do not appear in the abstracts or the press releases.

The "bottom lines" of some of the largest of the many RCTs on statins are shown in Figure 3-6. OK, it is a fussy figure, but give it time. The first column gives the name of the RCT as an acronym. The second column gives the generic name of the drug used in each RCT. Both the previous section and Appendix D will let you see which is which by trade name. The "Time" column gives the duration of the RCT. The "RR" column shows the relative risk of all-cause death. The next two columns give the actual absolute percentages of control (placebo) group patients still alive at the end of the trial, and of the drugged (treated) patients still alive. This is almost never shown in the media, yet this is what gives a clear picture of how minor the effects of the drugs are. Using these two figures, the change in absolute risk (AR) during the trial is shown — always a much smaller number than the RR, thus never used in advertising. The AR/year is obtained by dividing the AR by the number of years in the RCT. It is very small in all the trials. The number needed to treat (NNT) to prevent one death per year of treatment is in the last column, and it is large, being the reciprocal of the AR/year.

The first thing that can be seen at the top of this mass of numbers in Figure 3-6 is that lovastatin shortened lives in the EXCEL and AFCAPS trials. Their NNTs are actually the number of patients that had to be treated with drugs in order to kill one per year of treatment! While many of the RRs for the other statin drugs are statistically significant, because of the huge number of subjects in each trial, the absolute risk (AR) reductions are quite small, especially in the ALLHAT trial. Determining the mean of absolute risk reduction per year (AR/yr) from taking the statin drugs, we see that the mean value for all 11 RCTs is -0.28% per year. This means that your improved chance of not dying in 1 year while you are taking a statin drug is 1 in 357. These are not impressive odds. The mean trial duration in Figure 3-6 is 4.1 years, a far shorter duration than the recommendations intended to induce people to take statins for 20-50 years. Since TC levels go right back up again when these drugs are stopped, they are supposed to be continued forever once they are begun.

The HPS trial utilizing simvastatin (Zocor) was huge, with over 20,000 subjects in all. The reduction in RR of all-cause mortality was 12% (RR=0.88), but this amounts to only an absolute risk

Figure 3-6: Results of RCTs on Statin Drugs on All-Cause Mortality

| Acronym of RCT | Drug Used | Time (years) | RR (%) | Controls Alive (%) | Treated Alive (%) | AR (%) | AR/yr (%) | NNT /yr |
|---|---|---|---|---|---|---|---|---|
| EXCEL | lovastatin | 1 | +150 | 99.7 | 99.5 | +0.3 | +0.3 | 333* |
| AFCAPS | lovastatin | 5.2 | +3.9 | 97.7 | 97.6 | +0.09 | +0.02 | 5000* |
| 4S | simvastatin | 5.4 | -29 | 88.5 | 91.8 | -3.3 | -0.61 | 167 |
| HPS | simvastatin | 5 | -12 | 85.3 | 87.1 | -1.8 | -0.36 | 278 |
| WOSCOPS | pravastatin | 4.4 | -22 | 95.9 | 96.8 | -0.9 | -0.2 | 500 |
| PROSPER | pravastatin | 3 | -1.9 | 89.5 | 89.7 | -0.2 | -0.07 | 1429 |
| LIPID | pravastatin | 6.1 | -22 | 85.9 | 89 | -3.1 | -0.51 | 196 |
| CARE | pravastatin | 5 | -8 | 90.6 | 91.4 | -0.77 | -0.15 | 667 |
| ALLHAT-LLT | pravastatin | 6 | -0.01 ns | 84.7 | 85.1 | -0.6 | -0.1 | 1000 |
| FLORIDA | fluvastatin | 1 | -35 | 96.0 | 97.3 | -1.3 | -1.3 | 77 |
| ASCOT | atorvastatin | 3.3 | -12 | 95.9 | 96.4 | -0.5 | -0.15 | 667 |

RR = relative risk of death with treatment.  AR = absolute risk of death with treatment.

NNT/yr = number of patients needed to treat for 1 year to prevent 1 death (*to cause 1 death).

Data from U. Ravnskov, 2000, pp200-201 and e-mail of 2003, ALLHAT-LLT (ALLHAT, 2002), and FLORIDA (Liema et al., 2002).  HPS data from Collins et al., 2002.

(AR) reduction of 0.36% per year. The result usually quoted for patients is a RR reduction of 24%, but this is for mostly non-fatal cardiovascular events (stroke and MI). This mostly male trial, with only 18% female, as is typical, had no separate results for all-cause mortality in women (Collins et al., 2002).

Using the AR/yr of -0.15% for Lipitor in the ASCOT trial in Figure 3-6, your improved chance not to die in 1 year would be 1 in 667. The cost of a month's supply of Lipitor (atorvastatin) at 40 mg/day is $125 in the USA, or $1500/year, or $1,000,000 to prevent one death among 667 people taking this type of drug *for 1 year*. Again, this was based on a trial the drug's maker chose to report. Trials are chosen by their sponsors for the best results. The duration is chosen for best results.

Of 3 older trials reporting gender-specific mortality, there was a 1% decrease, a 12% increase, and a 57% increase in women, so the omission of gender-specific data in the HPS and in other trials can have serious consequences for women (Criqui & Golomb, 2004). If women are included in an RCT on a statin drug, the percentage of them is low, so that the known bad effects in women will not make the overall trial result negative for the statin. Usually results for women are  not reported separately.

"Medical articles" prepared as sales aids for statin drugs still present the results of certain trials as very positive, with minimal side-effects (Grundy, 1997). For example, the drop in RR of total mortality in the WOSCOPS trial of 22% (Figure 3-6) used in advertising is never accompanied by the news that this amounts to a drop of only 0.2% per year in absolute terms.

*****

Researchers at the University of Sheffield took a hard look at the earlier RCTs: AFCAPS, 4S, LIPID, WOSCOPS and CARE. They reported that statin use could be associated with an *increase* in mortality of 1% in 10 years. "This would be sufficiently large to negate statins' beneficial effect on CVD mortality in patients with a [fatal] CVD event risk of less than 13% over a 10 year period." "Patients' absolute risk of CVD should be calculated before starting statin treatment for primary prevention." (Jackson et al., 2001). It has already been shown (above and in Myth 2) that the usual calculations based on TC or LDL are not really predictive. TG/HDL, which is more predictive, is seldom used. All this indicates no meaningful benefit for primary prevention of mortality from CVD from statin drugs.

*****

In the ASCOT-LLA trial (Sever at al., 2003) on hypertensive subjects with average or lower TC, there was no change in the all-cause death rate vs. placebo after 3.5 years; however there was a 10% higher incidence of the arbitrarily defined primary endpoint of non-fatal MI plus fatal CVD among the 19% women in the trial, similar to the detrimental effect of aspirin in women (Kauffman, 2002). This was reported in the medical paper on the trial only by a data point in a Figure. No comment on this was found anywhere else in the paper (Sever et al., 2003). The slight reduction in AR/year of 0.15% was obtained mainly from the effect of Lipitor™ on the 81% men in the trial.

*****

What about secondary prevention? The surest indication of risk of a future fatal myocardial infarction (MI or heart attack) is having a non-fatal one (NFMI). The 16-week study with atorvastatin cited above (Schwartz et al., 2001) was on survivors of  MI or angina attacks admitted to hospitals. Here was a group for which treatment could truly be called secondary. This Myocardial Ischemia

Reduction with Aggressive Cholesterol Lowering (MIRACL) study actually showed no change in mortality or second MI rate.

In detail, this RCT on the effects of 80 mg/day of atorvastatin or placebo on 3,086 patients in hospital after angina or non-fatal MI and followed for 16 weeks, had the following conclusions in the abstract of the journal article: "For patients with acute coronary syndrome, lipid-lowering therapy with atorvastatin, 80 mg/day, reduces recurrent ischemic [clotting] events in the first 16 weeks, mostly recurrent symptomatic ischemia requiring re-hospitalization." Actually this is true. However, there was no change in the death rate, and no significant change in either the re-infarction rate or need for resuscitation from cardiac arrest. There was a statistically significant drop in chest pain requiring rehospitalization. The risk ratio plot was unusual in not having a vertical bar at the 1.00 point, making the outcomes hard to visualize from this figure. An example of such a bar may be seen in Figure 1-2. The discussion did not give any comparisons with alternate treatments, for example, that five weeks of aspirin would give significantly lower reinfarction and all-cause mortality rates in men. The standard treatment for angina pain, nitro compounds, such as Nitrodur™, was not compared with atorvastatin, either. Failure to make such obvious comparisons is poor medical science at best.

*****

Repetitive physician-prompting of patients to take their statin drugs was evaluated. Patients who had such serious CVD as to be admitted to a coronary care unit, were prompted to take their statin drugs vs. a similar control group who were not prompted. After 2 years, 14% who were prompted died vs. 12% of controls who were not; this was not statistically significant (Hilleman et al, 2001). This study was sponsored by Bristol-Myers and the American Association of Colleges of Pharmacy.

*****

In fact, a recent meta-analysis on 44 trials of atorvastatin reported no change whatever in the all-cause death rate for subjects on atorvastatin or other statins compared with those on placebo, not even by 1% (Newman et al, 2003). What is different here is that the mean duration of the trials was only 1 year. The benefits of statins, such as they are, are known to begin only after 1-2 years (Jackevicius et al., 2002).

*****

The studies sponsored by the drug makers are their own property. They run many more trials than they report on publicly, and only the best results are made public, some of these appearing as research papers in peer-reviewed medical journals (Robinson, 2001). So it is quite possible that there is no life extension on the whole from taking statin drugs, even in men. The evidence indicates that statins in general will not increase lifespan. The best of the statins in the sickest of patients might prolong life a few weeks or months (Kauffman, 2001), but at the cost of severe side-effects, which will be described later. And *not* by lowering TC or LDL.

## Do Statin Drugs Prevent Non-Fatal Heart Attacks?

The short answer is yes, but not by much (see Figure 3-7). Look at the column of control subjects who had a non-fatal MI (NFMI). All the statin trial patients were sicker than the PHS trial physicians, of whom only 1.93% of the controls had a non-fatal MI. Nevertheless, the biggest relative risk reduction in NFMI in the trials in Figure 3-7 was accomplished by Bufferin in the PHS trial, RR = 0.41 (-59%). Leaving out the 4S and FLORIDA trials, which are outliers, the typical statin trial reduced the AR of NFMI by 0.33% per year, which happens also to be the value for Lipitor in the ASCOT trial. This means that taking a statin drug lowers your chances of having an NFMI by 1/300 per year. Should you or your health insurer be paying for such a tiny reduction? The cost of a month's supply of Lipitor (atorvastatin) at 40 mg/day is $125/month, or $1500/year, or $450,000 to prevent one NFMI for just one year. About $1.67/month or $20/year of Bufferin or of Bayer aspirin with buffer and enteric coating at 81 mg/day will accomplish about the same thing with fewer side-effects, at least in men. Does the advertising for statin drugs seem a little overdone?

Oddly enough the FDA has been almost as realistic about Lipitor as about aspirin. In 2001 the FDA ordered Pfizer to stop promoting Lipitor as a treatment for CVD, noting that it had not been established as a preventive for CVD, or effective in reducing the rates of fatal MI or NFMI. It may only be promoted as a cholesterol-lowering drug. (http://www.fda.gov/cder/warn/2001/9607.pdf) Oh, well, no agency is perfect!

The physician-prompting trial with statins noted above did much better on the very sick patients involved, all with serious CVD to start. After 2 years about 56% of the control patients suffered some *non-fatal* cardiac event vs. 34% on statins; this was very significant. There was no change in the number of rescusitated cardiac arrests or strokes (Hilleman et al, 2001). This agrees with the results in the 4S and LIPID trials in which the patients were the sickest to start with.

## Do Statin Drugs Prevent Stroke?

Recent claims that statins reduce the risk of stroke, both fatal and non-fatal, fell into the trap of using relative and not absolute risks (Rosendorff, 1998). In the ALLHAT trial 94.7% of subjects on pravastatin did not have any stroke, while 94.2% on placebo did not; of course this was not significant. In the HPS trial 96.4% of the subjects on simvastatin did not have a non-fatal stroke, while 95.1% on placebo did not; significant; but what about that huge dropout rate? Also in HPS 99.1% of the subjects on simvastatin did not have a fatal stroke, while 98.8% on placebo did not; not significant. In the ASCOT trial 98.3% of the subjects on atorvastatin did not have any stroke, while 97.6% on placebo did not; while this was statistically significant, it amounts to a reduction of only 0.21% per year (NNT = 476, thus $714,000 to prevent one mostly non-fatal stroke for a single year).

## Do Statin Drugs Prevent Damage to the Retina of the Eye?

Two studies claimed that statin drug use prevented maculopathy, a progressive retinal disorder that causes untreatable blindness in the elderly. A careful study showed no evidence of such protection in statin users of <1 month, 1-12 months, or >12 months (Leeuwen et al., 2003).

## Do Statin Drugs Work by Lowering Cholesterol?

By now you may not care about the details of such mediocre benefits of the statin drugs. But every single research paper on those RCTs emphasizes how much TC or LDL are lowered by the statin drug. Typically this is 20% for TC and 28% for LDL for the older statin drugs (LaRosa, 1999) and 27% and 41% with atorvastatin (Newman, 2003). Based on the claims of Big Pharma repeated by so many MDs, one would think that lowering TC and LDL levels to those of a 20-year old would have a more dramatic effect on lowering heart attack rates and extending life than what is seen in Figures 3-6 and 3-7. One would be wrong.

Uffe Ravnskov, MD, PhD, noticed that, in a report on the CARE trial, the probability that the % change in LDL by pravastatin was responsible for the outcome of slightly lower heart attack rates

Figure 3-7: Results of RCTs on Statin Drugs on Non-Fatal Heart Attack (NFMI)

| Acronym of RCT | Drug Used | Time (years) | RR (%) | Controls NFMI (%) | Treated NFMI (%) | AR (%) | AR/yr (%) |
|---|---|---|---|---|---|---|---|
| AFCAPS | lovastatin | 5.2 | -38 | 5.5 | 3.5 | -2.0 | -0.38 |
| 4S | simvastatin | 5.4 | -30 | 22.6 | 13.9 | -6.7 | -1.24 |
| WOSCOPS | pravastatin | 4.4 | -22 | 6.2 | 4.3 | -1.8 | -0.41 |
| PROSPER | pravastatin | 3.1 | -12 | 8.7 | 7.7 | -1.0 | -0.32 |
| LIPID | pravastatin | 6.1 | -27 | 10.3 | 7.4 | -2.9 | -0.48 |
| CARE | pravastatin | 5 | -22 | 8.3 | 6.5 | -1.8 | -0.36 |
| ALLHAT-LLT | pravastatin | 6 | -2 | 4.8 | 4.7 | -0.1 | -0.017 |
| FLORIDA | fluvastatin | 1 | +68 | 4.7 | 7.9 | +3.2 | +3.2 |
| ASCOT | atorvastatin | 3.3 | -37 | 3.0 | 1.9 | -1.1 | -0.33 |
| PHS | Bufferin | 7.0 | -59 | 1.93 | 1.17 | -0.76 | -0.11 |

Data from U. Ravnskov, 2002, pp200-201, except ALLHAT-LLT, which includes fatal CVD (ALLHAT, 2002), FLORIDA (Liema et al., 2002), PROSPER (Blauw et al., 2002), ASCOT, which includes fatal CVD (Sever et al., 2003) and PHS (PHS, 1989). RR = relative risk of non-fatal MI with treatment. AR = absolute risk of non-fatal MI with treatment.

was only 24%. Using the absolute change in LDL level, the probability was 3% (Ravnskov, 2002a). To be considered significant, these numbers would have to be ≥95%.

Jørgen Vesti Nielsen, MD, looked at the figures on the website of a report on the HPS trial. The reduction in risk of any "unwanted cardiovascular event" was not consistently related to the initial level of LDL (Figure 3-8). Note that there was more risk with LDL <116 mg/dL (7.4%) than the middle level (6.3%). Note that the reduced risk of an event with statin is greater at the lower initial

**Figure 3-8. Risk of any unwanted cardiovascular event with pravastatin treatment relative to inital LDL levels**

| LDL Level Before Treatment (mg/dL) | AR of Event on Placebo (%) | AR of Event on Statin (%) | AR Reduction on Statin (%) |
|---|---|---|---|
| <116 | 7.4 | 5.9 | 1.5 |
| 116-135 | 6.3 | 4.7 | 1.6 |
| >135 | 11.9 | 9.3 | 2.6 |

From Nielsen, 2001.

LDL level than at the middle (normal) initial levels of LDL. This is not a logical cause-and-effect dose-response curve. Because TC or LDL lowering in trials before the statins appeared all caused higher mortality, it is clear that statins do not reduce MI rates by lowering TC or LDL, but by some other method (Nielsen, 2001).

The Japan Lipid Intervention Trial (J-LIT), a primary prevention trial utilizing simvastatin was carried out on 47,300 Japanese patients. Since they are more sensitive to statin drugs than occidentals, the dose was 5 mg/day for 90% and 10 mg/day for 10%. All were followed for 6 years including those who stopped the drug, which was open-labeled. There was no placebo group. Figure 3-9 A shows that those whose TC was *most reduced* had the *highest* all-cause death rate. The statin makers often stress that the main "benefit" of statins is to reduce LDL rather than TC. As shown in Figure 3-9 B, those with *lowest* achieved levels of LDL also had the *highest* all-cause death rate. Obviously, there is no reason to reduce TC below 250, or LDL below 130 mg/dL. Note that the Y-axis is cut off at 94% in A and 96% in B. The absolute differences are quite small, only 0.61% per year from best-to-worst levels of TC, and only 0.30% per year from best-to-worst levels of LDL. Here is the best evidence yet that the tiny gains in lifespan shown in other trials on statin drugs with placebo groups are not due to TC or LDL lowering (Matsuzaki, et al., 2002).

A recent study from the LDS Hospital and University of Utah, Salt Lake City, confirmed that statin use improved the survival rate among 651 patients, 75% male, with ≥70% blockage in at least 1 coronary artery when infection by cytomegalovirus was present, and more so, when inflammation was severe. There was no survival benefit when both were absent. This finding strongly supports the hypothesis that cholesterol lowering was irrelevant (Horne et al., 2003).

It is now understood that statins operate to lower heart attack rates by mechanisms other than cholesterol lowering, such as limiting production of the eicosanoids thromboxane A2 and B2, just as aspirin does (Ottoboni & Ottoboni, 2002, pp49-50). In a person taking aspirin, the addition of a statin drug does not push A2 levels much lower (Schmitz & Torzewski, 2002, p71). Thromboxane A2 raises blood pressure and promotes blood clotting. Thromboxane B2 causes inflammation and CVD.

Here is still more evidence that the change in levels of TC and LDL are not predictive of of the modest, but statistically valid benefits of statin drugs.

Since earlier non-statin drug treatments that lowered TC always gave higher death rates, measuring TC is clearly a useless surrogate endpoint, as has long been recognized (Fleming & DeMets, 1996). Therefore, the physicians who try to maintain credibility among their peers and feel ethical by prescribing statins "only to patients who need them" invariably make that determination by looking at the patients' TC and LDL levels, which are irrelevant to evaluating their health at a given age range, unless these levels are too *low*. This also means that there is no way to determine "the optimum dose", either. The trials in Figures 3-6 and 3-7 used different doses of whichever statin drug was "on trial".

## Will Taking Statin Drugs Make You Feel Better?

Generally not

There is no evidence for an improvement in general feeling of well-being when one is taking a statin drug; quite the contrary. Side-effects are usually said by the drug makers to affect 2-6% of patients. In fact, the 1996 PDR lists a total of 19% of patients on simvastatin with side-effects, about the same as for placebo. Yet 17% of the subjects quit simvastatin during the 5-year HPS trial (Collins et al., 2002). What if they had been forced to continue? My guess is that the HPS trial would have had less positive results, or even negative ones.

A recent meta-analysis on trials of atorvastatin noted side-effects in 65% of patients vs. 45% on placebo during a mean trial duration of 1 year (Newman et al, 2003).

In 1996 the Editor-in-Chief of the *American Journal of Cardiology* reported that 50% of "patients" prescribed a statin drug quit in 1 year, and that only 25% continued for 2 years (Roberts, 1996). What other reason could be responsible for such high dropout rates except adverse effects?

In a paper in the *Journal of the American Medical Association,* in which the head author admits to receiving honoraria from Bayer, Merck and Pfizer, the main theme is a lamentation on the fraction of elderly "patients" who do not adhere to their statin prescriptions for 2 years, and thus fail to receive the "benefits" (Jackevicius et al., 2002). Of people prescribed a statin for primary prevention of CVD, only 25.4% continued for more than 2 years. Of people prescribed a statin for secondary prevention of CVD, among those with chronic CVD but apparently without an NFMI, only 36.1% continued for more than 2 years. Among those who apparently had an NFMI, only 40.1% continued for more than 2 years. Sixty percent (100 — 40) is a high quit rate for people in fear for their lives. The authors tried to find some commonality among quitters and users, but the distress of side-effects was not considered. So of the "patients" in the worst shape, it seems obvious that 60-64% suffered side-effects, not that different from the crude value of 65% found by Newman et al. These percents are a long way from the "2-6%" claimed by drug makers.

Earlier, all articles on clinical trials assessing adherence to statin drugs were reviewed and categorized by patient population. The rates of non adherence and discontinuation were reported. Overall, levels of discontinuation reported in clinical trials (6-31%) and lipid clinics (2-38%) are similar, with unselected populations consistently reporting higher rates (15-78%). Again, side-effects as the probable reason were ignored (Tsuyuki & Bungard, 2001). Incidentally, a comment on the exaggeration of the benefits of statins by these authors was published in the same journal (Kauffman, 2001).

The recent shootout between pravastatin at 40 mg/day and atorvastatin at 80 mg/day has had all the favorable publicity the Pfizer Co. could have dreamt about. The pro-atorvastatin results of the

Figure 3-9. Cholesterol Levels Achieved vs. % Alive After 6 Years
of 5 mg/day of Simvastatin in Japanese Patients in the J-LIT Study
(from data in Matsuzaki M et al., 2002)

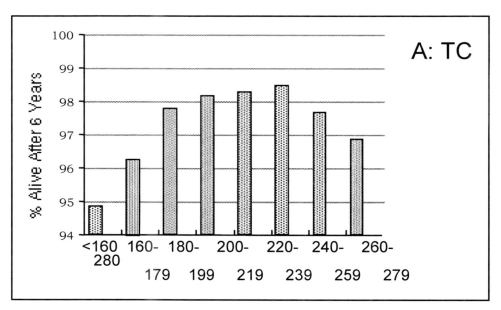

TotalCholesterol Levels Achieved

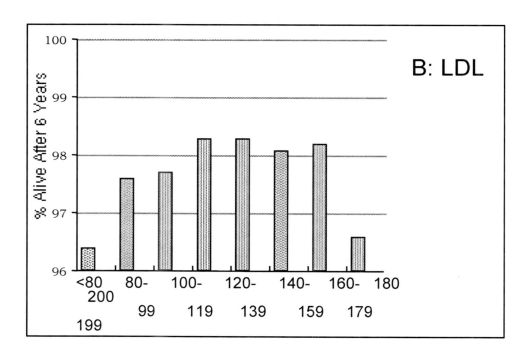

Pravastatin or Atorvastatin Evaluation and Infection Therapy—Thrombolysis in Myocardial Infarction 22 (PROVE IT—TIMI 22) trial generated press releases and editorials more appropriate to a school newspaper reporting on a rock concert (Cannon et al, 2004). The editors of the New York Times were completely taken in by the claims of benefit supposedly due to cholesterol lowering, and worried mainly about the staggering cost if every adult over 40 in the USA took atorvastatin (Anon., 2004). Incidentally, this would be $210 billion per year. An experienced medical writer at the New York Times was taken in by the combined end-point used, a combination of all-cause death *and* any major cardiovascular event, including chest pain, and the *relative* difference between the two drugs — 26% lower RR favoring atorvastatin (Kolata, 2004). What actually happened is that 33% of patients discontinued pravastatin and 30% discontinued atorvastatin after 2 years due to adverse events or other reasons. These staggering withdrawal rates somehow eluded the press releases. There was no placebo or control group in this well-randomized group of 4162 patients, 4/5 male as usual, mean age 58, who had just been hospitalized for a cardiac event. As for benefits, after 2 years, the all-cause death rate was 3.2% with pravastatin vs. 2.2% with atorvastatin, a gain of 0.5% absolute per year with the latter. As for the mostly non-fatal combined end-point so ballyhooed, 26% of patients on pravastatin had one vs. 22% on atorvastatin after 2.5 years, a gain of 1.6% absolute per year for the latter. As shown in the previous section, the degree of cholesterol reduction was probably irrelevant. Too bad Bufferin™ was not included in the trial.

The serious side effects of statins are cancer, constipation, erectile dysfunction, myalgia, myopathy, polyneuropathy, rhabdomyolysis, liver and kidney damage, congestive heart failure and amnesia. These will not make you feel better. Euphoria is not among them. A typical user will observe pain in many joints (myalgia), swelling of the legs, twinges in fingers and limbs (polyneuropathy), painful muscles (myalgia) and weakness (myopathy), (Cohen, 2001, pp90-91).

*****

"BOSTON, Sept. 28 /PRNewswire/ -- Consumers today filed the first-of-its-kind nationwide class-action lawsuit against Pfizer (NYSE: PFE), claiming the world's largest drug company misled consumers into using its anti-cholesterol drug Lipitor despite the absence of evidence from clinical trials that these drugs are of any benefit to large segments of the population. According to Steve Berman, the lead attorney for the proposed class, Pfizer promoted Lipitor by claiming it prevents heart disease in women and the elderly, where no clinical test has established such a benefit. In fact, according to the complaint, women without heart disease taking Lipitor actually developed 10 percent more heart attacks than women treated with a placebo.

"The lawsuit alleges that Pfizer engaged in a massive campaign to convince both doctors and patients that Lipitor is a beneficial treatment for nearly everyone with elevated cholesterol, even though no studies have shown it to be effective for women and those over 65 years of age who do not already have heart disease or diabetes.

"Normally, drugs become widely used as treatments for patients only when a well-designed clinical trial finds that the drug is safe and effective for patients of the same type and age. No such trial has shown that Lipitor helps the elderly or females without prior heart disease. "We believe Pfizer intentionally ignored the scientific evidence -- and lack thereof -- and launched a multi-million dollar ad campaign designed to push the drug to anyone they could convince to buy it," Berman said. "We intend to prove that Pfizer pocketed billions in sales to those who do not benefit from Lipitor."

## Cancer in rodents on statins

All members of the 2 most popular classes of anti-cholesterol drugs known in 1994, the statins and the fibrates, caused cancer in rodents at levels of exposure found in humans. The authors of this literature survey suggested that these classes of drugs should be avoided except in patients at high short-term risk of CVD (Newman & Hulley, 1996).

## Breast cancer in the CARE trial

In the CARE trial there was an absolute risk of breast cancer of 0.3% in women on placebo and 4.5% on pravastatin. In the typical manner in which benefit of drugs is expressed, the RR = 1500% for breast cancer; this, of course, is not a benefit (Ravnskov, 2000, p210).

## New cancer incidence in the PROSPER trial

In the PROSPER trial on elderly individuals, new cancer diagnoses were more frequent on pravastatin than on placebo (RR = 1.25, $p = 0.02$, thus significant). Cancer deaths were more frequent also (RR = 1.28, $p = 0.082$), but not considered significant with that higher $p$ value (Shepherd et al., 2002).

## Muscle breakdown

Using FDA data that resulted in the removal of cerivastatin from the US market, Sidney Wolfe, MD, of Public Citizen found 772 cases of rhabdomyolysis over a 39-month period, 72 fatal. Rhabdomyolysis is a breakdown (a lysis) of muscle tissue. The proteins then travel to the kidneys and can cause them to fail. Just 20 cases were caused by cerivastatin, which the FDA caused to be withdrawn from the US market in 2001; there were 52 deaths from other statins that remain on the market. Both Wolfe and Julian Whitaker, MD, separately petitioned the FDA to put a Black Box warning on all remaining statins. By now you can guess whether the FDA did it.

Even pro-statin pharmacologists have published that statins can induce one of the muscle-damaging conditions [myalgia (pain), myositis (inflammation), myopathy (weakness) and rhabdomyolysis (breakdown)] in up to 7% of people taking statins (Ucar et al, 2000).

And now rosuvastatin (Crestor) is on the USA market despite being the only statin that caused life-threatening rhabdomyolysis in pre-approval clinical trials along with elevations of protein in urine. So much so that the proposed 80 mg dose of rosuvastatin was abandoned, and the 40 mg dose is to be sold with special restrictions. Public Citizen made a presentation to the FDA on 9 July 2003 opposing the approval of this drug in any dose (Wolfe, 2003).

## Neuropathy from statin drugs

Elias Ragi, MD, Royal Devon and Exeter Hospital, England, reported in an electronic posting to the *British Medical Journal* on 12 Nov 2001 that he had observed patients 52-80 years old, 80% male, on statins who appeared to have, in addition to myopathy, a loss of coordination in the lower limbs. This was found to be due to neuropathy as determined by nerve conduction studies. The statins involved about equally were simvastatin, pravastatin, atorvastatin and cerivastatin.

A case-control study was performed on the 465,000 inhabitants of Funen county, Denmark. The 166 cases of polyneuropathy found showed a RR = 3.7 for statin use for all cases (35 definite, 54 probable, 77 possible), and for the 35 definite cases RR = 14.2 for statin use (Gaist et al., 2002). Granted, just 1 case per 5500 statin users was found. Much more harm was done when the statin was taken for more than 2 years rather than less. One can only wonder what the rate will be after 20-50 years of use, what Big Pharma lusts for.

Cognitive functioning affected by statin drugs

Treatment with lovastatin for 6 months caused small performance decrements in attention and psychomotor speed compared with placebo ($p < 0.04$), but did not cause psychological distress (Muldoon et al., 2000). This is a very short test period. The onset of statin-induced dementia in all published case reports did not occur until 9-12 months after subjects began to take the statin, or increased its dose. A longer-term (4-year) study on pravastatin at 40 mg/day showed no difference in attention span between treatment and control groups (King et al, 2003).

However, Muldoon persisted, using simvastatin (Zocor), 10 and 40 mg daily against placebo in 3 groups of about 94 subjects each, to see any effect on cognitive functioning by use of standard tests before and after 6 months on simvastatin. Here the power of the placebo emerged in a strange way. Usually subjects on placebo improve, and subjects on active treatment, whatever it is, have to improve significantly more than the ones on placebo to say that the active treatment works better. What happened in this trial is that the placebo group improved and the simvastatin groups were unchanged ($p = 0.002$). The subjects were 35-70 years old (mean 54) and had moderate "hypercholesterolemia", thus they were about 20 years younger than the typical swallower of simvastatin (Muldoon et al., 2004). We assume that people of mean age 74 would be more seriously damaged by simvastatin.

At the Bronx, NY, Veterans Administration Medical Center, a 51 year old male taking simvastatin for 1 year experienced short-term memory loss that worsened over 3 months to an extreme level. He was switched to pravastatin at 40 mg/day, which resolved the memory-loss problem in a month (Orsi et al., 2001). But this turned out not to be an isolated incident.

A group at Duke University Medical Center, Durham, NC, searched the literature from November, 1997 to February, 2002 to find 60 cases of statin-induced memory loss, of which 36 were due to simvastatin, 23 to atorvastatin and 1 to pravastatin. In 25 patients who discontinued the statin, 14 noted improvement. Of 4 who were rechallenged, all had memory loss again (Wagstaff et al., 2003).

At the University of Mississippi Medical Center a 67-year-old caucasian female with NIDDM was seen after 1 year of atorvastatin at 10 mg/day, then 2 months at 20 mg/day. By then she showed lassitude, memory problems and possibly depression. Discontinuation of atorvastatin resolved the problems in 1 month.

A 68-year-old caucasian female with well-controlled hypertension and a long habit of exercise on 5 days a week was started on 10 mg/day of atorvastatin. After 9 months, her daughter noticed extreme memory and intelligence loss. Stopping atorvastatin resolved the problems in a week. When she was restarted on atorvastatin a month later, the problems returned in 3 weeks. Again the responsible drug was discontinued, and the problems diminished. Simvastatin at 20 mg/day was begun. After 7 weeks the memory and intelligence loss were back along with weakness and pain. Discontinuation resolved all symptoms in 3 weeks. Incredibly, the authors of this study concluded: "The statin drug class will continue as a cornerstone of dyslipidemia therapy to achieve therapeutic goals and thereby reduce risks for cardiovascular and cerebral vascular disease [CVD and stroke]." (King et al, 2003). As was shown above, the risk reduction for CVD and stroke provided by statins is too small to warrant their use *even if they had no side-effects.*

Duane Graveline, MD, MPH, former astronaut, suffered global amnesia from atorvastatin himself, twice. The effect was so devastating that he wrote a book about it: *Lipitor Thief of Memory*, that appeared in early 2004 (http://www.Spacedoc.net/Lipitor_thief_of_memory.html). This is when he learned about the cholesterol scam, regretted having prescribed statins to so many of his patients when he had a general practice, and raised the alarm of sudden-onset amnesia in pilots or other machine operators. A newer version of this book (2005) is called: *Statin Drug Side-Effects: the misguided war on cholesterol.*

Congenital abnormalities from statins

Mothers may not feel so good knowing that infants exposed to statins *in utero* are at risk of developing congenital abnormalities, such as limb and central nervous system defects. Robin Edison et al. at the Medical Genetics branch of the NIH identified clusters of these normally rare abnormalities far in excess of expectations (Anon., 2003).

Erectile dysfunction caused by statin drugs

Since cholesterol is necessary for the synthesis of testosterone, the effects of statins on testosterone levels have been the subject of several investigations, most with negative results. One study noted that high-dose simvastatin directly suppressed testosterone synthesis by inhibiting a key enzyme near the end of the synthesis. This study reported on eight subjects who were found by the Netherlands Pharmacovigilance Centre to have had erectile dysfunction caused by statin drugs (de Graaf et al., 2004).

Congestive heart failure from statin drugs

By 1990, as noted above, it had been found that lovastatin lowered serum levels of coenzyme Q10, and that this caused cardiomyopathy, also called congestive heart failure (CHF). Dropping the dose of statin, or stopping it, and/or administering up to 200 mg of Q10 per day reversed the severity of the CHF in all of a small number of patients (Folkers et al., 1990). All statins lower Q10 levels in the proportion that they lower TC (Langsjoen & Langsjoen, 1998). On 5 Sep 2001 Prof. Gian Paul Littarru, on behalf of the International Coenzyme Q10 Association (http://wwwcsi.unian.it/coenzymeQ/) sent a position paper to the FDA, asking it to consider limiting the use of statins or advising the co-administration of Q10 with them, as was actually disclosed in US patents by Merck in 1990. The Association thought that the myalgia and rhabdomyolysis were due to decreases in Q10 concentration. A Q10 trial for halting CHF with excellent results was described in Myth 1.

Chronic fatigue from Zocor

Tom Scherer, a civil rights activist, was started on simvastatin (Zocor in the USA) and developed myalgia and chronic fatigue. He e-mailed on 28 Jul 04 that he had obtained data from the FDA under the Freedom of Information Act (and congressional intercession proved necessary) on adverse event reports actually reported from Nov. 1997 to May 14, 2004 on simvastatin. The data showed 11,589 individual adverse event reports, of which over 416 resulted in death. There were more than 4 adverse events per patient — 49,350 in all. It is believed that only 5% of the adverse effects of drugs are actually reported to the FDA (Cohen, 2001, p5).

Confusion and vertigo from statins

"Within three days of starting 10 mg of Lipitor [daily], Marlene, a healthy, active sixty-four-year old, became increasingly dizzy and confused, fell down several steps, and required emergency care. These symptoms disappeared within forty-eight hours of stopping the drug. Marlene's doctor then prescribed a standard dose of Zocor, which caused side-effects, and then Pravachol, which did the same. Fed up, Marlene quit treatment." (Cohen, 2005). While this is merely an anecdote, plenty of evidence given earlier shows that this result is not rare.

## Summing Up

The benefits of the statin drugs in reducing mortality are exaggerated (Figure 3-6), being only about 0.3% per year from the most favorable trials reported. This is not as great as the benefits of omega-3 supplements (see Myth 1). Indeed lovastatin (Mevacor) increased the all-cause mortality rate in its two reported trials.

Among male hospital patients with advanced coronary artery blockage, angina, or NFMI survivors, who actually show measurable signs of cytomegalovirus infection or inflammation, the newer statin drugs may provide a mortality benefit in the range of what a 5-week course of aspirin in men provides (see Myth 1).

In reducing the rate of mostly non-fatal heart attacks (Figure 3-7) and strokes, the statins have minor benefits in the range of those shown by long-term Bufferin in men.

Women are under-represented in most of the trials. The overall deleterious effect of atorvastatin in women in the ASCOT and other trials bodes ill for those who take it because of medical advice, or who fell for the TV ads and actually asked for it. There was no significant drop in the death rate for women on pravastatin in the LIPID trial, and people in this trial did have pre-existing NFMI or angina (LIPID, 1998). Pregnant women should avoid all statins to minimize chances for congenital defects in their infants.

People with almost any level of TC or LDL should not take statins. Those who have high TG levels or symptoms of CVD or CHF should take a look at Myths 1, 2 and 4 for non-toxic approaches that deal with underlying causes. Elevated TC or LDL can be a sign of defense against inflammation, infection, or cancer.

The victims of familial hypercholesterolemia (FH) are too few in number for any trials to have been run, so it is not known even if these would benefit from statins.

People who take statins, despite all the evidence against them, are advised to take enough coenzyme Q10 in addition to bring the measured levels of Q10 in serum back up to normal. For those with CHF, taking Q10 alone would be very beneficial (see Myth 1).

Cerivastatin, lovastatin (now available OTC) and rosuvastatin appear to be the most dangerous of the statins, but none are really as safe as they are claimed to be.

The side-effects of all the statins appear to be underplayed by their makers; but must be more serious than commonly believed, since up to 75% of people starting statins stop taking them within two years, even while thinking that the lower TC and LDL levels caused by the statins must be beneficial. This is confirmed by the difficulty in obtaining adverse effect data from the FDA.

The tendency of drug makers to make public the results of only the most favorable trials indicates that even the minor benefits described above might be exaggerated. To make sure there is no profit for those who deal in cholesterol-lowering drugs, resist the nonsense that "high" cholesterol levels are dangerous. They are not nearly as dangerous as low cholesterol levels. Your physician may have been wined, dined and paid up to $2000 to start just one patient, you, on a statin drug.

Statins are the drug class most likely to bankrupt Medicare, Medicaid and other insurance plans without any significant benefits. It is up to you not to ask for them, not to take them if offered, and to inform your loved ones to do the same.

## Myth 3 Acknowledgments

The help of many members of the International Cholesterol Skeptics Group (www.THINCS.org) is greatly appreciated, both for providing citations and enlightening discussion, and especially from its founder, Uffe Ravnskov. John

Lehmann (www.DrugIntel.com), Leslie Ann Bowman of the University of the Sciences in Philadelphia and Frances E. H. Pane, MSLS, edited this chapter. Editorial aid was also obtained from Duane Graveline, MD, Barry A. Cullen, BS, and Anne M. Klinkner, BS. Very valuable information was obtained from Tom Scherer.

## Myth 3 References

ALLHAT (2002). Major Outcomes in Moderately Hypercholesterolemic, Hypertensive Patients Randomized to Pravastatin vs Usual Care. *Journal of the American Medical Association* 288:2998-3007.

Anon. (2003). Statins linked to congenital defects. *Lancet* 362(9396):1635.

Anon. (2004). Extra-Low Cholesterol. New York Times, March 10, pA26.

Allred, J. B. (1993). Lowering Serum Cholesterol: Who Benefits? *Journal of Nutrition* 123:1453-1459.

Buydens-Branchey, L., Branchey, M. (2003). Association Between Low Plasma Levels of Cholesterol and Relapse in Cocaine Addicts. *Psychosomatic Medicine* 65:86-91.

Cannon CP, Braunwald E, McCabe CH, et al. (2004). Intensive versus Moderate Lipid Lowering with Statins after Acute Coronary Syndromes. *New England Journal of Medicine* 350(15):1495-1504.

Cohen JS (2001). *Over Dose. The Case Against the drug Companies.* New York, NY: Tarcher/Putnam.

Cohen JS (2005). *What You Must Know About Statin Drugs and Their Natural Alternatives,* Garden City Park, NY: Square One Publishers, pp 91, 93.

Collins R, Armitage J, Parish S, Sleight P, Peto R (2002). MRC/BHF Heart Protection Study of cholesterol lowering with simvastatin in 20 536 high-risk individuals: a randomised placebo-controlled trial. *Lancet* 360(9326):7-21.

Criqui MH, Golomb BA (2004). Editorial Comment. Low and lowered cholesterol and total mortality. *Journal of the American College of Cardiology* 44:1009-1010.

Dagenais GR, Ahmed Z, Robitaille NM, et al. (1990). Total and coronary heart disease mortality in relation to major risk factors--Quebec cardiovascular study. *Canadian Journal of Cardiology* 6(2):59-65.

Fleming TR, DeMets DL. (1996). Surrogate end points in clinical trials: are we being misled? *Annals of Internal Medicine* 125:605-613.

Folkers, K., Langsjoen, P., Willis, R. et al. (1990). Lovastatin decreases coenzyme Q10 levels in humans. *Proceedings National Academy of Sciences* 87:8931-8934.

Forette B, Tortrat D, Wolmark Y (1989). Cholesterol as risk factor for mortality in elderly women. *Lancet* 1:868-870.

Gaist D, Jeppesen U, Andersen M et al. (2002). Statins and Risk of Polyneuropathy. *Neurology* 58:1333-1337.

Golomb B (1998). Cholesterol and Violence: Is There a Connection? *Annals of Internal Medicine* 128:478-487.

de Graaf L, Brouwers HPM, Diemont WL (2004). Is decreased libido associated with the use of HMG-CoA-reductase inhibitors? *British Journal of Clinical Pharmacology* 58(3):326-328.

Grundy SM (1997). Lipid Abnormalities and Coronary Heart Disease. *Clinical Symposia,* 49(4):1-32.

Hecht HS, Superko HR (2001). Electron Beam Tomography and National Cholesterol Education Program Guidelines in Asymptomatic Women. *Journal of the American College of Cardiology* 37:506-1511.

Hecht HS, Harman SM (2003). Relation of Response of Subclinical Atherosclerosis Detected by Electron Beam Tomography to Baseline Low-Density Lipoprotein Cholesterol Levels. *American Journal of Cardiology* 93:101-103.

Hecht MM (2004-2005). The Cholesterol Scam. Challenging the Cholesterol Myth. *21st Century Science and Technology,* Winter, 17(4):42-44.

Hilleman DE, Monaghan MS, Ashby CL et al. (2001). Physician-Prompting Statin Therapy Intervention Improves Outcomes in Patients with Coronary Heart Disease. *Pharmacotherapy* 21(11):1415-1421.

Horne BD, Muhlstein JB, Carlquist JF, et al. (2003). Statin Therapy Interacts With Cytomegalovirus Seropositivity and High C-Reactive Protein in Reducing Mortality Among Patients With Angiographically Significant Coronary Disease. *Circulation* 107:1-6.

Horwich TB, Hamilton MA, Maclellan WR, Fonarow GC (2002). Low Serum Cholesterol Is Associated With Marked Increase in Mortality In Advanced Heart Failure. *Journal of Cardiac Failure* 8(4):216-224.

Jackevicius CA, Mamdani M, Tu JV (2002). Adherence With Statin Therapy in Elderly Patients With and Without Acute Coronary Syndromes. *Journal of the American Medical Association* 288:462-467.

Jackson PR, Wallis EJ, Haq IU, Ramsay LE (2001). Statins for primary prevention: at what coronary risk is safety assured? *British Journal of Pharmacology* 52:439-446.

Jacobs D, Blackburn H, Higgins M, et al. (1992). Report of the Conference on Low Blood Cholesterol: Mortality Associations. *Circulation* 86:1046-1060.

Kauffman JM (2001). Do Hypolipidemic Drugs Lower Medical Expenses? *Pharmacotherapy* 22 (12):1583.

Kauffman JM (2002). Aspirin Study Flawed, Letter to Editor, *J. Scientific Exploration* 16(2), 247-249.

King DS, Wilburn AJ, Wofford MR et al. (2003). Cognitive Impairment Associated with Atorvastatin and Simvastatin. *Pharmacotherapy* 23(12):1663-1667.

Kmietowicz Z (1998). Cholesterol screening is not worthwhile. *British Medical Journal* 316:725.

Kolata, G. (1985). Heart Panel's Conclusions Questioned. *Science* 227, 40-41.

Kolata G (2004). New Conclusions on Cholesterol. *New York Times,* March 9, pA1.

Langsjoen PH, Langsjoen AM (1998). Coenzyme Q10 In Cardiovascular Disease With Emphasis On Heart Failure and Myocardial Ischaemia. *Pacific Heart Journal* 7(3):160-168.

LaRosa JC (1996). Cholesterol Agonistics. *Annals of Internal Medicine* 124:505-508.

LaRosa JC (1999). Effect of Stains on Risk of Coronary Disease. *Journal of the American Medical Association* 282:2340-2346.

van Leeuwen R, Vingerling JR, Hofman A, deJong PTVM, Sticker BHC (2003). Cholesterol lowering drugs and risk of age related maculopathy: prospective cohort study with cumulative exposure measurement. *British Medical Journal* 326:255-256.

Liema AH, van Bovenb AJ, Veegerb NGJM, et al. (2002). Effect of fluvastatin on ischaemia following acute myocardial infarction: a randomized trial. *European Heart Journal* 23(24):1931-1937.

LIPID (1998). Prevention of Cardiovascular Events and Death with Pravastatin in Patients with Coronary Heart Disease and a Broad Range of Cholesterol Levels. *New England Journal of Medicine* 339:1349-1357.

Liu Y, Coresh J, Eustace JA, et al. (2004). Association Between Cholesterol Level and Mortality in Dialysis Patients. Role of Inflammation and Malnutrition. *Journal of the American Medical Association* 291(4):451-459.

Mann, G. V. (1977). Diet-Heart: End of an Era. *New England Journal of Medicine* 297(12):644-650.

Matsuzaki M, Kita T, Mabuchi H, et al. (2002). Large Scale Cohort Study of the Relationship Between Serum Cholesterol Concentration and Coronary Events with Low-Dose Simvastatin Therapy in Japanese Patients with Hypercholesterolemia. *Circulation Journal* 66:1087-1095.

Mauch DH, Nagler K, Schumacher S, Goritz C, Muller EC, Otto A, Pfrieger FW (2001). CNS synaptogenesis promoted by glia-derived cholesterol. *Science* 294(5545):1354-7.

Moore,T.J (1989). *Heart Failure,* New York, NY: Random House.

Newman, TB, Hulley, SB (1996). *Journal of the American Medical Association* 275:55-60.

Newman CB, Palmer G, Silbershatz H, Szarek M. (2003). Safety of Atorvastatin Derived from Analysis of 44 Completed Trials in 9,416 Patients. *American Journal of Cardiol*ogy 92:670-6.

Muldoon MF, Barger SD, Ryan CM, et al. (2000). Effects of Lovastatin on Cognitive Function and Psychological Well-Being. *American Journal of Medicine* 108:538-547.

Muldoon MF, Ryan CM, Sereika SM, Flory JD, Manuck SB (2004). Randomized Trial of the Effects of Simvastatin on Cognitive Functioning in Hypercholesterolemic Adults. *American Journal of Medicine* 117:823-829.

Nielsen JV (2001). Serum lipid lowering and risk reduction? Where is the connection? *British Medical Journal Rapid Response,* 19 Nov 01, to Kmietowicz Z (2001). Statins are the new aspirin, Oxford researchers say. *British Medical Journal* 323:1145.

Orsi A, Sherman O, Woldeselassie Z (2001). Simvastatin-Associated Memory Loss. *Pharmacotherapy* 21(6):767-769.

Ottoboni A, Ottoboni F (2002). *The Modern Nutritional Diseases: heart disease, stroke, type-2 diabetes, obesity, cancer, and how to prevent them.* Sparks, NV: Vincente Books.

Pekkanen, J., Nissinen, A., Punsar, S., Karvonen, M. J. (1989). Serum Cholesterol and Risk of Accidental or Violent Death in a 25-Year Follow-Up. *Archives of Internal Medicine* 149:1589-1591.

PHS 89: Steering Committee of the Physicians Health Study Research Group, *The New England Journal of Medicine* 321:129-135 (1989).

Raggi P, Cooil B, Callister TQ (2001). Use use of electron beam tomography to develop models for prediction of hard coronary events. *American Heart Journal* 141:375-82.

Rauchhaus M, Clark AL, Doehner W, et al., (2003). The relationship between cholesterol and survival in patients with chronic heart failure. *Journal of the American College of Cardiology* 42(11):1933-1940.

Ravnskov U (2000). *The Cholesterol Myths: Exposing the Fallacy that Saturated Fat and Cholesterol Cause Heart Disease,* Washington, DC: New Trends Publishing.

Ravnskov U (2002a). Is atherosclerosis caused by high cholesterol? *Quarterly Journal of Medicine* 95:397-403.

Ravnskov U (2003). High cholesterol may protect against infections and atherosclerosis. *Quarterly Journal of Medicine* 96:927-934.

Roberts WC (1996). The underused miracle drugs: the statin drugs are to atherosclerosis what penicillin was to infectious disease. *American Journal of Cardiology* 78:377-8.

Robinson J (2001). *Prescription Games. Money, Ego, and Power Inside the Global Pharmaceutical Industry,* Toronto, Ontario: McClelland & Stewart, pp63-82.

Rosendorff C (1998). Statins for prevention of stroke. *Lancet* 351:1002.

Schmitz G, Torzewski M, Eds. (2002). *HMG-CoA Reductase Inhibitors,* Boston, MA: Birkhauser.

Schupf N, Costa R, Luchsinger J, et al. (2005). Relationship Between Plasma Lipids and All-Cause Mortality in Nondemented Elderly. *Journal of the American Geriatrics Society* 53:219-226.

Schwartz GG, Olsson AG, Ezekowitz MD, et al. (2001). Effects of Atorvastatin on Early Recurrent Ischemic Events in Acute Coronary Syndromes. *Journal of the American Medical Association* 285:1711-1718.

Sever PS, Dahlof B, Poulter NR et al. (2003). Prevention of coronary and stroke events with atorvastatin in hypertensive patients who have average or lower-than-average cholesterol concentrations, in the Anglo-Scandinavian Cardiac Outcomes Trial—Lipid Lowering Arm (ASCOT-LLA): a multicentre randomised controlled trial. *Lancet* 361:1149-1158.

Sharp SJ, Pocock SJ (1997). Time Trends in Serum Cholesterol before Cancer Death. *Epidemiology* 8:132-136.

Shepherd J, Blauw GJ, Murphy MB et al., (2002). Pravastatin in elderly individuals at risk of vascular disease (PROSPER): a randomised controlled trial. *Lancet* 360(9346):1623-30.

Stehbens WE (2001). Coronary Heart Disease, Hypercholesterolemia, and Atherosclerosis II. Misrepresented Data. *Experimental and Molecular Pathology* 70:120-139.

Sutter MC (1994). Blood cholesterol is *not* causally related to atherosclerosis. *Cardiovascular Research* 28:575.

Tsuyuki RT, Bungard TJ (2001). Poor adherence with hypolipidemic drugs: a lost opportunity. *Pharmacotherapy* May, 21(5):576-82.

Ucar M, Mjörndal T, Dahlqvist R (2000). *Drug Safety* 22(6):441-457.

Ulmer H, Kelleher C, Diem G, Concin H (2004). Why Eve is not Adam: prospective follow-up in 149650 women and men of cholesterol and other risk factors related to cardiovascular and all-cause mortality. *Journal of Womens Health* (Larchmt) Jan-Feb;13(1):41-53..

Wagstaff LR, Mitton MW, McLendon Arvik B, Doraiswamy PM (2003). Statin-Associated Memory Loss: Analysis of 60 Case Reports and Review of the Literature. *Pharmacotherapy,* 23(7):871-880.

Weverling-Rijnsberger WE, Blauw GJ, Lagaay AM, Knook DL, Meinders AE (1997). Total cholesterol and risk of mortality in the oldest old. *Lancet* 350:1119-1123.

Wolfe SM (2003). Do Not Use! Rosuvastatin (Crestor) — A New But More Dangerous Cholesterol-Lowering "Statin" Drug. *Worst Pills Best Pills News* 9(10):73-76.

Yusuf S, Hawken S, Ôunpuu S, et al. (2004). Effect of potentially modifiable risk factors associated with myocardial infarction in 52 countries (the INTERHEART study): case-control study. *Lancet* 364:937-952.

Zureik M, Courbon D, Ducimetiére P (1997). Decline in Serum Cholesterol and the Risk of Death from Cancer. *Epidemiology* 8:137-143.

# Myth 4: Nearly Everyone Over 50 Should Take Drugs For High Blood Pressure

## The Oldest Myth

Over 100 years ago the blood pressure cuff joined the stethoscope as one of the most commonly used devices in a physician's "tool kit".

But only by the mid 20th century did the terms systolic and diastolic blood pressure begin to become commonplace in our society. As a 6-year-old child of the 1930s depression, Duane Graveline, MD, MPH, remembers his grandmother's blood pressure of some 300 over 100 "maxing out" old Dr. Piette's newfangled sphygmomanometer, much to his amusement, for she lived well into her nineties, finally passing of cancer. The medical community then was of the belief that elevations of blood pressure were a normal part of the aging process and did not consider these elevations a significant risk to health (Vlasses, 1985).

Back in those days if you survived infections and accidents, most of you were going to die from heart attacks and strokes and the rest from cancer and that was it! Then along came the Framingham study and the promise that much of this tendency for death from heart attacks and strokes, at least, was preventable if we could just control our blood pressures. Although this focus obviously was on just premature deaths, this truism was hardly noted in the uproar of a society noisily responsive to the possibility of stealing years of life from the grim reaper. The drug industry liked it, the doctors liked it and the public liked it. So began our national focus on lowering blood pressure, the evolution of hundreds of drugs designed to lower blood pressures, and the beginning of a still-growing, multi-billion dollar business.

Abnormally high blood pressures, usually in the elderly, became associated with the likelihood of mortality or of strokes, which are often debilitating or fatal. This was one of the early findings of the Framingham Study in the 1950s. Much useless advice was given to hypertensive patients about making changes in lifestyle, and still is, except for the sound advice to give up smoking.

About 50 years ago the first prescription drugs appeared for lowering blood pressure, and newer "antihypertensive" drugs are widely prescribed today. The logic seems so simple — if high blood pressure is bad, lowering it will be good, and people taking the drugs will have fewer strokes and live longer. As you will see, this is true only for people with very high blood pressures, the top 10%. What mainstream medicine ignores is that the side-effects of the drugs are so bad that 20-60% of people taking them stop within 3 years. Collateral damage is so extreme for many people that no increase in lifespan is obtained, or the cause of death is changed to something like congestive heart failure (CHF), which is not normally blamed on high blood pressure. When your body increases its blood pressure there is a reason — to maintain a good supply of oxygen and nutrients to all organs. The direct brute force approach of using drugs to lower blood pressure by dilating arteries or veins, weakening the heart, or increasing urination rarely does anything of overall value.

Read on to see how this Myth developed!

## Measuring Blood Pressure

Since the publication in 1628 of *Movement of the Heart and Blood in Animals* by William Harvey in England, it has been understood that the heart pumps blood carrying oxygen and nutrients to the aorta and other arteries. These branch into smaller arteries, and finally into tiny capillaries, from which the cells exchange oxygen and nutrients for carbon dioxide and waste materials. The capillaries collect waste and join into larger and larger veins to conduct the blood back to the heart, some going to the liver for waste detoxification, then to the heart where it is then pumped to the lungs to exchange carbon dioxide for oxygen. You can check on this and other details of the circulatory system in any general Biology text.

To analyze cardiovascular problems, it would probably be best to know the volume of blood moving per minute; however, the only non-invasive measurement related to flow rate is the blood pressure (BP). Since this is simple to measure, it has been a mainstay of physicians for over 100 years. The original, and still common form of device for the measurement is called a blood pressure cuff or sphygmomanometer, in which the differences between the actual heights in millimeters (mm) of columns of mercury (Hg) in a U-tube are read on a linear scale to give the BP, which is always expressed as mm Hg. While liquid mercury is not at all hazardous except under peculiar conditions of spillage, where it drains into a floor or ceiling and vaporizes, the much more durable and portable dial gauge types are now more common and almost as accurate. The dial gauges are also calibrated in mm Hg.

The sensor of a stethoscope is placed over the brachial artery just above the inside elbow, and may be just under the BP cuff, which is wrapped around the upper arm above the elbow. The cuff is pumped up by a squeeze-ball with a check valve to 20 mm Hg above the highest reading expected. The valve on the squeeze ball is unscrewed slightly to make the pressure drop by 2-3 mm Hg per second. When the squashed artery is released just enough for a pulsating sound to be heard, the corresponding pressure reading is called the systolic blood pressure (SBP). Dropping the pressure further finally opens the artery fully so that no more pulsation is heard; this lower pressure is called the diastolic blood pressure (DBP). The proper technique for accurate measurement is taught early in medical school, but seldom followed, often because of time constraints on the physician or nurse.

Patients' fears can raise readings, which can be reduced by relaxation in the office, or home readings can be taken by most adults with good hearing and average dexterity. The left arm is supposed to give more meaningful readings than the right. The arm should be supported by a table at the height of the heart for a seated patient with the elbow bent. Multiple readings, but only 3-4 at a sitting on the same arm, should give 2-3 repeatable values. The cuff size must be correct. A full bladder, a recent meal, smoking tobacco or drinking alcohol all influence the readings. Both numbers are important (Black et al., 2001, pp1561-2). In 30-40% of patients whose DBP exceeds 90 mm Hg, repeat readings taken soon after will be well below this value. These patients are supposed to be told that their BP is *borderline elevated* and should be checked at least annually (Kaplan, 2001, p845). Of course most patients told this will become anxious and soon actually have borderline elevated BP, and become targets for BP drugs.

Elevated BP is called hypertension; lowered is called hypotension.

Home measurements of BP tend to run 12 mm Hg lower for SBP and 7 mm Hg lower for DBP (often written as 12/7 mm Hg) lower than office measurements, whether done at home by sphygmomanometer or one of the newer automatic devices, whose output is called ambulatory blood pressure measurement (ABPM), (Black et al., 2001, pp1561-4). Because one may be subjected to expensive drugs with adverse side-effects based on a difference of 2 mmHg in BP measurement, it is important to be convinced that the values are accurate.

There are no symptoms of high blood pressure unless it is very high, above 200/100, seen in 5-8% of old people. This is understood to mean a SBP of 200 mm Hg and a DBP of 100 mm Hg. Changes in the retinas of the eyes and strokes are symptoms of high BP. Low blood pressure will cause ringing in the ears or fainting, possibly at levels below 60/30. Partially blocked carotid (neck) arteries may cause these same symptoms at higher BPs.

## How High is Hypertension?

BP has some parallels with cholesterol levels. One is that BP also rises naturally with age (Table 4-1). Note that it rises more in older females than in older males, yet females live longer. The "normal" values that physicians are supposed to tell us to strive to achieve, 120/80 mm Hg, are in fact observed in only 25% of adult males for SBP (Figure 4-0a) and in 36% of adult males for DBP (Figure 4-0b).

Table 4-1a: Normal Mean Arterial Blood Pressure Readings by Age and Sex. SBP/DBP in mm Hg

| Age | Female | Male |
|-----|--------|------|
| 1 | 90/54 | 90/56 |
| 6 | 97/57 | 97/58 |
| 12 | 107/66 | 108/65 |
| 18 | 113/67 | 122/71 |
| 21-30 | 115/75 | 131/79 |
| 31-40 | 118/78 | 126/82 |
| 41-50 | 122/79 | 127/83 |
| 51-60 | — | 128/83 |

Adapted from Lentner, 1990. Mostly caucasians USA.

Table 4-1b: Normal Mean Arterial Blood Pressure Readings by Age and Sex. SBP/DBP in mm Hg

| Age | Female | Male |
|-----|--------|------|
| 20-34 | 117/75 | 126/79 |
| 35-49 | 126/80 | 131/83 |
| 50-64 | 141/85 | 140/85 |
| 65 | 153/85 | 149/84 |

Adapted from Ulmer et al., 2004. Austrians.

Since fear, excitement or exertion make both heart rate and BP rise, it is clear that your body can make adjustments to the need for the nutrients in blood, and can change the amount of blood flowing by changing the pressure, among other ways. Your body is cleverly programmed to compensate for stress and changes in position in this manner, and your BP is not supposed to remain constant under all conditions.

One thing that old Dr. Piette found when he started using his new blood pressure cuff was that everyone had a different pressure. It was just like heights and weights and about every other thing he measured in people, even their blood sugars – no one had the same value. Some would be high, some would be low and most would be somewhere in the middle. A century before there was a fellow good with numbers by the name of Gauss who even had this tendency named for him – the so-called Gaussian frequency distribution pattern. It looked just like the outline of the bell in the church tower, hence the name "bell curve". Plot the measurement (blood pressure, height, weight - whatever) on the horizontal axis and the percent of people with that measurement on the vertical axis and out comes as a bell shaped curve as in Figures 4-0, a and b.

Figure 4-0a. Systolic Blood Pressure Distribution in 350,000
Adult Males in MRFIT Trial (Based on Kaplan, 2001, p942).

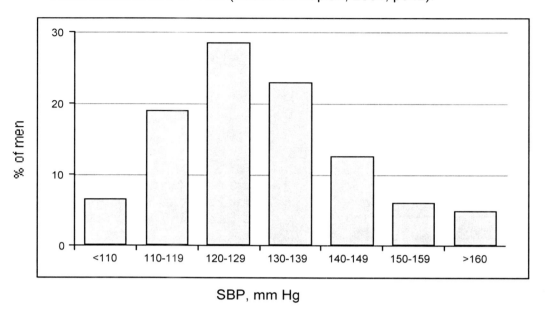

SBP, mm Hg

A few guys with plenty of your income tax to spend and not much else to do, apparently, took the blood pressures of 350,000 adult males and plotted the frequency distribution of their systolic and diastolic pressures separately. The systolic pressure is the pressure peak with each beat of the heart (systole) and the diastolic pressure is the basal pressure that is in the blood vessels even during relaxation of the heart (diastole). The result was the bell shaped frequency distribution curves (Figures 4-0, a and b). The third of a million participants in this study were not pre-selected, representing run of the mill, off the street, normal systolic and diastolic blood pressure values of fellow human beings.

Figure 4-0b. Diastolic Blood Pressure Distribution in 350,000
Adult Males in MRFIT Trial (Based on Kaplan, 2001, p942).

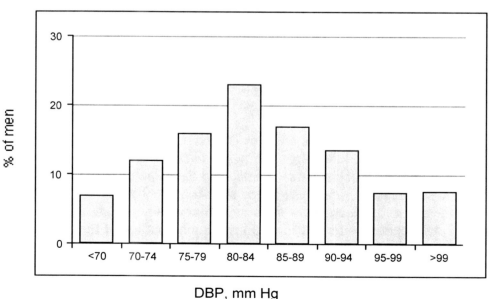

DBP, mm Hg

Additional research revealed that blood pressures tend to rise naturally with age in both men and women so that a 120 systolic blood pressure of a 20-year old (roughly 100 plus the age) becomes 140 in a forty year old and 160 in a 60 year old. This reality is presented in Tables 4-1 a and b for both systolic and diastolic pressures and had been known to all practicing physicians for many years. Even Dr. Piette soon learned about the 100 plus your age rule and it took much more than a 180/95 in an octogenarian to get his attention. He didn't have any blood pressure pills then so it didn't make much difference anyhow. What could he counsel? Avoid exertion!

Meanwhile scientists involved with our famous Framingham study had made the astounding correlation that the higher the systolic blood pressures of their Framingham community study patients the higher their all cause death rates. Figure 4-1 presents the data they reported to the medical and

Figure 4-1. Spurious Framingham Study Age-Adjusted All-Cause Death Rates vs. Systolic Blood Pressure (SBP) for Men Aged 45-74. Smooth curve was generated by a simple automatic curve-fitting program as shown. Data points were not the actual SBP values, but actually the ones used by the program to generate the curve. Note the smoothly increasing "risk". Adapted from Port et al., 2000a.

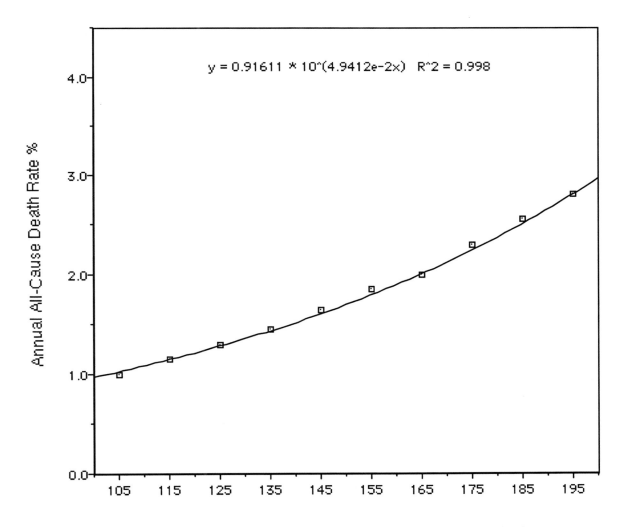

$y = 0.91611 * 10^{(4.9412e-2x)}$   $R^2 = 0.998$

Systolic Blood Pressure in mm Hg at Beginning of Each Year

109

scientific community, information that soon would radically change medical philosophy with respect to the treatment of high blood pressure. Their thinking went something like this: Since blood pressure elevation is associated with increased all-cause death rates, lowering of blood pressures by whatever means could only be good for humanity and the race to do it was on. They said that mortality increased in "a continuous and graded manner" with increased BP. The pharmaceutical industry loved it – this focus was to make them billions. The medical community loved it – it was so good for business and seemed ethically correct. The patients sort of loved it – they thought they were stealing time from the grim reaper.

So now the question arises, just how high is high BP? High enough to treat? Despite our past many decades of accepting the 100 plus your age, more or less, today's medical textbooks are warring over exact values and new national standards come out every few years placing the desirable blood pressure target values ever lower. Is good medical practice fueling this war or might it just be the multi-billion dollar pharmaceutical industry? For to lower the target value 5 points on the BP scale can mean $billions more in drug sales.

Most sources agree that SBP and DBP are equally important in defining hypertension and that the decision has been arbitrary on what levels should be treated. In the 1970s the limits were 160/95 mm Hg for resting BP, which will be seen to have been pretty reasonable for people under 50 years old. However, like the downward adjustments for "acceptable" cholesterol levels (see Myth 3), the "acceptable" BP values are now <140/90 mm Hg, according to one of the major Cardiology texts, which does caution that treatment should depend on factors besides the BP values. This text gives a list of the organizations in agreement on this value, which corresponds with about <133/84 mm Hg for home or ABPM readings. These organizations include the Sixth Joint National Committee on Prevention, Detection, Evaluation and Treatment of High Blood Pressure (JNC VI), the French Society of Hypertension, the American Society of Hypertension Ad Hoc Panel (ASH), the British Hypertension Society and the World Health Organization/International Society of Hypertension (Black et al., 2001, pp1554).

Another major Cardiology text is in agreement and lists the following stages of hypertension: Stage 1 means BP of >140-159/90-99, Stage 2 of BP >160-179/100-109, and the really ominous Stage 3 of BP ≥180/≥110 mm Hg for all adults aged ≥18 (Kaplan, 2001, p944).

The definitive monograph used by pharmacologists and medicinal chemists, called Goodman & Gilman, agrees with 140/90 (Oates & Brown, 2001, p871).

The definitive monograph used by pharmacists, Remington's, agreed with a DBP of >90, but only for persons ≤35 years old; and used a DBP of >95 for those >35 years old (Harvey & Withrow, 1990, p831). This allowance for age will be seen as unusually perceptive.

Our Public Citizen's Health Research Group strongly advises consideration of age in determining whether or not treatment is justified, suggesting before the year 2000 that in the elderly only pressures equal to or above 180/100 might be treated beneficially with drugs (Wolfe & Sasich, 1999, pp46-49).

The risks of hypertension are said to be hemorrhagic stroke, coronary artery disease, peripheral vascular disease, congestive heart failure (CHF), sudden cardiac death, kidney failure, and premature death. The amount of risk is said to increase progressively as BP values exceed 120/80 and is based on findings of the Framingham Study (Black et al., 2001, pp1554-5). The actual values of SBP in adult males enrolled in the MRFIT trial are shown in Figure 4-0a, and of DBP in Figure 4-0b.

How all-cause mortality is supposedly related to blood pressure is shown in Figure 4-1. But according to mathematics Professors Sidney Port and Robert Jennrich of UCLA and 3 colleagues who are cardiologists or physiologists, this curve was obtained by a simple curve-fitting routine to the data for all-cause death rate vs. SBP. What is shown is the age-adjusted death rate, seemingly 1-3% per year, against the SBP at the beginning of each year (Port et al, 2000a). The line is the regression line of a simple exponential curve-fit. The 10 data points are a fiction, being the points used by the computer to generate the line! Port et al. showed that the line in Figure 4-1 is an artifact of an early curve-fitting program for computers!

When the actual death rates were dug out of the original Framingham Study report by Port and plotted against SBP the result is quite different (Figure 4-2). The same curve as in Fig. 4-1 is drawn through the actual data, and is a poor fit as shown by the low $R^2$ value of 0.7. Port et al. found that there was no simple way to fit the data, and used 2 curves with different equations for each. It can be

Figure 4-2. Actual Framingham Study Age-Adjusted All-Cause Death Rates vs. Systolic Blood Pressure (SBP) for Men Aged 45-74. Same curve fit as in Fig. 4-1. Note uneven relationship of risk to SBP and lack of curve fit. Adapted from Port et al., 2000a.

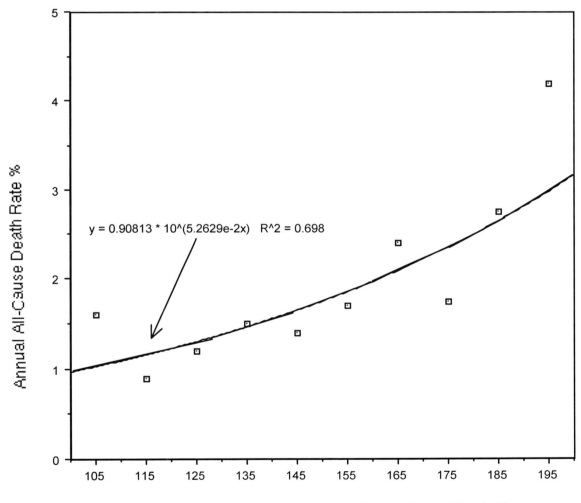

$$y = 0.90813 * 10^{\wedge}(5.2629e\text{-}2x) \quad R^{\wedge}2 = 0.698$$

Systolic Blood Pressure in mm Hg at Beginning of Each Year

seen that serious risk elevation begins at an SBP of 165 mm Hg if one is conservative, and at 185 mm Hg if one is not. A similar situation with DBP was found in the same way (Port et al., 2000b). By e-mail of 18 Jan 04 Prof. Port expressed his belief that the data point at 175 was a fluke, while I think it just as likely that the point at 165 is a fluke. Either way, there was some justification for the old cut at

111

160 mm Hg SBP, and certainly none for 140, or striving for 120 at any age. (For the mathematically inclined, a third-order polynomial fit gave $R^2 = 0.87$, a far better fit.) Looking at the data in Fig. 4-2, one would think that the curve would continue to rise as blood pressures decreased below an SBP of 105, because very low BP results in death, often from congestive heart failure (CHF).

What Port et al. actually found was that risk of death rose by about 1% per year at the 90th percentile (the top 10%) of SBP for men aged 45-74 compared with men in the 20th percentile (the bottom 20%) of BP (Figure 4-3). This corresponds with an SBP of 159 for men 45-54, 173 for men

Figure 4-3. Framingham Study All-Cause Death Rates vs. Percentile of Systolic Blood Pressure (SBP) for Men Aged 45-74 Years. Adapted from Port et al., 2000a.

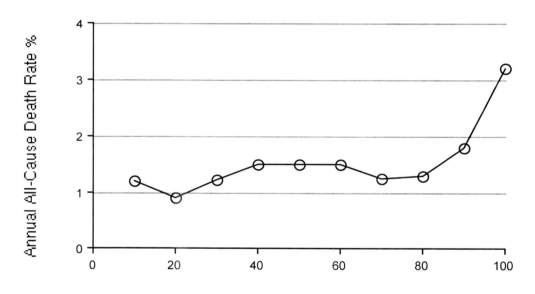

Percentile of Systolic Blood Pressure

55-64 and 184 for men 65-74; 165 for women 45-54, 183 for women 55-64 and 190 for women 65-74 (see Table 4-2). People with SBP lower than these levels for each age and sex should not be treated for high BP since they are not really at risk, contrary to the messages of the Big Pharma detail women. The higher pressures for women are accompanied by lower death rates when compared with those men with the same SBP and age. It is of some interest also that men with the *lowest* SBPs did *not* have the *lowest* death rate. Note from Figure 4-0a that men with SBP ≥160 represent only 5% of that population. But what Port et al. have shown so well is that the SBP indicating risk from hypertension rises with age, so the SBP that is high enough to indicate a benefit of treatment also rises with age as given above.

From Goodman & Gilman: "Robust evidence from multiple controlled trials indicates that pharmacological treatment of patients with diastolic pressures [DBP] of 95 mm Hg or greater will reduce morbidity, disability, and mortality from cardiovascular disease" (Oates & Brown, 2001, p871). This means that the evidence for a benefit of treating people whose DBP is <95 is *not* robust. From Figure 4-0b one can see that 15% of men have DBP ≥95. With no allowance for age in people ≥45 years old, it appears that only men with DBP >95 should be treated, and this will be 15% at most.

Table 4-2: Arterial Systolic Blood Pressure in mm Hg. Readings by Age and Sex in the 90th Percentile that might benefit from Treatment.*

| Age | Female | Male |
|---|---|---|
| 45-54 | 165 | 159 |
| 55-64 | 183 | 173 |
| 65-74 | 190 | 184 |

\*       From Port et al, 2000a.  Mostly caucasians USA.

When allowance for age is made according to Port et al., it is probable that only 5% of men should be treated for hypertension.  Since women are less damaged by higher BP, an equally small fraction should be treated. The authors of the monograph in Goodman & Gilman failed to allow for the effect of age on the risk posed by elevated BP.

The first report on the value of BP drugs in 1967, from the Veterans Administration Cooperative Trial, was on patients whose DBP was 115-129 mm Hg (Vlasses, 1985). This is an exceedingly high value to be found in only 1-2% of patients of advanced age, as shown in Figure 4-0b. The belief that antihypertensive drugs are more valuable than they are probably stems from the results of this early trial, which were favorable in these extremely hypertensive patients.

Trials to be described later will confirm that only very high BPs should be treated, and even then, the benefits are worthwhile but small.

## What Causes Hypertension?

Hypertension is not a disease, but is a physical finding, usually a symptom of some other problem, which may or may not be identified.  Hypertension is determined by cardiac output and peripheral resistance, the resistance to blood flow in the arteries, etc. Peripheral resistance is inversely proportional to the fourth power of the internal radius of the blood vessels, so tiny decreases in the opening size (lumen) by plaques (CVD) will raise BP a lot.  Physical activity and emotions cause blood pressure to rise, but only temporarily.  Afro-Americans at any age have twice the incidence of hypertension as Caucasians.

"Secondary Hypertension" accounts for only 2-6% of all cases.  It was given this name because it is secondary to some identifiable cause.  One such cause is atherosclerosis of the arteries in the kidneys.  Decreased blood flow is sensed by the kidneys, which release renin, an enzyme which can cleave or split certain proteins or peptides (short proteins made from a few or a few dozen amino acids).  Renin cleaves angiotensinogen to angiotensin I, a peptide, which is converted in the blood vessels of the lungs by an enzyme to angiotensin II, a shorter peptide.  This explanation is necessary for some understanding of why certain of the antihypertension drugs work.  Angiotensin II constricts blood vessels, raising BP, and stimulates aldosterone (a steroid hormone) production, and this substance causes retention of sodium ion and the excretion of potassium. Both of these moves raise BP. Note how the decreased blood flow is compensated for by an increase in BP.  Interfering with this natural process cannot possibly be a 100% benefit.  Other kidney problems can occur.

Endocrine disorders can raise BP by overproduction of aldosterone or thyroid hormones (Freston & Bosso, 1990, p671). Foods containing certain essential fatty acids (omega-3) are converted into good eicosanoids (such as prostaglandin $E_1$, a vasodilator that lowers blood pressure) in the presence of glucagon, the fat-metabolizing hormone. Other essential fatty acids (omega-6) are partially converted into bad eicosanoids (such as thromboxane $A_2$, a vasoconstrictor that raises blood pressure) in the presence of insulin, the fat-building hormone. Thromboxane $A_2$ stimulates the growth of cells in arterial walls to form the lesions of atherosclerosis (see Myth 2).

"Systolic hypertension" (without diastolic) is seen when cardiac output increases to compensate for anemia, fever, beriberi, aortic valve defects, hyperactive thyroid gland, and/or stiff blood vessels, which may be a result of atherosclerosis.

When an actual cause is identified and can be treated directly, hypertension may be reduced as a consequence, with an overall benefit to the patient.

The other 94-98% of cases of hypertension whose causes are not yet known are called primary, idiopathic, fixed or essential. This is an arrogant display of medical bluff stemming from ignorance when hypertension of no known cause is re-named "Essential Hypertension". Untreated severe hypertension leads to many kinds of damage. If a resulting stroke (ischemic due to clots, or hemorrhagic due to a burst or leaky artery) is not fatal, the heart will weaken (CHF), especially its left ventricle, and the actual cause of death will be due to the effects of low blood pressure (Freston & Bosso, 1990, p671).

Uffe Ravnskov, MD, PhD, brought to my attention by e-mail in early 2004, that there is a small group of people with extremely high BP, above 200/100, called "Malignant Hypertension" that is associated with retinal changes and familial hypercholesterolemia (see Myths 2 and 3). He thinks that only members of this group are the ones who may benefit from antihypertensive drug treatment, but has not seen a study that directly addressed this extreme condition. He will not prescribe antihypertensive drugs for patients with lower BPs than 200/100.

Very probably some of that 94-98% hypertension of no known cause is caused by prescription drugs. A few recent examples are the antiarthritis drugs leflunamide (Arava™), rofecoxib (Vioxx™); the antimigraine drugs almotriptan (Axert™), frovatriptan (Frova™), naratriptan (Amerge™), and rizatriptan (Maxalt™), which cause the blood vessels including the coronary arteries, to contract; and the anti-incontinence drugs oxybutynin (Ditropan™) and tolterodine (Detrol™), (Wolfe & Sasich, 2002). In addition, the widely-used ibuprofen (Motrin™) can nullify the effects of the widely-used antihypertensive diuretic hydrochlorothiazide (Diuril™), (Cohen, 2001, p114).

In a case-control study, 9411 patients ≥65 years old in the New Jersey Medicaid program who were taking nonaspirin nonsteroidal antiinflammatory drugs (NSAIDs) such as ibuprofen (Motrin™), naproxen (Aleve™), etc., were matched with a similar number of controls who were not. Those taking NSAIDs had a RR = 1.66, that is, 1 2/3 the chance of being started on antihypertensive drugs. This finding was very statistically significant, and strongly dependent on the dose of the NSAIDs (Gurwitz et al., 1994). So that's how arthritis can lead to high BPs! What should one do? Try a low-carb diet to beat the arthritis (see Myth 2).

In a retrospective study on the elderly (mean age 76.5), it was found that their RR = 1.8 for CHF after they were started on rofecoxib (Vioxx™) compared with no NSAID use. The authors wrote: "...none of the funding for this study was provided by any pharmaceutical company." (Mamdani et al., 2004).

Smoking tobacco will raise SBP by 20 mm Hg within 4 minutes (Kaplan, 2001, p977). Whether the rise itself is damaging, or the increase in CVD-related mortality is due to some other type of toxicity of nicotine or other components in the smoke is not clear.

## Lifestyle Modifications as First-Line Defense against Hypertension

Smoking: All cardiologists and MDs will recommend stopping smoking, an effective move toward reducing hypertension.

Exercise: For all patients with hypertension who have no specific condition that would make exercise inapplicable or unsafe, a major cardiology text cites a recommendation from the JNC VI for an increase in physical activity (Black et al., 2001, p1573). The other major cardiology text recommends exercise for *all* hypertensive patients (Kaplan, 2001, p976,978). Actually, it was known over 20 years ago that for the vast majority of hypertensive people around the world that exercise is inadequate and ineffective as a primary treatment. Even vigorous exercise performed 3 or 4 times a week does not result in any BP lowering, and is known to cause sudden death (see Myth 6 and Solomon, 1984, pp71-72).

Salt: Most MDs will recommend lowering salt intake despite the very persuasive evidence showing that will BP go down in only 1/5 of people, that it will go up in 1/5, and that 3/5 will be almost unaffected. Overall, in the gigantic Intersalt trial, there was very little effect of salt on BP, much less than the hypertensive effects of alcohol or obesity, while greater potassium intake was hypotensive (Elliott et al., 1988). Alterations in salt intake from the biologically determined set-point of about 10 g per day for adults, an intake that is not hedonistic abuse, by 10-fold either way produce only marginal changes in BP on average (Folkow, 2003). One must try altering salt intake on an individual basis to find its effect on BP. In listing sodium (ion), FDA food labels are presuming facts not in evidence, and are misleading and counterproductive.

Fish oils: Fish consumption or taking omega-3 supplements (see Myths 1 and 2) is beneficial, but not entirely because of any effect on blood pressure, but because the rate of sudden cardiac death is reduced by prevention of heart arrhythmias.

Diet: Reports on the Dietary Approaches to Stop Hypertension (DASH) trial, sponsored by the NHLBI, emphasize eating fruits and vegetables regardless of GI and GL (Obarzarnek et al., 2001). The supposed benefits were lower intake of cholesterol and saturated fats; such benefits were shown to be nonexistent in Myth 2. Fiber has no direct effect on BP, but micronutrients associated with fiber such as vitamin B6 may have long-term benefits, as would the macronutrients magnesium and potassium ions in fruits and vegetables. Some researchers have accepted that the main benefit of the DASH diet is the increase in magnesium intake (Cohen, 2004, p61). The typical lowering of BP in the DASH trial subjects was 2.8/1.1 mm Hg (Black et al., 2001, p1575), an almost laughable result which is still taken seriously by many.

Diabetes: As shown in Myth 2, the most frequent precursor to hypertension is NIDDM, from which about 80% of the sufferers are abdominally obese, and for whom the only effective diet is a low-carb one. This means that they should *avoid* high-GI and -GL fruits and vegetables — even the beloved banana! A 10 kg reduction of body weight, easily accomplished with a low-carb diet, reduces BP by about 10/8 mm Hg (Black et al., 2001, p1574), as much as many antihypertensive drugs do, and without the bad side-effects. In another study, a similar weight loss was reported to result in a BP reduction of 16/13 mm Hg (Kaplan, 2001, pp976-977).

Some of this parallels the cholesterol situation because the most likely diets to be recommended do not work! After the inevitable failure of conventional diet advice, antihypertensive drugs are prescribed — even for people over 80 years old and for children as young as 3 years old! This sort of advice, clearly at odds with the lack of testing of antihypertensive drugs in the elderly or in children, and the absence of any real beneficial effect for most adults, as described below, has even appeared in a Sunday Supplement, *Parade,* on 8 Aug 04, masquerading as "Medical News That Matters" (Rosenfeld, 2004). Well, it matters for Big Pharma profits, I guess.

## How Do Antihypertensive Drugs Work?

In general, the drugs work by reducing the amount of fluid in the body, by relaxing the arteries, or by making the heart pump slower or with less force. The effects can be quite indirect, for example, by inhibiting production of thromboxane $A_2$, a vasoconstrictor that raises blood pressure. Examples of the more common drug classes only are given, mostly from Oates & Brown, 2001, p871-895.

Diuretics: Amazingly, the exact mechanism by which diuretics lower BP by increasing urination is not certain. Initially, the drugs decrease extracellular volume and cardiac output, but the latter returns to pretreatment levels. Laboratory experiments have shown that diuretics do not relax the muscles of blood vessels directly, but mimic the supposed effect of salt reduction. Examples are hydrochlorothiazide (Diuril™) and chlorthalidone (Hygroton™). These drugs also cause loss of potassium ion, which is a serious side-effect. The potassium-sparing diuretics such as amiloride (Moduretic™), triamterene (Dyrenium™) and spironolactone (Aldactone™) were introduced to prevent this loss, but these have their own serious side-effects, and have not taken over from the older diuretics. Neither type are magnesium-sparing, and the low magnesium levels are associated with heart arrhythmias, high blood pressure, headaches, diabetes, muscle cramps, and even ringing in the ears (tinnitus), (Cohen, 2004).

Vasodilators: One of the earliest and the only one still in common use, hydralazine (Apresoline™) causes direct relaxation of the smooth muscles of arteries, but not of veins. It is now usually used in combination with other drugs, especially diuretics and beta-blockers. Its desirable effects are accompanied by stimulation of the sympathetic nervous system, which results in increased heartbeat rate. Increased renin activity, which causes blood vessel contraction and fluid retention, is dealt with by diuretics.

Beta-Blockers: Of the many cellular "switches" in your body that respond to tiny concentrations of messenger molecules, ones called "beta-receptors" in the heart stimulated a faster heartbeat when switched on. After this 1948 discovery, James Whyte Black, a British physician and physiologist realized that a drug molecule that could target this type of receptor and bind to them might relieve the pain of angina. The result was propranolol (Inderal™), which is still in wide use, along with half a dozen others whose names end in -lol, and new ones including carvedilol (Coreg™), which do indeed prevent angina pain, prevent heart attacks and lower BP. The problem with these and other drugs is that, trying as hard as they can to design a drug molecule that targets only the proper receptor, medicinal chemists usually cannot allow for effects on the same receptor in other locations, or other receptors found anywhere in the body (Moore, 1998, pp36-41). Hence this class of drugs is infamous for engendering "postural hypotension", the tendency to faint when rising from a lying or sitting position.

Calcium Channel Blockers: Also called $Ca^{2+}$-channel antagonists, these newer drugs were very popular in the 1980s-1990s. Examples are verapamil (Calan™), diltiazem (Cardizem™), amlodipine (Norvasc™), felodipine (Plendil™), isradipine (Dynacirc™), nicardipine (Cardene™), nifedipine (Adalat™ and Procardia™), and nisoldipine (Sular™). Hypertension of no other cause is usually caused by stiffness of the blood vessels. Since contraction of their smooth muscle is dependent on the concentration of $Ca^{+2}$ (calcium ion), decreasing the amount of calcium ion that can enter these muscle cells from the blood relaxes the smooth muscle of the arteries, decreasing resistance to blood flow, and lowering the blood pressure. An enzyme that causes smooth muscle contraction is activated by calcium ion, so less calcium causes less contraction. The "channel" is the route calcium takes through the cell membrane. (The balancing ion, magnesium, is the natural calcium channel blocker, and ingesting it as food or supplements along with potassium ion lowers BP and does not cause side-effects.) The drugs whose names end in -ipine, the dihydropyridines, may also cause rapid heartbeat as a side-effect. Long-term use of the calcium channel blockers causes damage to the heart's left ventricle, and does not improve survival in MI survivors or diabetics, but worsens it. Calcium channel blockers are no longer considered to be the best initial drug treatment for hypertension except in the elderly and Afro-Americans. It is now understood that the rapid-acting calcium channel blockers (ones whose names end in -ipine) should be used, if at all, only in a slow-release formulation to avoid rapid oscillation in BP and other side-effects. Beta-blockers and diuretics are often administered concurrently with calcium channel blockers. The calcium channel blockers have many undesirable interactions with other types of drugs. So the inital enthusiasm for calcium channel blockers had cooled considerably by the late 1990s.

ACE Inhibitors: The conversion of angiotensin I to angiotensin II by an enzyme, angiotensin converting enzyme (ACE), was another logical target for the medicinal chemists (see above). Lowering resistance of blood vessels by limiting the amount of angiotensin II is the mode of action. The first "successful" drug to result was captopril (Capoten™), quickly followed by enalapril (Vasotec™), and half a dozen others whose names end in -pril. These drugs have special advantages for diabetic patients, slowing the kidney damage of diabetes. Given after a first MI the ACE inhibitors reduce morbidity and mortality a little. Nothing is "free" in the drug business, it seems, and the oddball side-effect for which these drugs are infamous is a dry, hacking, persistent cough. About 10% of patients stop using this type of drug for this reason, and another 15% who cough continue anyhow. The ACE inhibitors, which cause retention of potassium, work "well" in combination with the older diuretics, which cause loss of potassium, permitting lower doses of each to be used.

Angiotensin II-Receptor Antagonists: Also called $AT_1$-Receptor Antagonists, these newest of the major antihypertensive drug groups prevent angiotensin II from causing contraction of smooth muscle in blood vessels. They also act as diuretics, reducing plasma volume, and are less likely than ACE inhibitors to cause thickening of cell walls in the cardiovascular system. And all this without the cough! However, there are other side-effects, the main one being dizziness (Wolfe & Sasich, 1999, pp90-91). In patients in whom blood pressure is highly dependent on the concentration of angiotensin II, hypotension may result, or liver and kidney damage or heart failure. Examples are losartan (Cozaar™), candesartan (Atacand™), irbesartan (Avapro™) and valsartan (Diovan™). There are at least a dozen others whose generic names end in -sartan. Like the ACE inhibitors, these $AT_1$ drugs are less effective in Afro-Americans and some other groups. One may speculate that both classes of antihypertensive drugs may provide some of their benefit by raising serum potassium ion levels.

*****

All types of antihypertensive drugs have effects beyond lowering BP, and all their modes of action are not always understood. Lowering BP is always a stress on the body, which tries to maintain a good supply of oxygen and nutrients to vital organs by keeping BP as high as necessary. Interfering with this natural process is asking for trouble. The only method of assessing the value of antihypertensive drugs is to run RCTs long enough to determine all-cause mortality and quality-of-life after several years on a given drug in a large enough group of patients. A dropout rate of over 5% above the placebo dropout rate is a sure sign of failure, even if BP is lowered by the desired amount.

So how can expensive drugs under patent protection be used ethically after a 3-5 year clinical trial when they are expected to be taken for 30-40 years? Drug patents last 20 years, and half of this may be lost even with present trial durations and approval delays. Some ethical solution to this dilemma is still needed.

# Results of Clinical Trials of Antihypertensive Drugs

What do patients expect from antihypertensive drugs? Lowered BP is usually not felt unless it is extreme (hypotension). Do physicians say how many more years one will live, on average? Or how much the absolute risk of stroke, CVD, CHF or MI will be reduced? A patient has the right to be told, for example, that her chance of all stroke, over a 5-year period, let us say, is reduced from 10% to 2%. This would be a good reason to stick with a drug, even one with side-effects, assuming the all-cause death rate was lower, or at least not higher. Or a patient would want to hear how many years longer she would live by taking a particular drug or combination of drugs.

The first and most prominent table in one of the big cardiology texts is designed to convince physicians of the great benefits of certain antihypertensive drugs by showing reductions in the relative risk (RR) of cardiovascular problems and death (Figure 4-4). The results of about 20 randomized clinical trials (RCTs) are combined as a meta-analysis, and at first glance, the results look very impressive. Cardiologists from the time they are students actually believe that such results are iron-clad proof that "high" BP should be treated with drugs.

Bear in mind, however, that the same problem exists as with the statin drugs — only the trials with the best results are published, so this data represent the maximum possible benefit of the drugs used. First, it shows that high-dose diuretics prevent half of all stroke (RR = 0.49), a seemingly impressive result. Next, it seems that high-dose diuretics prevent 5/6 of all diagnosed congestive heart failure (CHF), another seemingly impressive result (RR = 0.17). On the downside, the results in Figure 4-4 for coronary heart disease (CVD) and for all-cause death (mortality) are not statistically significant when the drug choices were high-dose diuretics or beta-blockers. There is no table of the corresponding *absolute* benefits in this text (Kaplan, 2001, pp973-974).

With the benefit of the absolute numbers of events observed in Figure 4-4 as well as the number of participants in each group of trials, both provided in the caption of Figure 4-4, the absolute benefits were calculated, and are shown in Figure 4-5. It actually turned out that high-dose diuretics prevented only 0.8% of strokes over the average trial duration of about 5 years. The RR = 0.17 with high-dose diuretics for CHF represented a mere 0.2% (absolute) drop in diagnoses of CHF. When the results were examined in this more realistic manner, low-dose diuretic was by far the most effective of the 3 regimens. This could be the basis for the present recommendations to start hypertensive patients on low-dose diuretics. The problem is that the number needed to treat (NNT) to prevent one event in every case was high, from 42 to ∞ to prevent a single undesired event or end-point, and for mortality the NNT was 50-1000 to prevent a single death. As a very rough approximation, suppose 500 patients must be treated for 5 years to prevent 1 death during that period of 2500 patient-years. Then 1/2500 is 0.004 years or 1.5 days of average duration of life gained (ADLG) after 5 years of treatment when the NNT = 500. Is this worth what Big Pharma charges for BP drugs under patent? Or even generics?

A more recent meta-analysis of 9 trials, involving 62,605 patients in all, compared different types of antihypertensive drugs, and new and old drugs of similar classes. But the trials had no placebo control groups and no all-cause death rates that were reported in the meta-analysis. All that the authors could claim is that calcium channel blockers were the most effective in prevention of stroke, and that the newer drugs were poorer than the older ones (Staessen et al., 2001).

\*\*\*\*\*

A number of individual key trials of antihypertensive drugs will now be discussed. All of these discussions are based on articles published in peer-reviewed medical journals normally considered to have the highest reputation. For most of the trials, a brief description of the results will be given in the first paragraph. A detailed description will follow in the next paragraph, so those who are interested

## Figure 4-4. Results of a Meta-Analysis of RCTs of Antihypertensive Drugs. Reproduced from a Cardiology Text (Kaplan, 2001, p973).

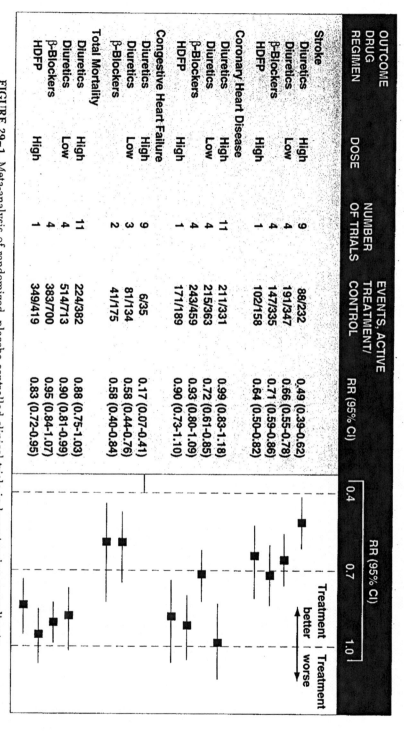

| OUTCOME DRUG REGIMEN | DOSE | NUMBER OF TRIALS | EVENTS, ACTIVE TREATMENT/ CONTROL | RR (95% CI) |
|---|---|---|---|---|
| **Stroke** | | | | |
| Diuretics | High | 9 | 88/232 | 0.49 (0.39–0.62) |
| Diuretics | Low | 4 | 191/347 | 0.66 (0.55–0.78) |
| β-Blockers | | 4 | 147/335 | 0.71 (0.59–0.86) |
| HDFP | High | 1 | 102/158 | 0.64 (0.50–0.82) |
| **Coronary Heart Disease** | | | | |
| Diuretics | High | 11 | 211/331 | 0.99 (0.83–1.18) |
| Diuretics | Low | 4 | 215/363 | 0.72 (0.61–0.85) |
| β-Blockers | | 4 | 243/459 | 0.93 (0.80–1.09) |
| HDFP | High | 1 | 171/189 | 0.90 (0.73–1.10) |
| **Congestive Heart Failure** | | | | |
| Diuretics | High | 9 | 6/35 | 0.17 (0.07–0.41) |
| Diuretics | Low | 3 | 81/134 | 0.58 (0.44–0.76) |
| β-Blockers | | 2 | 41/175 | 0.58 (0.40–0.84) |
| **Total Mortality** | | | | |
| Diuretics | High | 11 | 224/382 | 0.88 (0.75–1.03) |
| Diuretics | Low | 4 | 514/713 | 0.90 (0.81–0.99) |
| β-Blockers | | 4 | 383/700 | 0.95 (0.84–1.07) |
| HDFP | High | 1 | 349/419 | 0.83 (0.72–0.95) |

**FIGURE 29–1.** Meta-analysis of randomized, placebo-controlled clinical trials in hypertension according to first-line treatment strategy. Trials indicate number of trials with at least one endpoint of interest. For these comparisons, the numbers of participants randomized to active treatment and placebo, respectively, were 7768 and 12,075 for high-dose diuretic therapy, 4305 and 5116 for low-dose diuretic therapy, and 6736 and 12,147 for beta-blocker therapy. Because the Medical Research Council trials included two active arms, the placebo group is included twice in these totals (for diuretic comparison and for beta-blocker comparison). The total numbers of participants randomized to active and control therapy were 24,294 and 23,926, respectively. RR = relative risk; CI = confidence interval; HDFP = Hypertension Detection and Follow-up Program. (Data from Psaty BM, Smith NL, Siscovick DS, et al: Health outcomes associated with antihypertensive therapies used as first-line agents. JAMA 277:739, 1997.)

119

Figure 4-5.  Realistic Interpretation of the Results of the Meta-Analysis of
Antihypertensive Drug Trials in Figure 4-4.

| End-Point | % NO Event | | | |
| Drugs | Drug | Control | Difference | NNT* |
| --- | --- | --- | --- | --- |
| **Stroke** | | | | |
| Diuretics, high dose | 98.9 | 98.1 | 0.8 | 125 |
| Diuretics, low dose | 95.6 | 93.2 | 2.4 | 42 |
| Beta-Blockers | 97.8 | 97.2 | 0.6 | 167 |
| **CVD** | | | | |
| Diuretics, high dose | 97.3 | 97.3 | 0.0 | ∞ |
| Diuretics, low dose | 95.0 | 92.9 | 2.1 | 48 |
| Beta-Blockers | 96.4 | 96.2 | 0.2 | 500 |
| **CHF** | | | | |
| Diuretics, high dose | 99.9 | 99.7 | 0.2 | 500 |
| Diuretics, low dose | 98.2 | 97.4 | 0.6 | 167 |
| Beta-Blockers | 99.4 | 98.6 | 0.8 | 125 |
| **Mortality** | | | | |
| Diuretics, high dose | 97.1 | 96.8 | 0.3 | 333 |
| Diuretics, low dose | 88.1 | 86.1 | 2.0 | 50 |
| Beta-Blockers | 94.3 | 94.2 | 0.1 | 1000 |

*NNT = number needed to treat to prevent 1 event during trial duration of
several years.  Crude NNT = 100/Difference

can understand how minor results are often magnified in the abstracts of the articles, almost always by using relative risk (RR) reductions and non-fatal outcomes of drug treatments. These abstracts are usually the bases of press releases and promotional information, and often the only part of the article that is easily obtainable on PubMed or other search engines for medical papers. Key data on the magnitude of side-effects, on the dropout rates of the trials, and on mortality are usually not to be found in the abstracts, but in the body of the paper, either in text or in tables.

*****

The Medical Research Council (MRC) of the UK sponsored a trial that compared the diuretic bendrofluazide (also called bendroflumethazide) with the beta-blocker propranolol and with placebo for the treatment of "mild hypertension". The trial lasted 5.5 years and included both sexes of ages 35-64 at the beginning (baseline) of the trial. Benefits on reducing all-cause mortality and all stroke were negligible. The number-need-to-treat to prevent 1 event (NNT) during this trial ranged from 556 for the effect of diuretic on stroke to 10,000 for the effect of diuretic on all-cause mortality (see Figure 4-6).

There were about 2350 subjects on each drug and about 4500 on placebo, a big trial. The mean baseline BP values were 158/98 for men and 165/99 for women. Compared with any BP reduction with placebo, the diuretic reduced BP by 11/6 more for men and by 15/6 more for women; while the beta-blocker reduced BP by 9/6 more for men and by 10/4 more for women. From Figure 4-6 one can see that both all-cause mortality and stroke reduction were very small and unrelated to the degree of BP reduction, another indication that any beneficial effects of beta-blockers, at least on mortality, may not be related to their effect on BP. The actual benefits were negligible, with very high NNT values. All the mortality benefits were in men in whom 0.11% more survived with drug treatment (NNT = 909), while 0.09% *fewer* treated women survived, another parallel to the sex-related effects of both aspirin and statins. This study has a clear picture of withdrawals due to adverse events: 5% of men or women withdrew from placebo, 20% of each withdrew from beta-blocker, and 23% of men and 13% of women withdrew from diuretic. One is tempted to speculate that, if withdrawal had been forbidden, and the patients had been forced to continue to take drugs or placebo (unethical, of course) that the death rates for drug treatment would have been far higher. The authors note that there was no benefit of treatment on the rates of coronary events (non-fatal MI, angina, etc.), and they were realistic on the overall absence of any value of treatment (MRC, 1985).

Figure 4-6. Realistic Interpretation of the Results of the Medical Research Council (MRC) of the UK Trial of Treatment of Mild Hypertension with with Diuretic or Beta-Blocker for 5.5 Years (Adapted from MRC, 1985).

| End-Point | % NO Event | | | |
| Drugs | Drug | Placebo | Difference | NNT* |
| --- | --- | --- | --- | --- |
| Mortality | | | | |
| Diuretic** | 99.40 | 99.41 | 0.01 | 10,000 |
| Beta-Blocker*** | 99.45 | 99.41 | 0.04 | 2,500 |
| All Stroke | | | | |
| Diuretic** | 99.92 | 99.74 | 0.18 | 556 |
| Beta-Blocker*** | 99.81 | 99.74 | 0.07 | 1,429 |

*NNT = number needed to treat to prevent 1 event during trial duration of several years.  Crude NNT = 100/Difference.  **bendrofluazide  ***propranolol

Here then is the result of a well-done trial that showed no benefit of drug treatment in subjects with baseline BP that Big Pharma now says "must be treated".

***** *

Men Born in 1914 was a prospective study on 484 men 68 years old at baseline living in Malmö, Sweden, and followed for 10 years. Of these, 113 men were taking one or more common antihypertensive drugs; 68 used 1 drug, 39 used 2, and 6 used 3 drugs. Two-thirds of the men with "severe" hypertension did not take any BP drugs. Men with DBP ≤ 90 mm Hg at baseline were much worse off with drug treatment. Those with DBP > 90 were slightly worse off.

Diuretics (mainly thiazides) were taken by 72 men, beta-blockers by 64, hydralazine by 18, calcium channel blockers by 4, an alpha-blocker by 2, and 3 men took some other type. The end-point was any ischemic cardiac event, in this case, myocardial infarction (MI, heart attack) or CHF, both fatal and non-fatal. Men taking antihypertensive drugs had a cardiac-event-free rate of 65%, while those men not on medication had an 82% event-free rate! The population group was divided into those above and below a DBP of 90 mm Hg. Of the 267 men with baseline DBP ≤90, the crude or adjusted RR = 4 *with* treatment! Of the 217 men with baseline DBP >90, the crude RR = 2 *with* treatment, and when adjusted for BMI, smoking, TC, etc., the RR = 1.1. Not only was treatment actually detrimental for all of these men as a group, but the currently recommended DBP for treatment, 90 mm Hg, has no basis whatever here. The authors were frank and realistic about these results. Funding for this study was from the Swedish National Corporation of Pharmacies, the Bank of Sweden, the Swedish Heart and Lung Foundation, and the National Institute for Public Health (Merlo et al., 1996).

\*\*\*\*\*

The same primary end-points, any ischemic cardiac event, in this case, MI or CHF, both fatal and non-fatal, were counted in the BP arm of the huge Anti-Hypertensive and Lipid-Lowering Treatment to Prevent Heart Attack Trial (ALLHAT, 2002), in which there was *no* placebo group, ignoring the poor results of trials *with* placebo groups as demonstrated above. The subjects actually had normal BPs for their average age of 67 (see Table 4-1). This trial was intended to compare treatment with diuretic, calcium channel blocker, or angiotensin converting enzyme (ACE) inhibitor. No differences in all-cause mortality, fatal CVD or non-fatal MI were observed, and only minor ones for stroke rates and hospitalizations. Yet this trial report was used to promote diuretics as the first type of drug to be used for hypertension treatment, even in people who are not really hypertensive!

Participants, 47% female, a mean of 67 years old at baseline, had mean BP of 146/84 at baseline and one additional risk factor for CVD such as smoking, previous MI, high BMI (a mean of 30), NIDDM or others. The object of the trial was to compare the outcomes of 15,255 subjects on a diuretic (chlorthalidone) with those of 9,048 subjects on a calcium channel blocker (amlodipine, Norvasc™), and 9,054 subjects on an angiotensin converting enzyme (ACE) inhibitor (lisinopril, Prinivil™ or Zestril™) for the control of blood pressure, followed for a mean of 4.9 years. The diuretic lowered BP to a mean of 140/75; the calcium channel blocker to 135/75 and ACE-I to 136/75. There were minor differences in stroke rates (1% absolute, lisinopril best) and in hospitalizations for "heart failure" (2% absolute, amlodipine best). The World Health Organization does not think older adults should use chlorthalidone because the risk of serious side effects is so high (Wolfe & Sasich, 1999, p105). It did not have the most favorable effect on any outcome, even on BP at the doses given. Yet the authors wrote in the Conclusion of their Abstract in *JAMA:* "Thiazide-type diuretics are superior in preventing one or more major forms of CVD and are less expensive. They should be preferred for first-step anti-hypertensive therapy." Does this strike you as evidence-based medicine? The conclusion should have been, with attention to the results in earlier trials with controls or placebo, that *no* standard treatment with prescription anti-hypertensive agents is worthwhile for people who are not actually hypertensive for their ages (Table 4-1). This study was supported by the NHLBI ("Heart Institute") and Pfizer, Inc., maker of Norvasc.

\*\*\*\*\*

In contrast, the placebo-controlled, double-blinded trial with the very best results cited in a major cardiology text (Kaplan, 2001, p974) is the Swedish Trial in Old Patients (STOP) with hypertension (Dahlöf et al., 1991). The 1627 subjects of both sexes were 70-84 years old at the start, had mean BP = 195/102 at baseline, and were followed for 4 years at 116 health centers in Sweden. The drugs were a diuretic, or the same combined with a beta-blocker. After 4 years 89% of the drug-treated group were alive vs. 85% on placebo. This may not seem a great result, but it is the best of any of the trials discussed here or known to me.

The drugs were all taken once-daily: diuretic (25 mg hydrochlorthiazide), the same plus 2.5 mg of the beta-blocker amiloride, or 100 mg of the beta-blocker metoprolol, or 5 mg pindolol. The ending BP was 195/95 with placebo and 166/85 with drug treatment. There was no difference in any outcome for the first 6 months. At the end of 4 years 85% on placebo were alive vs. 89% of those treated, a difference of 1% per year absolute. At the end of 4 years 90% on placebo were free from all stroke vs. 96% of those treated, a difference of 1.5% per year absolute. Results were not separated by sex. The authors did not calculate the dropout rate, but it could be calculated from the numbers said to have dropped out; it was 7% of the treatment group and 6% of the placebo group. The authors' conclusions were: "We conclude that antihypertensive treatment in hypertensive men and women aged 70-84 confers highly significant and clinically relevant reductions in cardiovascular morbidity and mortality as well as in total mortality." This study was supported by what are now Astra/Zeneca, Merck, Novartis and the Swedish County Councils. If the minimal results of this very best trial are thought to be worthwhile, it is worth noting that, in this trial, the subjects who obtained these benefits were at about the 95th percentile of BP, since their baseline SBP was greater than what is shown in the last line of Table 4-2. All the other individual trials cited in this chapter were on subjects with mostly non-threatening BP levels, according to the findings of Sidney Port et al., as discussed earlier.

*****

The second Swedish Trial in Old Patients (STOP-2) showed that ACE inhibitors and calcium channel blockers were no better than diuretics or beta-blockers in subjects with baseline BP of 194/98 (Pahor et al., 2000).

*****

So has any research group found out how much BP lowering is best? A more recent international RCT sought to compare the degree of DBP reduction with the usual outcomes (stroke, MI, etc.) — the Hypertension Optimal Treatment (HOT) trial (Hansson et al., 1998). The goal was to compare the outcomes of lowering DBP in 3 groups of similar patients to different levels by use of different doses of a calcium channel blocker, with addition of other drugs if the calcium channel blocker alone could not bring down the DBP to the desired level. The outcome was the reverse of the expectation — patients with DBP lowered the most had the highest mortality, except those with diabetes. The differences in both cases were quite small.

Here about 19,000 subjects of mean age 61.5 years with mean DBP of 105 mm Hg were treated with the calcium channel blocker felodipine (Plendil™) in 3 equal sized groups: the first to have a target DBP of ≤90, the second ≤85, and the third tertile of ≤80 mm Hg. When felodipine alone could not achieve the goal, ACE inhibitors, beta-blockers, or diuretics or combinations were added. The achieved DBPs were 85, 83 and 81 respectively. There was no placebo. After an apparent mean trial duration of 4 years, the fraction alive in each tertile at the end was 97.0%, 96.9% and 96.7% respectively, the reverse order to what was expected! In patients with diabetes of unspecified type, the fraction alive in each tertile at the end was 94.0%, 94.2% and 96.6% respectively. This pathetic result was, at least, in the order expected, but was not likely to be a result of the antihypertensive effect of the drug. Why, then did the authors conclude that: "The principal results of the HOT study demonstrate the benefits of lowering blood pressure to 140 mm Hg systolic and 85 mm Hg diastolic or lower... Active lowering of blood pressure was particularly beneficial in the subgroup of patients with diabetes mellitus..."? The principal sponsor was Astra AB, Sweden, with support from Astra Merck USA, TEVA, Israel, and Hoechst, Argentina.

*****

123

You may be surprised to learn that there are large studies on the effects of antihypertensive drugs on subjects with average to low BP. The Cooperative North Scandinavian Enalapril Survival Study (CONSENSUS, 1987) examined the effects of enalapril (Vasotec™) on 127 patients with CHF in New York Heart Association (NYHA) class IV (the worst) with 126 similar patients on placebo, who were followed for up to 1 year. The baseline BP was 118/74 for enalapril subjects and 121/76 for placebo subjects, because of the weak pumping of the heart due to CHF. In the enalapril treatment group 64% were still alive, and in the placebo group 48% were still alive (p = 0.001). Because of the uneven follow-up times, the average duration of life gained was hard to calculate, but it was 8 months (Lubsen et al., 2000).

Now here is a solid result, but there was a confounder. In 49% of all the subjects a vasodilator (hydralazine, nitrates, prazosin) was also being used; among these, 58% of the treatment group survived vs. 52% of the placebo group. In the subjects not taking a vasodilator, 63% in the treatment group survived vs. 40% in the placebo group, proving the toxicity of the vasodilators in some patients and benefit in others. This trial was supported by Merck USA. Obviously, the beneficial effect of the enalapril was not due to any lowering of BP because it was dangerously low to begin with.

*****

A much larger trial of enalapril on 1285 subjects vs. placebo on 1284 subjects, 90% of whom were in NYHA classes II and III of CHF averaged 41.5 months of follow-up. This was the Studies of Left Ventricular Dysfunction (SOLVD, 1991) trial. Both groups were also taking other drugs in about the same proportions, and both had BP of 125/77 at baseline due to CHF. Survival was 65% in the enalapril group and 60% in the placebo group (*p* = 0.007), or 1.4% absolute better per year for treatment.

This allowed the authors to write: "The addition of enalapril to conventional therapy significantly reduced mortality and hospitalizations for heart failure in patients with chronic congestive heart failure and low ejection fractions." Well, the reduction in mortality was quite significant statistically, at least, if not that great in absolute terms. This study was supported by the NHLBI and Merck. The latter was said to have had no part in the conduct of or reporting on the study. What was really accomplished? The average duration of life gained was just 2 months! (Lubsen et al., 2000).

*****

For comparison with the coenzyme Q10 trial that follows, the enalapril group had 87% survival after 1 year, and the placebo group 84%. After 3 years the rates were 69% vs. 65%.

## Nutritional Supplements

What a pity that coenzyme Q10 was not compared with enalapril for those subjects with CHF. A RCT with 1 year of follow-up showed that subjects in NYHA classes III and IV (the most seriously ill) had a 95% survival with coenzyme Q10 and 93% on placebo. As in the SOLVD trial, non-fatal outcomes also favored treatment (Morisco et al., 1993). As noted in Myth 1, patients in NYHA classes III and IV followed for 3 years had 75% survival on Q10 and 25% without it. Q10 has no side-effects.

Many publications suggest benefit from L-carnitine, another inexpensive supplement, in a number of conditions, including both CVD and CHF. Clinical trial data in prevention of MI are promising and have prompted the initiation of a large-scale trial that will determine mortality (Schofield & Hill, 2001). This natural amino acid has no side effects.

Naturally occurring L-arginine is the source of nitric oxide, a potent vasodilator that lowers BP. Oral administration of it lowers BP somewhat and improves exercise capacity in patients with pulmonary hypotension (Nagaya et al., 2001). This natural amino acid also has no side effects at 0.5 g per 10 kg of body weight, about 3.5 g per day. More study is needed.

Many people respond to magnesium supplements. Magnesium deficiencies (hypomagnesemia) is the most common mineral deficiency. At least 4 studies (RCTs) whose results were published in peer-reviewed journals during the 1990s found that 400-600 mg/day of magnesium in soluble compounds lowered SBP by 8-9 mm Hg and DBP by 4-8 mm Hg, showing magnesium to be as effective as many of the prescription drugs (Cohen, 2004, pp25-26). Unlike prescription drugs, the magnesium conferred beneficial side-effects of fewer cramps or headaches as well as lower blood glucose levels. The reasons for contradictory results in other trials was too low a dose, or administration of a poorly absorbed form of magnesium. The magnesium oxide and hydroxide are poorly absorbed because they are not soluble enough. The citrate is poorly absorbed because it is too soluble, or too loosely bound to the magnesium. The aspartate or mixed amino acid chelates are the best forms. Ideally, 1-2 times as much potassium in the same capsule will improve the benefits.

## Nutrition

Since hypertension and CVD are so closely associated with prior diabetes, insulin resistance, or Syndrome X (Cohen, 2004, pp42-45), prevention of high blood glucose levels and insulin levels by diet is actually the best way to prevent or limit hypertension. Only low-carb diets will accomplish this. The low-fat diets so widely recommended actually make the situation worse by leading to diabetes (NIDDM) because they are high-carb diets (see Myth 2).

Many types of fruits, nuts and vegetables contain magnesium. Mother was right: eat your (low-GI) vegetables!

## How Bad are the Side-Effects of Antihypertensive Drugs?

In another parallel with the statin drugs, half of the users of antihypertensive drugs discontinue them within a year (Cohen, 2001, p109). In the Multicenter Isradipine Diuretic Atherosclerosis Study (MIDAS) 12.4% on isradipine (a calcium channel blocker) or hydrochlorothiazide (the diuretic) either with or without enalapril (an ACE inhibitor) quit within 1 year, and 18-20% quit within 3 years (Borhani et al., 1996). As noted above, 13-20% quit diuretic or beta-blocker in the MRC trial (MRC, 1985). The dropout rate was 34-39% in the STOP-2 trial, depending on the drug used, which included enalapril, atenolol (a beta-blocker) as well as felodipine and isradipine (calcium channel blockers). How extreme can the dropout rate be? In the Appropriate Blood Pressure Control in Diabetes (ABCD) trial where the baseline BP was only 156/98, it was 55% on enalapril and 60% on nisoldipine, a calcium channel blocker (Pahor et al., 2000).

One of the weirdest effects of ACE inhibitors, particularly the once-best-selling enalapril (Vasotec) was chronic coughing. The 1996 PDR lists the incidence of cough as 1.3% vs. 0.9% for placebo. According to Jay S. Cohen, MD, Merck claimed the frequency of cough was 2.2%, yet a study in 1989 showed that 10.5% of 209 people taking Vasotec quit because of a persistent, dry, severe cough within 3 months. Of those who did not quit, 15.5% of 187 reported coughing (Gibson, 1989). This is a total of 26% who complained of coughing. A later study showed that 3 other ACE inhibitors, lisinopril (Prinivil™, Zestril), ramipril (Altace™) and perindopril had about 3.5 times the incidence of cough of enalapril (Kubota et al., 1996). Simple calculation indicates that over 90% of patients taking these newer ACE inhibitors coughed.

Some of the earliest calcium channel blockers whose generic names ended in -ipine actually created a scandal when it was discovered that they increased the risk of MI, cancer or internal bleeding. In 1995 Public Citizen's Health Research Group filed a petition with the FDA to change the labeling of all calcium channel blockers to warn of the increased risk of MI and death. In 1996 the FDA stopped recommending nifedipine for treatment of high BP (Wolfe & Sasich, 1999, p77). If calcium channel blockers injure only 0.5% of the 7,000,000 people taking them in a recent year, that amounts to 35,000 annual casualties for a drug class whose benefits are minimal at best (Moore, 1998, 24-27). As noted above, slow-release formulations and slower-acting calcium channel blockers are available, but the benefits are miniscule to negative. In a meta-analysis of RCTs encompassing 28,000 subjects, intermediate-acting or slow-acting calcium channel blockers were compared with diuretics, beta-blockers, and ACE inhibitors. Subjects on calcium channel blockers were more likely to have acute MI ($RR = 1.26$, $p = 0.0003$), to have CHF ($RR = 1.25$, $p = 0.005$) and other heart problems such as arrhythmias ($RR = 1.10$, $p = 0.018$), albeit there was no difference in the rate of strokes (Pahor et al., 2000). The industry response was typical: defend the drugs at any cost. The cover-up was successful. Were you aware of it?

Treatment with a combination of diuretic and beta-blocker raises serum glucose by 7 mg/dL, TC by 5 mg/dL, and TG by 21 mg/dL, while potassium drops 0.4 mEq/L (Hall, 1996). These changes are in the undesired directions. Well, maybe not TC. Nearly all of the common antihypertensive drugs raise serum glucose. The common beta-blockers mask hypoglycemia (Bernstein, 2003, p453-454). If hypotension is mistaken for hypoglycemia and given emergency treatment, death could result. The thiazide diuretics also raise homocysteine levels (McCully, 2000, p129); see Myth 2.

The potassium-sparing diuretics such as amiloride (Moduretic™), triamterene (Dyrenium™) and spironolactone (Aldactone™) were introduced to prevent potassium loss, but these have their own serious side-effects, namely kidney failure, kidney stones, muscle paralysis, mental confusion, and interference with red blood cell production. So serious are these effects that the Public Citizen Health Research Group recommends not using them at all (Wolfe & Sasich, 1999, pp57,99).

The main side-effects of $AT_1$-receptor antagonists are dizziness and hypotension. The latter may be caused by all types of antihypertensive drugs. A serious form is called postural hypotension. People taking antihypertensive drugs are often warned to arise from bed in stages with pauses. An all-to-common scenario is that a person awakens at night with an urgent need to urinate or defecate, so does not pause. Fainting (syncope) follows, often leading to a fall of the type that causes broken hips in the elderly. How many physicians would connect antihypertensive drugs with broken hips? Not that many. They would recommend Fosamax™ or its congeners to prevent the next fracture despite lack of evidence for any more benefit than higher bone densities on scans; but this story is for another time.

Withdrawal of subjects due to adverse effects is probably the reason why any benefit at all is reported for the subjects remaining in most of the trials. When you see the term "the drug was well-tolerated" it means only that more than half of the subjects remained in the trials of the drug. Since these trials are usually a few years in duration, we do not know how many patients would tolerate a particular drug or combination for 30 years, which is the duration that a patient begun on a drug at age 50 would have to endure all side effects, assuming she lived to the age of 80.

Does Big Pharma lie about side-effects? One method of avoiding direct falsehood is to have a "run-in period" during the clinical trials. Any patients who are "non-compliant" with the drug regimen (or moan about the side-effects) are eliminated from the main trials.


## Bottom Line on Blood Pressure Control

Trials (RCTs) of antihypertensive drugs not sponsored by drug manufacturers or which have a placebo arm show minor or no benefits of antihypertensive drugs unless untreated BP is extremely high. Recent RCTs run with no placebo leave great doubt about the overall benefit of treatment, as well as on the level of BP that should be treated, compared with no drug treatment at all. People with SBP higher than the 90th percentile for their age and sex as shown in Table 4-2 might benefit somewhat from treatment as shown in the STOP trial.

Even very reputable journals continue to publish articles discussing the choice of antihypertensive drugs with which to begin treatment of "high" BP and CHF, and in what order to add more drugs. Because of the adverse effects of all antihypertensive drugs, it does make sense to use small doses of as many as 5 types of antihypertensive drugs in combination, but only for extremely high BP, above the 90% percentile for age and sex (Table 4-2). Drug purveyors ignore the lack of benefit in most people with SBP below the 90th percentile, and studiously ignore the beneficial effects of low-carbohydrate diets and certain supplements (Erdman, 2003; Lechat, 2003).

The association of high BP with NIDDM is tight; of NIDDM with obesity very high; and the association of excessive carbohydrate and *trans* fat consumption with obesity is high. These relationships show how a low-carbohydrate diet might lower BP. As noted above and in Myth 2, the low-fat or DASH diets promoted by the AHA, NHLBI and others, which are invariably high-carb diets, cannot succeed.

Drug use should be considered only for the extremely hypertensive (top 10%) only after a low-carbohydrate diet and supplements such as L-arginine, magnesium and fish oil have been tried. Partial success with such a diet and supplements may allow much lower doses of drugs to be used, minimizing side-effects.

The effect of reducing salt consumption on BP should be checked on each individual since only 1/5th have been shown to benefit.

Newer classes of drugs for old conditions are usually promoted as being better in some way. This is possible because the selectivity of the newer drug for its intended receptors may be so much greater that lower doses may be given than of its predecessors, producing fewer side effects. What is always true is that some of these promotions are meant to switch patients to the drugs still covered by patents. This maintains profit levels, because these drugs are more expensive until competition from low-cost "generics" begins when the patent expires. Drug makers have a serious conflict of interest in trying to balance the interests of employees and shareholders against the interests of patients. More than once a newer class of drug for lowering BP has proven to be either no more effective, or less effective, or more dangerous, or both. This has been shown to be true for both the ACE inhibitor and calcium channel blocker classes of antihypertensive drugs (Staessen et al., 2001; Pahor et al., 2000).

Cardiologists usually believe what colleagues and cardiology texts tell them. From one major text: "...few other aspects of clinical practice have as strong an evidence base as does the treatment of hypertension" (Kaplan, 2001, p972). And medicinal chemists and pharmacologists will see in Goodman & Gilman: "Effective antihypertensive therapy [meaning drugs] will almost completely prevent the hemorrhagic strokes, cardiac failure, and renal insufficiency due to hypertension." (Oates & Brown, 2001, p872). The evidence presented in this chapter refutes these baseless conceits.

Myth 4 Acknowledgments

The help of many members of the International Cholesterol Skeptics Group (www.THINCS.org) is greatly appreciated, both for providing citations and enlightening discussion, and especially from its founder, Uffe Ravnskov, MD, PhD. John Lehmann (www.DrugIntel.com) and Leslie Ann Bowman, AMLS, of the University of the Sciences in Philadelphia, Duane Graveline, MD, MPH, and Frances E. H. Pane, MSLS, edited this chapter. Editorial aid was also obtained from Jane M. Orient, MD, FACP, Fred Ottoboni, PhD, MPH and Alice Ottoboni, PhD.

## Myth 4 References

ALLHAT (2002). Major outcomes in high-risk hypertensive patients randomized to angiotensin-converting enzyme inhibitor or calcium channel blocker vs. diuretic. *JAMA* 288:2981-2997.

Bernstein RK (2003). *Dr. Bernstein's Diabetes Solution.* Boston, MA: Little, Brown.

Black HR, Backris GL, Elliott WJ (2001). Hypertension: Epidemiology, Pathophysiology, Diagnosis and Treatment in *Hurst's The Heart,* 10th ed., Fuster V et al., Eds., New York, NY: McGraw-Hill.

Borhani NO, Mercuri M, Borhani PA, et al. (1996). Final Outcome Results of the Multicenter Isradipine Diuretic Atherosclerosis Study (MIDAS). *JAMA* 276:785-791.

Cohen JS (2001). *Overdose: the Case Against the Drug Companies.* New York, N.Y: Tarcher/Putnam.

Cohen JS (2004). *The Magnesium Solution for High Blood Pressure. How to Use Magnesium to Help Prevent & Relieve Hypertension Naturally,* Garden City Park, NY: Square One Publishing.

CONSENSUS (1987). Effects of Enalapril on Mortality in Severe Congestive Heart Failure. *New England Journal of Medicine* 316:1429-1435.

Dahlöf B, Lindholm LH, Hansson L, et al. (1991). Morbidity and mortality in the Swedish Trial in Old Patients (STOP-hypertension). *Lancet* 338:1281-1285.

Elliott P, et al. (1988). Intersalt: an international study of electrolyte excretion and blood pressure. Results for 24 hour urinary sodium and potassium excretion. *British Medical Journal* 297:319-328.

Erdman E (2003). Pharmacotherapy for chronic heart failure: when to use which drug and at which dose? *European Heart Journal* 5, S-I:164-168.

Folkow B (2003). Salt and blood pressure - centenarian bone of contention. *Läkartidningen 100*:3142-3147.

Freston JW, Bosso JA (1990). Diseases: Manifestations and Pathophysiology in *Remington's Pharmaceutical Sciences,* 18th ed., Gennaro AR, Ed., Easton, PA: Mack.

Gibson GR (1989). Enalapril-Induced Caugh. *Archives of Internal Medicine* 149:2701-2703.

Gurwitz JH, Avorn J, Bohn RL, Glynn RJ, Monane M, Mogun H (1994). Initiation of antihypertensive treatment during nonsteroidal anti-inflammatory drug therapy.*JAMA* 272(10):781-6.

Hall WD (1996). Management of Systolic Hypertension in the Elderly. *Seminars in Nephrology* 16(4):299-308.

Hansson L, Zanchetti A, Carruthers SG, et al. (1998). Effects of intensive blood-pressure lowering and low-dose aspirin in patients with hypertension:principal results of the Hypertension Optimal Treatment (HOT) randomised trial. *Lancet* 351:1755-1762.

Harvey SC, Withrow CD (1990). Cardiovascular Drugs in *Remington's Pharmaceutical Sciences,* 18th ed., Gennaro AR, Ed., Easton, PA: Mack.

Kaplan NM (2001). Hypertensive and Atherosclerotic Cardiovascular Disease in *Heart Disease: A Textbook of Cardiovascular Medicine,* 6th ed., Braunwald E et al., Eds., Philadelphia, PA: W. B. Saunders.

Kubota K, Kubota N, Pearce GL, Inman WHW (1996). ACE-inhibitor-incuded cough, an adverse drug reaction unrecognised for several years: studies in Prescription-Event Monitoring. *European Journal of Pharmacology* 49:431-437.

Lechat P (2003). Therapeutic strategies in heart failure: what is the optimal sequence of drug therapy? *European Heart Journal* 5, S-I:169-174.

Lubsen J, Hoes A, Grobbee D (2000). Implications of trial results: the potentially misleading notions of number needed to treat and average duration of life gained. *Lancet* 356:1757-1759.

Mamdani M, Juurlink DN, Lee DS, et al. (2004). Cyclo-oxygenase-2 inhibitors versus non-selective non-steroidal antiinflammatory drugs and congestive heart failure outcomes in elderly patients: a population-based cohort study. *Lancet* 363:1751-1756.

McCully KS, McCully M (2000). *The Heart Revolution: The Extraordinary Discovery that Laid the Cholesterol Myth to Rest.* New York, NY: Harper/Perennial.

Merlo J, Ranstam J, Liedholm H, et al. (1996). Incidence of myocardial infarction in elderly men being treated with anti-hypertensive drugs: population-based cohort study. *British Medical Journal* 313:457-461.

Moore TJ (1998). *Prescription for Disaster.* New York, NY:Simon & Schuster.

Morisco C, Trimarco B, Condorelli M (1993). Effect of coenzyme Q10 therapy in patients with congestive heart failure: a long-term multicenter randomized study. *Clinical Investigations* 71:S134-S136.

MRC (1985). MRC trial of treatment of mild hypertension: principal results. *British Medical Journal* 291:97-104.

Nagaya N, Uematsu M, Oya H, et al. (2001). Short-term Oral Administration of L-Arginine Improves Hemodynamics and Exercise Capacity in Patients with Precapillary Pulmonary Hypertension. *American Journal of Respiratory Critical Care Medicine* 163:887-891.

Oates JA, Brown NJ (2001). Antihypertensive Agents and the Therapy of Hypertension in *Goodman and Gilman's the Pharmacological Basis of Therapeutics,* 10th ed., Hardman JG et al., Eds. New York, NY: McGraw-Hill.

Obarzarnek E, Sacks FM, Vollmer WM, et al. (2001). Effects on blood lipids of a blood pressure-lowering diet: the Dietary Approaches to Stop Hypertension (DASH) Trial. American *Journal of Clinical Nutrition* 74:80-89.

Pahor M, Psaty BM, Alderman MH et al. (2000). Health outcomes associated with calcium antagonists compared with other first-line antihypertensive therapies: a meta-analysis of randomised controlled trials. *Lancet* 356(9246):1949-1954.

Port S, Demer L, Jennrich R, Walter D, Garfinkel A (2000a). Systolic blood pressure and mortality. *Lancet* 355:T175-180.

Port S, Garfinkel A, Boyle N (2000b). There is a non-linear relationship between mortality and blood pressure. *European Heart Journal* 21:1635-1638.

Rosenfeld I (2004). High Blood Pressure in Kids. *Parade* 8 Aug 04, p18.

Schofield RS, Hill JA (2001). Role of metabolically active drugs in the management of ischemic heart disease. *American Journal of Cardiovascular Drugs* 1(1):23-35.

Solomon HA (1984). *The Exercise Myth.* Orlando, FL: Harcourt Brace Jovanovich.

Staessen JA, Wang J-G, Thijs L (2001). Cardiovascular protection and blood pressure reduction: a meta-analysis. *Lancet* 358:1305-1315.

Vlasses PH (1985). Hypertension. Current and Future Concepts in Treatment. *American Journal of Pharmacy* 157:9-22.

Wolfe SM, Sasich LD (1999). *Worst Pills Best Pills.* New York, N.Y.: Pocket Books.

Wolfe SM, Sasich LD (2002). *Worst Pills, Best Pills, Companion for Use with the 1999 Edition,* Washington, DC: Public Citizen Health Research Group.

# Myth 5: A Drink a Day Keeps the Doctor Away.

A Synopsis by Spacedoc

Shortly after my internship at Walter Reed Army Medical Center in 1955, another myth was added to my growing repertoire of what every young doctor should know. The first had been the misguided promulgation of our national low fat/low cholesterol diet to our young and tender minds. The second had been the high-carb diabetic diet mandated by the American Diabetes Association in diabetes management. The third was from WRAMC on merits of daily or moderate alcohol consumption in curtailing the risk of cardiovascular disease. Even young, tender minds occasionally have meritorious thoughts and my own at that time, were, "How could this be?"

Having acquired a fair amount of pharmacology and physiology over the years, I have remained skeptical of these claims despite the glowingly positive reports of supposedly competently done research studies. And now Joel M. Kauffman has done what very few have the time, inclination and background to do – he has done a much needed in-depth review of these studies and challenged their validity.

When I was undertaking the study of Biostatistics at Johns Hopkins in 1957 we had a saying as we sat at our mechanical calculators pulling the cranks, "Figures don't lie but liars figure." We realized that misrepresentation of statistical information rarely was intentional but, in our young minds then, those twisting the data whether intentional or not, were liars, at least in the functional sense. So when nationally known researchers publish in national journals that we can reduce the probability of dying from a heart attack by 60% simply by drinking wine regularly, this wins the author of the article a life long supply of wine from the appreciative manufacturers, gets the immediate attention of our public almost as if it were in the National Enquirer and is about as true as whatever else we find in the Enquirer.

Dr. Kauffman has reviewed several epidemiological studies on the relationship of alcohol consumption to cardiovascular disease and found almost all studies were "fatally flawed" in basing their findings on this specific endpoint without all-cause mortality. Since we all are destined to die, a reduction in specific death rate from heart disease while increasing deaths from accidental injury is hardly a net gain. Most of these studies failed to show total death rates, so they gave a misleading view of the benefit (or loss) associated with alcohol consumption. One of the few studies not flawed was that reported in 2001 by Theobald et al. of the Karolinska Institute. The all-cause death rates are included in the study on this group of some 28,000 volunteers followed for up to 20 years and the results are sobering (pardon the pun). End result was neither benefit nor gain – whether minimal drinker or moderate drinker the statistical difference is insignificant, but heavy drinkers beware!

So if you like the effect of moderate alcohol intake you may continue it, knowing that in so doing, you are not significantly hurting yourself. However, if you are not a drinker, please do not start because of any perceptions of health gains, for these are false.

---Duane Graveline, MD, MPH

Dr. Barnard's Advice on Drinking Alcohol

Christiaan Barnard, MD, who performed the world's first successful heart transplant operation, and over 150 heart surgeries since, wrote a book: *50 Ways to a Healthy Heart,* in which the following passages appear in Chapter 3, *Drink Red Wine:* "A person drinking two glasses of red wine per day is helping his heart." "...what is it about wine, beer and other alcoholic beverages that all of a sudden

130

they are treated like medicine? Well, they can keep you healthy and lengthen your life." "...more than 60 reliable research studies from around the world...have established the positive effects of red wine in particular." And he quotes Dr. David Goldberg: "If every North American would drink two glasses of red wine every day, heart disease would be reduced by 40% and $40 billion in medical costs could be saved every year." (Barnard, 2001, pp18-19).

As evidence in support of these recommendations, Dr. Barnard cited the findings of 4 studies with great enthusiasm:

• In 1926 the American biologist Raymond Pearl discovered that a person drinking 2 or 3 glasses of wine a day would reduce his chances of getting a heart attack by 40%.

• In a large-scale study in the 1970s the American cardiologist Arthur Klatsky was able to confirm that moderate alcohol consumption can reduce the risk of heart attacks.

• In 1990 the American Cancer Society reported that a study on 277,000 men showed that one alcoholic drink per day reduces the risk of heart disease by 25%.

• In 1995 the Danish Doctor Martin Gronbaek followed 13,000 people for 12 years. HIs report indicated that a person drinking wine regularly reduces the probability of dying from a heart attack by 60%. Beer lovers who consume 3-5 glasses per day reduced their chances of a heart attack by 30%, but beer had no positive effects on cancer. Whiskey or other hard liquors had almost no medical advantages compared with those who did not drink alcohol at all. (Barnard, 2001, pp19-20).

Eight more studies are cited, all without specific references, as was the case with the 4 above, that give benefits of drinking red wine, such as raising HDL levels or promoting an enzyme that dissolves clots, etc. Without references that can be checked, of what value are all those relative risks?

Based on the techniques of analysis of trials presented so far in this book, what is a rational person supposed to make of Dr. Barnard's well-meaning recommendations? Not a single one of his touts for wine or beer gives the all-cause death rate for various levels of alcohol consumption. If one does not die of cardiovascular disease (CVD) or congestive heart failure (CHF), one is most likely to die of cancer or stroke. It is unlikely that most people would prefer the latter pair of deaths as a consequence of choosing to imbibe alcohol. Even though Dr. Barnard's book focused on heart problems, he was sloppy at the least in ignoring other causes of death. Note also that relative risks are used throughout Dr. Barnard's writing: "...reduces the probability of dying from a heart attack by 60%" is a relative risk (RR) even without being given that name. Without absolute risks there is no possible way to decide whether to drink more or less alcohol. The most extreme RR reduction given, 60%, does not say what kind of wine, how much was consumed per day, or give separate results by sex. Dr. Barnard does not even give the volume of the wine glass he refers to so often. Wine glasses vary greatly in size. The most common size filled to a typical level contains 180 mL or 6 fluid ounces.

<u>What is the Advice of the Low-Carb Diet Book Authors on Drinking Alcohol?</u>

A quick look at Table 5-1 shows very little agreement. Beer is recommended by 5 of the 9 authors; wine by all of them with red specified by 3, and distilled spirits (hard liquor) by 4. Among those who recommend beer, the amount is 1-5 glasses per day; of wine 1/4 to "several" (4?) glasses per day, and of spirits 1-2 drinks per day. No wonder people who read more than 1 diet book give up in disgust!

But as pointed out in Myth 2, the carb content of drinks matters a lot to the carb-sensitive 3/4 of us. Typical beer contains 13 g of high-GI carb per 360 mL bottle or glass; ale and stout up to 18 g; but "lite" or diet beer 2.5-9 g. According to the operators of my local beer store, more than 1/3 of all beer sales are now diet beer. Only "dry" (low-sugar) wines such as dark red pinot noir contain about 6g

Table 5-1:  Advice on How Much Alcohol to Consume Daily
Given by Dr. Barnard and the Low-Carb Diet Book Authors*

| Author | Beer** (glasses) | Wine*** (glasses) | Spirits**** (drinks) |
|---|---|---|---|
| Barnard | 3-5 | 2 red | 0 |
| Atkins | ? | 1/4 | ? |
| Allan & Lutz | 1-2 | several | 0 |
| Bernstein | 1 | 1 | 1 |
| Eades & Eades | 1 | 1 | 1 |
| Groves | 0 | 1 | 1 |
| McCully | 0 | 1-2 red | 0 |
| Mercola | 0 | ? red | 0 |
| Ottoboni & Ottoboni | 1-2 | 1-2 | 1-2 |

*See Myth #2 for complete references to books on low-carb diets.
**May contain 4.5-7% alcohol and includes ale and stout.  A glass is 360 mL (12 fl oz) containing 20 mL alcohol (at 5.5%).
***A glass contains 180 mL (6 fl oz) containing 22 mL of alcohol; can be 30 mL for fortified wine.
****Typically 40% alcohol.  May be known as distilled spirits, hard liquor, whiskey, liqueurs or cordials.  A "drink" is 35 mL (1.25 fl oz) containing 14 mL of alcohol.

of carb per 180 mL glass, while many white or pink wines are far higher in carb, especially the ones called "dessert wines". There is a scale of sugar contents for sparkling wines, such as champagne, that shows how much sugar(s) content can vary (Table 5-2). It is interesting to see how dry a sparkling wine one should select for a low-carb diet. The common whiskeys do not contain much carb, but liqueurs and cordials may be very high in carb — 5-10 times the sugar content of dry wine. The common and thoughtless recommendations for moderate drinking of all kinds of alcoholic beverages, however well-meaning, including Dr. Barnard's, usually ignore this important factor.

The low-carb diet movement was not lost on all vintners. Without changing any carb contents, several vintners list it on the label of the bottle for a 5-ounce serving. My figures here are adjusted for the more common 6-ounce serving. Diageo Chateau & Estate Wines made a BV Coastal Estates 2002 chardonnay with 4 g of carbs. Sutter Home Family Vineyards made a 2002 sauvignon blanc with 3 g of carbs, a 2002 merlot with 5 g, and a white zinfandel with 10 g. More expensive wines are less likely to have their carb content listed. (Locke, 2004).

Table 5-2: Sugar(s) Content of Sparkling Wines and Other Common Drinks

| Type of Drink Sugar(s) Level | % Sugar(s) | Mass Sugar(s) in a 180 mL glass |
|---|---|---|
| Sparkling Wine (Champagne) | | |
| Brut Nature | 0.0 - 0.5 | 0.0 - 0.9 g |
| Brut | 0.5 - 1.5 | 0.9 - 2.7 |
| Extra Dry | 1.2 - 2.0 | 2.2 - 3.6 |
| Dry or Sec | 1.7 - 3.5 | 3.1 - 6.3 |
| Demi-Sec | 3.3 - 5.0 | 5.9 - 9.0 |
| Doux | > 5.0 | > 9.0 |
| Beer, Amstel Lite | 1.4 | 2.5 |
| Pinot Noir (Oregon, USA) | 3.3 | 6 |
| Welch's 100% Grape Juice | 17.5 | 31.5 |

The antioxidants in dark grapes are often promoted as the beneficial component rather than the alcohol content of wine. Advice to drink grape juice is deadly to carb-sensitive people because the high-GI sugar content of grape juice is so high — every bit as high as in a typical soda (Table 5-2). The serving size of Welch's 100% Grape Juice is 240 mL (8 fl oz). This contains 42 g of high-GI carbs, including 40 g of sugars, and would contain half of an entire day's carb ration for even a moderately carb-sensitive person (see Myth 2). Eating whole grapes may be the better way to take in the antioxidants. But are the antioxidants the true life-extenders? Was Dr. Barnard correct in writing that hard liquor had no medical benefits at all?

<u>What do the Epidemiological Trials on Drinking Alcohol Actually Show?</u>

Fully 34 early studies on alcohol consumption considered only cardiovascular disease (CVD) and congestive heart failure (CHF), concluding that the death rates from these conditions were reduced by alcohol consumption. Most of the studies investigated 0 - 3 drinks per day. Some studies of alcoholics showed lower CVD rates even with 12 - 24 drinks of whiskey per day. Dr. William Darby of Vanderbilt University, Nashville, TN, USA, found that 5 drinks per day of whiskey caused little if any damage to health in general. A book by the Royal College of Psychiatrists in London (UK) recommends a maximum of 8 drinks per day. Cirrhosis of the liver, according to a renowned expert on alcoholism, is contracted by only 0.11% of actual alcoholics, and is not their major cause of death (Smith, 1991, pp104,207-208). And what value have all these studies? None, because the effect of alcohol on *all causes* of death was not determined or not reported. Quality of life was not considered either.

Even Linus Pauling fixated on a single epidemiological study reported in 1955 (!) by Chope and Breslow showing that moderate drinkers (1-3 per day) were more "healthy" than non-drinkers or those consuming ≥4 drinks per day. "Healthy" was not defined, nor did Pauling verify that adjustments were made for age and socioeconomic class (Pauling, 1986, p39).

New Zealand case-control study, 1991

A more recent case-control study from New Zealand sought to correlate non-fatal heart attacks (NFMI) and fatal CVD with the frequency of drinking alcohol. The researchers depended on the recall of NFMI survivors as to how much alcohol consumption each had, and on the recall of next-of-kin on how much alcohol the non-survivors of CVD had. This was a retrospective study on free-living populations, both the stricken ones, and a matched control group, so there was no follow-up time given or needed. There were no differences in outcome related to the type of alcohol consumed (wine, beer, spirits), contrary to Dr. Barnard and others. HDL levels were raised or lowered in the same direction as the level of alcohol consumption. Adjusting the raw data for HDL levels weakened an already weak association, while adjusting for LDL levels made no difference. So the worthwhile adjustments made were for age, smoking, hypertension, social class, amount of exercise, and recent changes in drinking frequency.

From the Results section of the paper's Abstract: "After...[adjustments]...people in all categories of drinking (up to more than 56 drinks per week) had at least a 40% reduction in risk of fatal [CVD] and non-fatal coronary heart disease [better called non-fatal myocardial infarction, NFMI] compared with never drinkers." A quick look at their Table IV for men who drank 36-56 drinks per week showed RR = 0.58 for NFMI or fatal CVD, but the 95% CI values were 0.27-1.28 (see Introduction for explanation of CI). Thus this finding was not significant, since 1.28 is more than the value of RR = 1.00 for the never drinkers, the reference group. For women who drank 36-56 drinks per week the RR = 0.42 for NFMI or fatal CVD, but the 95% CI values were 0.04-4.4, so there was no significance at all to this finding (Jackson et al., 1991). The data in their Table IV were adjusted for age, smoking, hypertension (which may not have been relevant, see Myth 4), social class and exercise (which may not have been relevant, see Myth 6), and it did not provide or allow calculation of *absolute* changes in risks or benefits. This study also had the extreme flaw also found in the the studies cited by Dr. Barnard — no all-cause death rates were determined, easy as it would have been to do so, and so no one can make any rational decisions based on this study.

Australian observational study, 1997

One of the studies related to the World Health Organization's MONICA project, which monitored trends in CVD in more than 20 countries over 10 years, was an Australian study which fixated, as usual, on the incidence of NFMI and fatal CVD. While these outcomes were as useless as those of most of the other alcohol studies, because there were no all-cause death rates, something of value was learned. Compared with non-drinkers, those men who consumed 1-4 drinks daily on 5-6 days per week had a RR = 0.31 for any major coronary event; this was the most effective level of consumption. This amounted to absolute levels of 95.9% of non-drinkers with no event compared with 98.5% of moderate drinkers with no event, a gain of 0.26% per year.

Note how a RR of 0.31 for moderate drinkers seems so much more impressive than an absolute risk reduction of just 0.26% per year, just as it does for typical drugs for chronic conditions (see Myths 1, 3, 4). Occasional binge drinkers fared much worse by consuming the same weekly amount of alcohol during just 1 day. Women who consumed 1-2 drinks daily on 5-6 days per week had a RR = 0.33 for any major coronary event; this was the most effective level of consumption. This amounted to absolute levels of 96.8% of non-drinkers with no event compared with 99.2% of moderate drinkers with no event, a gain of 0.24% per year.

If alcohol were handled as a drug, the number needed to treat (NNT) would be 417 women to prevent 1 NFMI or fatal CVD event (combined) in 1 year. As is so common, the authors did not give any of the absolute results. All types of drinks were included (McElduff & Dobson, 1997). Their excuse for not recommending alcohol consumption at the most "beneficial" levels was not the lack of all-cause death rates in their data, or the lack of absolute risks, but the fear of abuse and alcoholism! Then why bother to waste money doing the study?

McElduff & Dobson also found that 1-2 drinks in the 24 hours preceding a NFMI lowered the RR to 0.74 in men and to 0.43 in women compared with that of non-drinkers. Contrarily, a more recent study found that use of alcohol within 24 hours of a NFMI had no effect on the infarct size, arrhythmias or CHF in 399 drinkers (83.5% male), in 3 medical centers in Boston, MA, USA (Mukamal et al., 1999). All types of drinks were included, and the type made no difference to the outcome. So there is no solid evidence that gulping alcohol in anticipation of a heart attack will do any good.

Scottish male drinkers, 21-year follow-up, 1999

A 21-year follow-up of the fate of 5766 Scottish men vs. their drinking habits was presented as relative risks only in a prospective cohort study. The raw data was adjusted for age, and then further adjusted for smoking, BMI, cholesterol, social class (1 of 6), father's social class (1 of 6), education, car use, siblings, angina, CVD, bronchitis, diastolic blood pressure (DBP) and others. Since there was no accounting for how the adjustment for cholesterol was done (see Myth 3) or how DBP was handled (see Myth 4), the adjusted figures are suspect. The authors concluded that total mortality was higher for men drinking more than 3 drinks per day, and that there was a strong positive correlation between stroke and alcohol consumption, rising to to a RR ≈ 2 for > 5 drinks per day vs. none.

The relation so often reported in the past with protection against CVD was very slight, with 87-91% of men not dying of it (Hart et al., 1999). Because the absolute numbers of men in each group of consumption was provided along with the absolute numbers of death for each, the results could be calculated in a more meaningful manner (Table 5-3). The slight protection of ≤ 2 drinks per day can be seen, peaking at 1-2 drinks per day as in other studies. However, the absolute percentages of men *not* dying from stroke (85% hemorrhagic plus 15% ischemic) were so high, 97-98% at all levels of alcohol intake, that there was no reason to reduce consumption to prevent stroke.

However, for non cardiovascular causes of death, the ones not given in the study, more than 1-2 drinks per day were more lethal, especially >5 drinks per day (Table 5-3). Here is an excellent example of how selection of only cardiovascular causes of death, as in all the studies cited by Dr. Barnard, can be dangerously misleading.

| Figure 5-3. Absolute Rates of Mortality of 5766 Scottish Men after 21 Years of Follw-Up vs. Amounts of Alcohol Consumed. (Calculated from raw data in Hart et al., 1999.) | | | | | | |
|---|---|---|---|---|---|---|
| Outcome | Drinks/Day | | | | | |
| | 0 | $\leq 1$ | 1-2 | 2-3 | 3-5 | > 5 |
| % Alive, Total | 73 | 75 | 75 | 68 | 66 | 63 |
| % No CHD Death | 89 | 89 | 91 | 87 | 88 | 87 |
| % No Stroke | 98 | 98 | 98 | 97 | 97 | 97 |

**Stockholm County, Sweden, 26-year follow-up, 2001**

Not all studies are "fatally" flawed, however. An unusually good one was reported in 2001 from the Karolinska Institute, Stockholm, Sweden (Theobald et al., 2001). All-cause death rates totaling 14% were separately determined for all common causes of death among 28,000 residents of Stockholm County, Sweden, who were 50.5% female and followed for up to 26 years. All subjects were grouped into tertiles of alcohol consumption. Low consumers drank < 4.5 drinks per week, moderate consumers had 4.5 - 12.5 drinks per week (near enough to 1-2 per day), and high consumers had > 12.5 drinks per week. Causes of death and main diagnoses during hospitalization were recorded according to standards of the World Health Organization. The autopsy rate was about 40% and the findings were taken into account by physicians who issued the death certificates.

Table 5-4 clearly shows that low and moderate consumers of alcohol have about the same all-cause death rate. Use of relative risks is accepted here because the absolute overall level of mortality was given at 14%, so one can calculate that a mortality RR of 1.48 would mean that 21% of the male high intake drinkers died. High consumers have an elevated all-cause death rate mainly due to accidents (falls, car crashes), poisoning and gastrointestinal illnesses (ulcers and bleeding from esophageal varicosities — swollen blood vessels that burst and are difficult to treat). All types of drinks were included. Moderate drinkers do not live significantly longer than low-level and non-drinkers. Male heavy drinkers were about 40% more likely to die, since their RR of mortality was 1.48 *and* the 95% CI range (1.36-1.61) does not cross the reference level of RR = 1.00. It is tempting to look at the low-intake RR of 0.69 for accidents and poisoning, but the CI range (0.44-1.09) *does* cross the value of 1.00, so this does not allow you to say that low alcohol intake makes people less accident-prone than moderate intake. High intake is another story, though.

Table 5-4. Mortality according to alcohol intake, from various diseases. The reference group were the moderate consumers whose RR = 1.00. Age-adjusted risk ratios (RR) with 95% confidence intervals (CI) are shown.

MEN

| | Alcohol Intake | |
| | Low | High |
| Diagnosis | RR (CI) | RR (CI) |
| --- | --- | --- |
| Total mortality | 1.09 (0.97-1.22) | 1.48 (1.36-1.61) |
| Coronary heart disease | 1.16 (0.95-1.42) | 1.10 (0.92-1.31) |
| Cerebrovascular disease | 1.31 (0.86-2.00) | 1.58 (1.12-2.22) |
| Cardiovascular diseases | 1.23 (1.05-1.44) | 1.28 (1.12-1.46) |
| Accidents/poisoning | 0.69 (0.44-1.09) | 2.10 (1.67-2.65) |
| Gastrointestinal diseases | 1.31 (0.62-2.83) | 4.65 (2.93-7.36) |

WOMEN

| | | |
| --- | --- | --- |
| Total mortality | 1.19 (1.07-1.32) | 1.40 (1.14-1.71) |
| Coronary heart disease | 1.18 (0.92-1.51) | 0.98 (0.53-1.81) |
| Cerebrovascular disease | 1.26 (0.90-1.75) | 1.19 (0.57-2.48) |
| Cardiovascular diseases | 1.25 (1.07-1.47) | 1.03 (0.70-1.51) |
| Accidents/poisoning | 1.09 (0.74-1.61) | 2.95 (1.82-4.78) |
| Gastrointestinal diseases | 1.42 (0.72-2.80) | 3.60 (1.40-9.24) |

Low alcohol intake was < 4.5 drinks per week.
Moderate intake was 4.5-12.5 drinks per week (1-2 per day).
High intake was > 12.5 drinks per week.

Adapted from Theobald et al., 2001.

Table 5-5. Hospitalizations according to alcohol intake, from various diseases. The reference group were the moderate consumers whose RR = 1.00. Age-adjusted risk ratios (RR) with 95% confidence intervals (CI) are shown.

### MEN

| | Alcohol Intake | |
| | Low | High |
| Diagnosis | RR (CI) | RR (CI) |
| --- | --- | --- |
| Total mortality | 0.98 (0.92-1.05) | 1.16 (1.10-1.22) |
| Coronary heart disease | 0.99 (0.84-1.18) | 1.11 (0.97-1.27) |
| Cerebrovascular disease | 1.03 (0.84-1.29) | 1.40 (1.19-1.65) |
| Cardiovascular diseases | 1.03 (0.93-1.14) | 1.25 (1.16-1.36) |
| Accidents/poisoning | 0.88 (0.77-1.00) | 1.37 (1.25-1.49) |
| Gastrointestinal diseases | 1.04 (0.62-2.83) | 1.21 (1.11-1.32) |

### WOMEN

| | | |
| --- | --- | --- |
| Total mortality | 0.95 (0.90-0.99) | 1.03 (0.95-1.11) |
| Coronary heart disease | 1.29 (1.07-1.54) | 0.97 (0.65-1.43) |
| Cerebrovascular disease | 1.14 (0.96-1.35) | 1.04 (0.73-1.48) |
| Cardiovascular diseases | 1.12 (1.03-1.21) | 1.05 (0.90-1.22) |
| Accidents/poisoning | 1.01 (0.92-1.10) | 1.48 (1.29-1.71) |
| Gastrointestinal diseases | 1.08 (0.99-1.18) | 0.98 (0.83-1.06) |

Low alcohol intake was < 4.5 drinks per week.
Moderate intake was 4.5-12.5 drinks per week (1-2 per day).
High intake was > 12.5 drinks per week.

Adapted from Theobald et al., 2001.

Table 5-5 on hospitalization rates shows that low-level and non-drinkers are no less healthy than moderate drinkers. Admissions of high alcohol consumers, both men and women, were significantly higher for accidents and poisoning. For men who were high alcohol consumers, hospital admissions for stroke ("cerebrovascular disease") and imminent mortality were higher.

Table 5-6 shows that there was a statistically significant, but not great difference in all-cancer levels that is inversely proportional to the tertiles of alcohol consumption. Only esophageal, pancreatic, bronchial and lung cancer rates are significantly higher in high-level drinkers, and the authors thought cancers in the latter pair were due to increased smoking levels in that group, for which no correction could be made. Tables 5-4, -5 and -6 are number-dense because the 95% confidence intervals (CI) are included. This was done so you could see how many of the 95% CI limits of both the low and high intake drinkers overlapped the reference value of 1.00 for the moderate drinkers. Overlap means the finding is not statistically significant. Some of the risks suffered by the heavy drinkers were quite significant, exposing the truth that some of the trials presented by Drs. Barnard and Pauling did not allow for confounders or have a long enough time period, or all-cause mortality. In general, rich people drink more, but also can afford better food and medical care.

Table 5-6. Cancer incidence according to alcohol intake, from various diseases. The reference group were the moderate consumers whose RR = 1.00. Age-adjusted risk ratios (RR) with 95% confidence intervals (CI) are shown. Both men and women.

| | Alcohol Intake | |
| | Low | High |
| Cancer Diagnosis — Type | RR (CI) | RR (CI) |
| --- | --- | --- |
| All types except leukemia | 0.79 (0.72-0.87) | 1.13 (1.01-1.25) |
| Leukemia | 0.93 (0.65-1.33) | 0.82 (0.54-1.24) |
| Esophagus and ventricle | 1.03 (0.60-1.76) | 1.95 (1.16-3.18) |
| Pancreas | 1.14 (0.62-2.09) | 1.91 (1.05-3.47) |
| Colon | 0.78 (0.53-1.16) | 0.96 (0.63-1.47) |
| Breast (females) | 0.87 (0.70-1.07) | 1.05 (0.73-1.51) |
| Pulmonary (bronchi and lung) | 0.72 (0.49-1.05) | 1.62 (1.19-2.22) |

Low alcohol intake was < 4.5 drinks per week.
Moderate intake was 4.5-12.5 drinks per week (1-2 per day).
High intake was > 12.5 drinks per week.

Adapted from Theobald et al., 2001.

Russian men in Novosibirsk, 9.5-year follow-up, 2002

Much harder to interpret was a prospective cohort study based in Novosibirsk, population 1.4 million, the third largest city in Russia. Examination of alcohol intake in 6502 men (no women), who were 25-64 years old at baseline and followed for a median of 9.5 years, included the all-cause death rate. An arbitrary set of six levels of consumption were considered: non-drinkers, <0.5 drink/day, 0.5-1.0, 1.0-1.5, 1.5-2.0 and >2.0 drinks per day. Even 2 drinks per day is quite moderate consumption compared with some of the higher levels reported in earlier studies. As you would expect, there was no significant difference in all-cause mortality in any of these groups, nor was there any for heart deaths or stroke deaths or "other causes". Binge drinking "only" doubled the risk of all-cause or heart deaths. It was not thought to be under-reported because even binge-drinking in Russian men does not bear a social stigma! So here, too, moderate drinking is no more healthy than non-drinking when the scatter (large CI intervals) in the data are considered (Malyutina et al., 2002).

## So What About Those Antioxidants in Red Wine?

The antioxidants are known by several names: flavonoids, phenols, polyphenols, etc. Assays confirm that the content of phenols in white wine are 0.01% by weight, and that in red wine are 0.1-0.2% (Singleton & Butzke, 1998). There was no evidence found in long-term trials of the effects of alcoholic beverage consumption in humans to indicate any specific benefit of any or all of the phenols on freedom from NFMI or lowered all-cause death rates. There is no agreement on which antioxidants in red wine are beneficial for the long term (Miller & Rice-Evans, 1995), and other components in wine may yet turn out to be more important for what small health benefit there may be.

In a study carried out in Aarhus University Hospital, Denmark, seven-week-old mice who were bred to be artificially atherosclerotic were randomized to receive water, red wine diluted 1:1 with water (to be 6% in alcohol content), 6% alcohol, or red wine powder in water. At the age of 26 weeks the mice were sacrificed and examined. All groups had advanced atherosclerosis in part of the aorta, and less advanced cases in another major blood vessel. This showed that for advanced and clinically relevant atherosclerosis in mice, neither alcohol nor the other components of wine made any difference (Bentzon et al., 2001).

One recent Australian study was also carried out on mice who were bred to be artificially atherosclerotic. This is not really similar to the development of atherosclerosis in humans. Some mice were given de-alcoholized red wine (DRW) and they were compared with control mice who were not. Several surrogate endpoints that involved assaying concentrations of this or that in serum were checked with inconclusive results. Lipid deposition in the aortas of mice given red wine was significantly (60%) less than in the controls after 26 weeks. For various and hard-to-explain reasons the authors concluded that the protective action of the antioxidant polyphenols (flavonoids) in de-alcoholized red wine was independent of any antioxidant action. They also noted that earlier studies showed inconclusive results on the effects of red wine or de-alcoholized red wine on LDL oxidation in humans and in animal models (Waddington et al., 2004).

In another study carried out in Australia, wine, red wine, or de-alcoholized red wine all worked equally well with vitamin E to prevent oxidation of fatty proteins *in vitro,* showing that the presence of alcohol was not needed to observe this effect. The DRW in artificially atherosclerotic mice decreased atherosclerosis somewhat after 24 weeks in only a part of the aorta of the mice so treated. An unusual observation was that mice treated with DRW had larger coenzyme Q9 and Q10 concentrations in their blood plasma, and triple the concentration of Q9 and Q10 in their aortic lipids (Stocker & O'Halloran, 2004).

Both studies are too short in duration and too far removed from human experience to be of any value in deciding what we should drink. Neither included mortality of any sort in the mice.

Table 5-7. Serum Antioxidant Capacity (SAOC) increases by Ingestion of Red Wine, White Wine or Vitamin C (from data in Whitehead et al., 1995.)

| Substance | Increases in SAOC after... | |
| --- | --- | --- |
| | 1 hour | 2 hours |
| Red Wine, 300 mL | 18% | 11% |
| White Wine, 300 mL | 4 | 7 |
| Vitamin C, 1 gram | 22 | 29 |

Table 5-8. Relative Antioxidant Capacity of Various Drinks. Adapted from Whitehead et al, 1995.

| Drink | Relative Antioxidant Capacity |
| --- | --- |
| Red wine (9 varieties) | 10-21, mean 15 |
| White wine (4 varieties) | 9-13, mean 11 |
| Apple Juice | 8 |
| Orange Juice | 2 |
| Grape Juice | 0.7 |

The study that seems to have been the basis for the sudden enthusiasm for red wine in the late 1990s was carried out, appropriately, in the Department of Pathology of the University of Birmingham, England, UK (Whitehead et al., 1995). People, not mice, were given either 300 mL of red wine (an amount that would inebriate this author), 300 mL of white wine, or 1 g of vitamin C. An accepted assay for the serum antioxidant capacity (SAOC) of the subjects was carried out 1 hour and 2 hours after ingestion of the wine or vitamin C with the results shown in Table 5-7. While the red wine increased antioxidant capacity more than the white wine, the increases were minor, and pale in comparison to the effect of 1 g of vitamin C after 2 hours. Of course, the vitamin C is much cheaper, does not intoxicate, and has fewer other side-effects than wine, or the sulfites added to most wine sold in the USA. How very odd, then, that not a single recommendation for red wine based on this study is accompanied by a much stronger one for vitamin C. Many other assays might have been carried out instead of SAOC; the choice was arbitrary. This study did, however, reveal another failing in grape juice (freshly squeezed in this case) — it has only 1/23 the antioxidant ability of a typical red wine (Table 5-8). Apple juice had over 1/2 the antioxidant ability of a typical red wine.

The abnormal publicity for the Whitehead et al. study began with a wildly enthusiastic editorial in the same journal, *Clinical Chemistry*, in which the antioxidant ability of vitamin C was acknowledged, yet the supposed virtues of wine alone were rhapsodized (Goldberg, 1995).

Short-term studies in mice and humans such as these, with only surrogate endpoints, cannot reasonably be extrapolated to a recommendation for long-term use of red wine to provide benefits in humans. Besides, the results are conflicting. Only the results of very long-term studies in humans as given above that include all-cause death rates can be the basis for medical advice of any value. Those studies do not show any worthwhile absolute benefit of moderate drinking even when a benefit is statistically significant. One must wonder whether the pervasive testimonials for drinking red wine or other alcoholic beverages stem from attempts to justify a lust for alcohol. Dr. Barnard's quotation of Dr. Goldberg on a 40% reduction in CVD by consumption of 2 glasses of red wine daily (a relative, not an absolute risk, and with mostly non-fatal end-points) was not based on a trial, but was lifted from an opinion in a book by another author.

How fascinating, then, to find that Chemistry Professor Joseph A.Vinson, University of Scranton, PA, assayed many foods for total antioxidant content, to find that the average red wine contained 200 mg of antioxidants per 100 mL, less than half of what he found in coffee — 433 mg per 100 mL (Vinson, 2005).

And by no means are any real benefits of phenolic antioxidants proven for real endpoints, such as mortality, even in test animals, let alone in humans.


### Summing Up

There is no evidence that moderate drinking of any common alcoholic beverage has worthwhile health benefits overall. At least there are no detriments except for the cost. If you do not already enjoy beer, wine or spirits, there is no reason for you to begin drinking in a vain attempt to obtain longer life. While the reductions of heart attacks and heart deaths brought about by moderate alcohol consumption are statistically significant, because of the number and size of the studies, the absolute effects are too small to matter much. The same finding exists for all-cause mortality.

On the other hand, if your alcohol consumption amounts to 1-2 drinks per day if you are a woman, or 1-4 drinks per day if you are a man, there is no non-financial reason to stop, so long as you are not driving if you are impaired by these amounts.

The sugar content of some beers, some wines, and of liqueurs and cordials can be serious impediments to maintaining a low-carb diet, which was shown in Myth 2 to be a great benefit to about 25% of us and a worthwhile benefit to 50% of us.

Advice to drink grape juice or even grape soda to obtain the antioxidants in red wine ignores the serious effects of the hyperglycemia and consequent hyperinsulinemia their sugar content will cause in many people. Moreover, the concentration of antioxidants in fresh grape juice, at least, is much lower than in any wine or in apple juice.

The antioxidants present in wine and beer may improve the values of assays of components in serum of mice and people, but not as much as vitamin C does. These assays merely give values for surrogate end points. Short-term studies in mice or humans utilizing surrogate end points are as valueless for determination of the effects of alcohol and other components of wine as they are for those of prescription drugs. Moreover, the very long-term epidemiological studies of alcohol consumption in humans include *all* the effects, good or bad, of *all* the substances found in *all* 3 main varieties of alcoholic drinks, including the effects of antioxidants in red wine.

Even the most famous people, Nobel Prize winners, may fall victims of common dogma.

Any *overall* benefit of moderate drinking is minor to non-existent. At least no harm is done.


## Myth 5 Acknowledgements

Frances E. H. Pane, MSLS, William Reinsmith, DA, Alice Ottoboni, PhD, and Fred Ottoboni, PhD, MPH, provided valuable editorial aid. Duane Graveline, MD, MPH, provided the basis for the Synopsis.

## Myth 5 References

Barnard C (2001). *50 Ways to a Healthy Heart.* London, England: Thorsons.

Bentzon JF, Skobenborg E, Moller J et al. (2001). Red wine does not reduce mature atherosclerosis in apolipoprotein E-deficient mice. *Circulation* 103(12):1681-1687.

Goldberg DM (1995). Does Wine Work? *Clinical Chemistry* 41(1):14-16.

Hart CI, Smith GD, Hole DJ, Hawthorne VM (1999). Alcohol consumption and mortality from all causes, coronary heart disease, and stroke: results from a prospective cohort study of Scottish men with 21 years of follow up. *British Medical Journal* 318:1725-1729.

Jackson R, Scragg R, Beaglehole R (1991). Alcohol consumption and risk of coronary heart disease. *British Medical Journal* 303:211-216.

Locke M (2004). Wine labels to give low-carb lowdown. *New York Times,* May 23, p D1.

Malyutina S, Bobak M, Kurilovitch S, Gafarov V, Simonova G, Nikitin Y, Marmot M (2002). Relation between heavy and binge drinking and all-cause and cardiovascular mortality in Novosibirsk, Russia: a prospective cohort study. *Lancet* 360:1448-1454.

McElduff P, Dobson AJ (1997). How much alcohol and how often? Population based case-control study of alcohol consumption and risk of a major coronary event. *British Medical Journal* 314:1159-1164.

Miller NJ, Rice-Evans CA (1995). Antioxidant Activity of Resveratrol in Red Wine. *Clinical Chemistry* 41(12):1789.

Pauling L (1986). *How to Live Longer and Feel Better.* New York, NY: Freeman.

Singleton VL, Butzke CE (1998). "Wine" in *Encyclopedia of Chemical Technology,* 4th ed., Howe-Grant M, Ed., New York, NY:Wiley, p745\.

Stocker R, O'Halloran RA (2004). Dealcoholized red wine decreases atherosclerosis in apolipoprotein E gene-deficient mice independently of inhibition of lipid peroxidation in the artery wall. *American Journal of Clinical Nutrition* 79(1):123-130.

Smith RE, Pinckney ER (1991). *The Cholesterol Conspiracy.* St. Louis, MO: Warren H. Green, Inc.

Theobald H, Johansson S-E, Bygren L-O, Engfeldt P (2001). The Effects of Alcohol Consumption on Mortality and Morbidity: A 26-Year Follow-Up Study. *Journal of Studies on Alcohol* 62:783-789.

Vinson JA (2005). E-mail of 28 Sep 05. Also see Schmid RE (2005). Study: Coffee top source of healthy [sic] antioxidants. *The Trentonian* Aug 29, p10.

Waddington E, Puddey IB, Croft KD (2004). Red wine polyphenolic compounds inhibit atherosclerosis in apolipoprotein E-deficient mice independently of effects on lipid peroxidation. *American Journal of Clinical Nutrition* 79(1):54-61.

Whitehead TP, Robinson D, Allaway S, Syms J, Hale A (1995). Effect of Red Wine Ingestion on the Antioxidant Capacity of Serum. *Clinical Chemistry* 41(1):32-35.

# Myth 6:  Exercise!  Run for your life!  No pain, no gain!

## Synopsis by Spacedoc

Just when I think Doctor Kauffman has exhausted the medical myth topics which have affected me, either personally or in my medical practice, another one emerges – this one in the form of Bruno Balke, PhD, physiologist at the USAF School of Aerospace Medicine beckoning me in 1958 with his finger and stern glance to accompany him on his mid-day run around the base. I had just been assigned to Bruno, one of Wernher Von Braun's cadre of rigid German scientists, for the next month. We were to study bed rest deconditioning, aka - couch potato assessment under the old medical adage "if you don't use it, you lose it". We would go from a two-week bed rest study to one of freely floating in a tank of water for one week.

Now we have proof from MIR and the International Space Station of Mother Earth's gravitational demands that, even with two hours of aggressive exercise daily, we barely are able to stand on our return to Earth, and that our poor bones are more those of an 80-year old woman than a of 30-year old hot-shot astronaut. Same with our couch potatoes defying Earth's gravitational demands hours on end so that even a trip to the refrigerator becomes a stressful event.

Bottom line - we on Earth have evolved muscles, bones and a circulatory system that makes strolling about easily tolerable, requiring barely noticeable effort. If, for any reason we do not maintain our anti-gravity gift of evolution, we lose it, making getting about uncomfortable and stressful. Aging is a major contributor to losing it, making reasonable efforts at exercise such as simply walking about a desirable goal for the elderly. For most of us this same principle holds – exercise sufficiently for routine needs. A balance must be struck. Why exercise for planet Jupiter when you likely are never going to leave planet Earth? The only reason I can think of for stress exercise is so you can more easily overtake some other poor confused masochistic soul. And the price society pays for jocks! Having lost several of my apparently healthy, young colleagues to sudden death during stress exercise, I cannot say I was surprised to read Kauffman's presentation devoted to this subject; but still it got my attention. And sudden death is only one of the prices paid for our running shoes hitting the pavement. Progressive deterioration of cartilage, ligaments and tendons is a problem of truly astronomical proportions, especially when you realize these effects may take years to manifest themselves.

Many years ago, in the midst of all the media hoopla about running for your lives, I recall the words of so many of my patients, "Doctor, I can't run. What am I going to do?" I knew then that our emphasis on stress exercise would be counterproductive and it was. It was then I stopped running and recommended walking to all of my patients including those with angina, emphysema and arthritis. No one was off the hook with those guidelines and it worked. I have found no reason in the last thirty years to change my philosophy. Doctor Kauffman's much needed literature review of this subject confirms my thoughts.

---Duane Graveline, MD, MPH

## Dr. Barnard's Advice on Exercise

Christiaan Barnard, MD, the famous heart surgeon, provides as good a target with his exercise advice as he did with his advice on alcohol:

"You can reach the ripe old age of 120 and even more.  Every hour of fast walking increases your life span by 60 minutes." But later: "Winston Churchill hated sport and lived to be 91. Millions injure themselves in some form of sporting activity every year." "In Germany alone the treatment of [sports] injuries costs over 27 billion marks every year. A large proportion of these injuries are the result of sporting accidents. So why exercise? Because there is no other way which can so easily lengthen our life expectancy." "Sport and exercise help the body in its battle against many illnesses: cancer, arthritis, osteoporosis, migraine, asthma, and stroke." "Exercise activates the body to produce endorphins, the so-called 'happiness hormones'." "Above all, sport and exercise are true miracle workers for the heart. Exercising reduces blood pressure and cholesterol levels, minimizes the possibility of weight gain, and can protect against diabetes — four of the main [sic] risk factors for heart and circulatory diseases."

"There is a good deal of evidence to support the fact that exercise is good for the heart. One of the most important studies was conducted on 10,269 graduates of the renowned Harvard University who were observed over an 8-year time span. The group who took part in two or three hours of endurance training per week had the best results. These graduates were found to have 60% less risk of dying from heart-related illnesses." (Barnard, 2001, pp175-177).

"The most important rule, however, is: if you are 40 years old and have never really exercised then it is advisable before you start a training program to first see a doctor. He or she can ascertain just how much exercise your heart can take. Remember: you can have a heart problem without knowing it and without it affecting your daily life. But as soon as you start with sport or exercise, this problem could become life-threatening." (Barnard, 2001, pp184).

Myth 4 gave evidence that exercise does not reduce blood pressure. When people believe it does, it may be because they have begun to take antihypertensive drugs simultaneously as part of the usual well-intentioned multifaceted attack on high blood pressure. Myths 2 and 3 showed that elevated cholesterol levels are not a danger, quite the opposite. Myth 2 showed that IDDM is a condition related to destruction of the insulin-making cells of the pancreas; and that NIDDM is a result of too much carbohydrate consumption in people with a genetic tendency to make too much insulin; neither can be prevented by exercise. Exercising to an extreme can prevent weight gain or promote weight loss, but often at the cost of other damage to be described later.

Now about those Harvard graduates: notice that Dr. Barnard used his usual relative risk presentation: "...60% less risk..." which means nothing when the absolute risk is unknown. Also Dr. Barnard, as usual, did not consider all-cause death rates: "...of dying from heart-related illnesses." When a Dr. Paffenberger analyzed the 16,936 questionnaires of supposedly healthy Harvard alumni graduating between 1916 and 1950 who had enrolled in this study, he estimated energy expenditure from the activities the respondents reported. Activities ranged from reading to squash, from doing nothing to long distance running and violent team games. The data seemed to indicate that high-level energy expenditure was protective against fatal and non-fatal cardiovascular disease (CVD), but that anything less than high-level energy output was of little or no protective value. A sober reexamination of the survey, which had relied on the graduates answering a questionnaire, showed that respondents were not dying off as fast as non-respondents; therefore, the respondents were a self-selected and not a representative group. Moreover, 1 of 5 respondents who claimed to have no heart disease actually did have CVD. It is quite logical that those who had CVD would have had lower activity levels, either because of symptom limitation such as pain, breathlessness or dizziness, or because of the many ill-defined factors that make sick people do less. Those who had CVD would indeed have increased mortality, but in the study it would be attributed to their inactivity (Solomon, 1984, pp50,56).

Dr. Barnard's best advice "...see a doctor..." contains a conundrum: people who are healthy might or might not benefit from exercise, but Dr. Barnard concedes that people with heart problems could be damaged by exercise. He unwittingly exposes the main logic flaw about exercise: those who are well enough to do strenuous exercise may do it and claim to feel even better. There is a strong placebo effect of believing it will do them good, which includes peer, spouse and boss pressure. Those who are not well enough to exercise strenuously will feel even worse than they might if they had not been pressured to exercise, because the prevailing myth is that they are somehow defective in will. In controlled trials of exercise, there may be a control group of subjects, but there cannot be a placebo group. All trials, therefore, are biased towards reporting benefits from exercise.

The problem with Dr. Barnard's best advice is that people who have no outward signs of CVD or CHF who do check with their physicians on whether they are healthy enough to engage in high energy-level exercise will usually get the "OK" if their heartbeat or EKGs are normal, and their blood pressures are below 140/90 mm Hg (see Myth 4). In diagnosing heart disease it has been common to have the patient undergo a stress test on a treadmill or stairs. Neither physicians nor physical therapists are aware of the significant numbers of false positives and false negatives from stress testing. These make stress testing of almost no additional value. Worse yet, stress tests caused about 9 casualties in 10,000 tests in 1 study, and 1 death in 3,500-10,000 tests was reported in other studies. EKG and BP measurements, along with a medical history, are sufficient to make a determination of heart disease (Solomon, 1984, pp24-43).

Still worse, a form of angiography utilizing a radioisotope, called "exercise radionuclide ventriculograms" was said to have high discrimination between patients with and without CVD, and could discern which ones "should have" bypass or other surgery. Eventually it was discovered that an elementary error had been committed in determining the specificity of the test: only the "sickest of the sick" and the "wellest of the well" had been included. Applied to a group of patients who were between the extremes, the test was no more specific than flipping a coin (Robin, 1984, pp74-75).

And do you see the logic of walking 1 hour to live 1 hour longer? Even if it is true?

## Levels of Exercise

The level of exercise that will be shown to be damaging is high energy-level exercise (Table 6-1). This includes such activities as fast dancing, running, jogging, handball, squash, tennis, long-distance cycling and heavy weight lifting, which will now be called "strenuous exercise". Most of these are performed to be aerobic, that is, intensely enough to cause sweating and panting. Strenuous exercise involves an energy output over 350 kcal/hour by common convention and will refer to any activity that occasionally causes sweating, pain, nausea, dizziness, etc. in people who are judged fit enough to do it. Medium-level exercises are not in the same class, such as fast walking, gardening, swimming, slow dancing, and hiking with a backpack on trails. Low-level exercise, such as walking on flat surfaces or lifting light weights or doing mild isometrics, is not usually stressful.

The goal of this chapter is not to debunk exercise altogether, but to show the dangers and adverse effects of strenuous exercise as compared with mild to medium or moderate exercise.

Some books on exercise, but not all of them, fail to note that the energy output of exercise is related to one's body weight. Some use a 154-lb (70 kg) male as the basis, and some use a 125-lb (57 kg) female. Another common failing is giving energy values as calories and not correctly as kilocalories (kcal, 1000 calories). Yet another quirk, not a failing, is that the energy expenditure in doing various types of exercise is not always given per hour, but per 30 minutes or per 20 minutes. In deciding on which exercise you will use and for how long, you should be careful to compare not just the kcal, but also the time span and body weight in the example given so as not to be misled.

146

Table 6-1. Energy Levels of Various Types of Activity for a 154-lb (70 kg) Person in kilocalories (kcal) per hour. Source: http://www.fpnotebook.com/SPO31.htm via http://www.cdc.gov/nccdphp/dnpa/physical

| Light | | Medium | | Strenuous (HELE) | |
|---|---|---|---|---|---|
| Lying or Sleeping | 80 | Yard Work | | Bicycling | |
| | | Gardening | 220 | 5.5 mph | 220 |
| Sitting | 100 | Power Mower | 250 | 11 mph | 440 |
| | | Push Mower* | 460 | 16.5 mph | 660 |
| Desk Work | 110 | | | | |
| | | Bowling | 270 | Dancing | |
| Driving | 120 | | | Slow | 300 |
| | | Golf | | Square | 350 |
| Fishing | 130 | Using Cart | 150 | Fast | 490 |
| | | Walking | 300 | | |
| Standing | 140 | | | Shoveling | 400 |
| | | Boating | | | |
| Housework | 180 | Canoe, 2.5 mph | 230 | Skating, 10 mph | 400 |
| | | Rowing, 2.5 mph | 300 | | |
| | | | | Skiing | |
| | | Swimming, .25 mph | 300 | Water | 460 |
| | | | | Downhill | 600 |
| | | Walking | | Cross-Country | 900 |
| | | 2 mph | 150 | | |
| | | 3 mph** | 240 | Raquet Sports | |
| | | 4 mph | 330 | Badminton | 350 |
| | | | | Tennis singles | 420 |
| | | | | Squash | 600 |
| | | | | Raquetball sing. | 775 |
| | | | | | |
| | | | | Running | |
| | | | | Jogging, 5 mph | 640 |
| | | | | Moderate, 6 mph | 750 |
| | | | | Fast, 10 mph | 1200 |

1 kcal = 4.2 kJ
1 mile = 1.6 km

*From McCully & McCully, see Myth #2.
**Calculated by interpolation.

### How did the Strenuous Exercise Exercise Myth Begin?

The specific belief that exercise prolongs your life because it prevents CVD was first promulgated by by Jeremy Morris in a 1953 study of London, England, transport workers. He analyzed the health records of 31,000 male transport workers aged 35-64 years at baseline. He divided them all into just 2 classes of energy expenditure, drivers and conductors. Conductors were an active group, helping old ladies on and off, charging here and there to collect fares, including up and down all the helical stairs in the London double-decker buses. The first results reported were that the conductors had less CVD than the drivers. When CVD did appear in the conductors, it was at later ages, was less severe, so the conductors lived longer. This study is often quoted to this day by the true believers. "Everybody knows" that "exercise is not an option" to be ignored.

But Morris and his colleagues were utterly honest, having listed other possible reasons than activity level for their findings. In 1956 he published that drivers and conductors were not similar people from the outset of their employment or the study. The bus drivers were fatter both in girth and weight and had higher blood pressure than the conductors *when they were hired.* In 1967 R. M. Oliver studied the physiques and "blood fats" of recruits for the jobs of bus driver and conductor before the activity of the job itself could affect the men. Again, the drivers were fatter and more sedentary than the conductors when applying for, or when each was assigned, to his type of job.

In the 1962 study of the American railroad industry, H. L. Taylor of the University of Minnesota School of Public Health analyzed records of 191,000 men, finding lower death rates in more active occupations in the industry and more CVD in men with sedentary occupations. On closer examination of this study report, lower *all-cause* death rates in more active people turned up *only* in workers of *certain age groups.* Lower death rates were observed *only* in those 60-64 years old, when the moderately active were compared with the least active. When the most active were compared with the least active, *all-cause* death rates were lower only in the age group 55-64. Even for CVD deaths, only certain age groups showed the correlation that "everybody knows" must be true, proving that such a weak correlation is not likely to be a cause. Switchmen, who are among the most active, had no statistically significant differences in all-cause death rates (higher) or CVD deaths (lower) than more sedentary workers (Solomon, 1984, pp49-54,57).

Linus Pauling cited a 1964 study on more than a million men and women, and reproduced a graph from the study report on the fate of 461,440 men followed for 2 years to determine death rate vs. exercise. The rates of death rise dramatically in inverse proportion to exercise level as commonly expected. At age 70 the death rates are 20/1000 for no exercise, 9/1000 for light, 5/1000 for medium and 4/1000 for heavy. This was said to correspond with 10-20 years more life for heavy exercisers. Pauling then went on to cite a study in which a 5-year life gain went to people who exercised moderately vs. those who did none, with no advantage to strenuous exercise (Pauling, 1986, p219). Pauling's recommendation was for moderate exercise.

A look at that 1964 article cited by Pauling confirmed that there was little difference on death rates in men between moderate and heavy exercisers. The author, E. C. Hammond, understood that the study had the usual problems with self-selection, with the more healthy men being willing and able to exercise more. He actually wrote: "It is generally thought that exercise is good for health. Conversely, ill health may reduce the ability or desire to indulge in exercise." He understood that he may have found a correlation that was not a cause, the common flaw in epidemiological studies (Hammond, 1964).

## The Early Data on the True "Benefits" of Exercise

In the 1969 Health Insurance Plan study, data were obtained by reviewing the medical records of 110,000 people enrolled in the plan. Most of those who met the criteria for CVD were specially examined and/or interviewed. These were found by questionnaire sent to a random 12% of the lot, of whom 83% responded, a good response rate. But only 156 patients had the special examination *and* the interview *and* answered the questionnaire, and the researchers found that exercise levels did not correspond well between the interview and the questionnaire, so they honestly advised caution in interpreting the results, which are not worth citing here. Other factors that could have contributed to CVD were not even considered.

A 1967 study on Indian railroad workers showed that mortality in sedentary clerks was *lower* than that of the physically active fitters.

148

A 1970 study of Italian railroad workers showed that neither all-cause death rates nor CVD deaths were related to their occupational physical activity. Yet 6 years later, an analysis of 172,459 workers found all-cause death rates higher, but with CVD death rates lower among men performing heavy work compared with moderate and sedentary workers. The heavy work group had more CHF.

In a 1976 study comparing several levels of activity of Finnish men, all-cause mortality was highest for men doing the most vigorous physical activity.

During the burst of enthusiasm for running in the 1970s the "Marathon Hypothesis" was promulgated by T. J. Bassler, MD, a pathologist in CA, USA, and a devoted marathoner. He wrote that marathon running conferred absolute protection against death from CVD! And that any person whose lifestyle allows completion of the 26-mile (42-km) race is immune to dying from CVD (all 6 studies from Solomon, 1984, pp50-51).

Yet the reality is that B.F. Waller and W. C. Roberts, MDs, of the NIH, Bethesda, MD, USA, examined 5 people who died while running. Two of them were marathoners, and none of whom had any overt evidence of CVD before their deaths. All 5 had severe CVD. T. D. Nokes and L. H. Opie, MDs, of South Africa reported evidence of CVD in 4 marathoners. Renu Virmani, MD, of the Armed Forces Institute of Pathology, Washington, DC, found that 6 of 10 marathoners she autopsied had died of CVD. She reviewed the literature to find that, of 57 dead runners, 43 of whom were joggers, CVD occurred in 77% of them and was the most frequent cause of death. She personally then examined 24 other runners, of whom 21 were joggers, of whom 13 died while jogging and 6 soon after, to find that 23 of the lot had severe CVD. P. D. Thompson, MD, of Stanford (CA) University Medical Center found that 13 of 18 jogging-related deaths were due to CVD; most had seen physicians regularly. J. B. Handler, MD, at the Naval Regional Medical Center, San Diego, CA, reported on a 48-year-old man who had no known coronary risk factors, was extremely fit, yet developed CVD after 8 years of running with a 99% blockage of 1 major coronary artery (Solomon, 1984, pp112-114).

Since the early evidence for primary prevention of CVD by exercise is almost non-existent, contradictory or statistically weak, what about secondary prevention? Can exercise prevent the arrhythmia that causes the sudden cardiac death of people with or without CVD? To repeat a bit of Myth 4: one major cardiology text cites a recommendation from the JNC VI for an increase in physical activity for all patients with hypertension who have no specific condition that would make exercise inapplicable or unsafe (Black et al., 2001, p1573). The other major cardiology text recommends exercise for *all* hypertensive patients (Kaplan, 2001, p976,978). Since the most common cause of hypertension is blocked arteries (CVD), the question is: will exercise unblock them? And the answer is: NO! Even the best-designed studies from 20 or more years ago showed no reduction in frequency or severity of heart attacks, no slowing of plaque formation, and no protection from sudden death.

For example, a 1975 report from Sweden covered 315 survivors of MIs who were randomly assigned either to an exercise training program or none. There was no evidence of an exercise influence on either the all-cause death rate or the rate of recurrent MIs.

A 1981 Canadian multicenter study included 733 men who survived an initial MI. Well-matched individuals were randomly assigned to either a strenuous exercise or low-intensity program for 4 years and followed for a total of 7 years. There was a 9.5% rate of repeat MI in the strenuous exercise group and 7.3% of repeat MI in the low-intensity program; this was not statistically significant.

A 1979 WHO study of 375 MI survivors who were randomly assigned to either a comprehensive intervention group including drugs and exercise, or to a control group showed no difference in survival after 5 years. There were more NFMIs in the intervention group, and no difference in either group's ability to do work. Believe it or not, the title of the paper in *The Lancet* was: Reduction [sic] in sudden deaths by a Multifactorial Intervention Programme After Acute Myocardial Infarction.

Reported in 1981, the US National Exercise and Heart Disease Project was scaled back from initially high enrollment to just 651 male patients who had had an NFMI and were assigned to exercise or not, then were followed for 3 years. Result: a barely statistically significant lowered risk of recurrent MI or all-cause death rates; the RR = 0.86 for age-adjusted all-cause mortality for those who exercised.

Several angiographic studies of blood flow did not show any difference brought about by exercise in blood flow in coronary arteries, development of collateral (new) arterial circulation or in progression of CVD, whether in athletes or others (all 6 examples from Solomon, 1984, pp63-67).

## More Recent Data on the "Benefits" of Exercise

Compulsive runners obtained a sense of self, a feeling of control over internal and external circumstances, and spouse or group approbation, the latter partly because of the use of a "uniform" of special clothes and shoes. It is not unusual for runners to lose 25% of their original weight, including nearly all the fat, down to 4-5% body fat, within months of beginning to run (Yates et al., 1983). Were there no side-effects, such as the ones described above as well as in a later section, these would be valuable achievements.

The runners in the Peachtree Road Race of 10 km held on 4 July 1980 in Atlanta, GA, were contacted 11 months later by mailed questionnaire. It seemed that 81% of men and 75% of women who smoked cigarettes before beginning a running program had stopped smoking. This alone, if typical, might explain many of the benefits of running. Weight loss of more than 5 kg was reported by 38% of the men and 16% of the women; the more obese lost more weight, certainly a great benefit (Koplan et al., 1982).

Examined further at 5, 10, 15 and 19-year intervals, those men from the US National Exercise and Heart Disease Project mentioned in the previous section had even fewer benefits of exercise; their RR = 0.92 for age-adjusted all-cause mortality for those who exercised, and was even less significant. CVD mortality was reduced more in the exercisers, but still was not significantly different. The unadjusted all-cause mortality in the exercise group steadily increased over time to a RR = 1.09, but was not significant. What looks more dramatic is that, after 16-19 years of follow-up, 51.4% of the exercise group died vs. 47.0% of the control group (Dorn et al., 1999).

In a 1-year study from the Department of Cardiology, University of Heidelberg, Germany, 45 men with stable angina were randomized to an intervention group participating in strenuous exercise. Of these, 29 lasted the full year. Of a control group of 43 at baseline, 33 lasted the full year. The amount of energy expended in exercise was determined by observation when it was done in group exercising, and by questionnaire. After 1 year the strenuous exercise group increased its oxygen uptake by 7% at the "ventilatory threshold", that is, the transition from aerobic to anaerobic status; while the control group dropped its oxygen uptake by 8%. Using before-and-after coronary angiography, the strenuous exercise group was shown to have reversed its CVD somewhat, while the control group worsened somewhat. Reversal of CVD was associated with leisure time physical activity involving an energy expenditure of 2,200 kcal/week, while halting progression of CVD was associated with an energy expenditure of 1,533 kcal/week. All this was in the Abstract of this article (Hambrecht et al., 1993). Better fitness with strenuous exercise seemed to have been achieved with less CVD, contrary to many of the earlier studies cited above; but see below under Dangers... for the complete and unnerving findings in this study.

Jumping to very recent studies, a prospective multicenter study in the USA on 73,743 postmenopausal women 50-79 years old, who were enrolled in the Women's Health Initiative Observational Study and followed for 3.2 years, compared walking with aerobics (strenuous exercise) to find the effect on the incidence of CVD. Excluded from the study were women who, upon initial examination, showed the presence of any medical condition with predicted survival of <3 years, or alcoholism, mental illness, dementia, lung disease needing oxygen, history of CVD, cancer, stroke, and those who were not ambulatory. Exercise activity level was determined by questionnaire. The level of exercise reported was used to divide the group into quintiles to reveal the results. From the Conclusions of the Abstract of this widely quoted and cited study: "These prospective data indicate that both walking and vigorous exercise are associated with substantial reductions in the incidence of cardiovascular events among postmenopausal women, irrespective of race or ethnic group, age, and body-mass-index. Prolonged sitting predicts increased cardiovascular risk" (Manson et al., 2002). The flaws in this study include non-randomization, since the women just reported on the amount of exercise they did; determination of exercise level by questionnaire; adjustments for a number of factors, including at least 3 of doubtful validity, such as the amount of saturated fat intake (see Myth 2); and the reporting of relative risks without absolute risks.

A more realistic interpretation of the results may be seen in Table 6-2. Just enough data was given by Manson et al. to make the calculation of absolute risk possible, and thus the key figures — the % in each quintile of exercise level, whether walking or aerobic, who had NO cardiovascular event (MI, sudden cardiac death, bypass surgery, stents, CHF, stroke) during the 3.2 year period. Since almost any amount of walking or aerobics in any of the top 4 quintiles gave about the same result compared with the lowest quintile, the only conclusion that can be drawn is that the women who had

Table 6-2. Realistic Results of Exercise Levels vs. CVD Incidence in Post-Menopausal Women Aged 50-79 at Entry and Followed for 3.2 Years (mean). Data from Manson et al., 2002.

|  | Quintile of Exercise Level | | | | |
|  | 1 (lowest) | 2 | 3 | 4 | 5 (highest) |
| --- | --- | --- | --- | --- | --- |
| Subjects (N) | 13,890 | 14,011 | 14,234 | 15,296 | 14,679 |
| **Walking** | | | | | |
| Number with CVD Event | 550 | 322 | 249 | 236 | 194 |
| % with NO CVD Event | 96.04 | 97.70 | 98.25 | 98.46 | 98.68 |
| **Aerobic Exercise** | | | | | |
| Number with CVD Event | 1,220 | 125 | 78 | 61 | 67 |
| % with NO CVD Event | 91.22 | 99.11 | 99.46 | 99.60 | 99.54 |

little to no exercise were very sick at baseline, despite some medical examination, and many exclusions at baseline. This is the lowest quintile in each group. In the top 4 quintiles there were minor benefits in proportion to the amount of walking. Moreover, while the energy expended in the top quintile of walking was twice that in the fourth quintile, and that was twice what was in the third quintile, and so on, the differences in outcome (number of events) were insignificantly different from the second through fifth quintiles. And for aerobics, while the energy output in each quintile was 2/3 of the next higher one, the differences in outcome were quite small in the top four quintiles (Table 6-2). The top quintile of strenuous exercise did not even have the fewest events among the top four. There were more than twice as many events in women who attempted minimal aerobics as in those who attempted minimal walking. Here is persuasive evidence that people not fit to do exercise are harmed by it. The lack of all-cause deaths may be forgiven because there would not have been enough for persuasive statistics, even for these authors.

Of course, there is no lack of articles on the benefits of exercise. A meta-analysis of 38 studies of the relationship between physical activity and all-cause mortality in women reported a mean RR = 0.66 for the women doing the most exercise vs. those doing the least (Oguma et al., 2002). The self-selection effect was not recognized. Only 23 of the studies reported any effect with statistical significance. All results were given as reduced RR with no absolute values at all, and no indication of how many years of life were gained. The benefits were said to be similar to those in men. It is likely that the true picture overall is similar to what is shown in Table 6-2.

A University of Colorado (USA) team found that a retrospective study on 138 men showed that those who did habitual aerobic-endurance exercise had less large artery (such as the aorta) stiffness than those who engaged in moderate activity or had a total lack of aerobic exercise; this is favorable. However, the thickness and mass of the left ventricle of the heart, which increase normally with age, accompanied by less pumping ability (CHF), was worsened by strenuous exercise, but not by moderate activity or a total lack of aerobic exercise. To confuse the issue, the authors called the no-aerobics group sedentary, but it was not (Gates et al., 2003).

A Belgian team of cardiologists found that arrhythmias and other abnormalities found by EKGs are common in athletes, but generally thought to be benign. The outcomes over 4.7 years (median) in 46 endurance athletes (80% cyclists, 45 male, median age 31 years) who had arrhythmias at baseline were observed. There were major arrhythmias in 18 with sudden death in 9 athletes, all cyclists, and in the younger ones at that (23 years old vs. 38 years old for survivors). Imagine — 20% dead in under 5 years in this young group! This outcome could not be predicted by any symptoms at baseline or non-invasive evaluation of arrhythmias. Endurance cycling was considered by these cardiologists to be more stressful than running (Heidbüchel et al., 2003).

A large number of recent studies report "favorable" effects of strenuous exercise by measurement of surrogate endpoints, from TC and LDL levels (Walsh et al., 2003) to resting heart rate (Carter et al., 2003) to improved blood flow, etc. All that is accomplished is to confirm that fitness is improved by strenuous exercise, not that longer life will result (Rosenwinkel et al., 2001).

Recently, studies have appeared purporting to show cognitive improvement in elderly women after aerobic exercise by means of magnetic resonance imaging of their brains, showing less loss of tissue densities in key areas, thus extending the benefits of aerobic exercise "beyond cardiovascular health" (Colcombe et al., 2003). This is merely another short-term study utilizing a surrogate endpoint, and it is of no value in making long-term decisions on how much to exercise.

One of those studies with a surrogate, yet pretty reasonable endpoint — following the change in thickness of the wall of a carotid artery by ultrasound — was carried out in Eastern Finland. Less thickening is the better outcome. Half of 140 middle-aged white men were assigned to an exercise group or to a control group and followed for 6 years. The exercise group became more fit as shown by a 20% increase in the ventilatory threshold. However, there was no difference found in carotid artery wall thickness between groups at the end of 6 years, and very little in favor of the exercise group at years 3 and 5. Of men not taking statin drugs (see Myth 3) there was less wall thickening at the end of 6 years in the exercise group by 0.05 mm, a minor change. Since there were reversals between the groups at years 2 and 4, there was no benefit overall in the exercise group in this time frame (Rauramaa et al., 2004).

By now you have been made aware that medical scientists usually approach a study with a pre-conceived notion of the outcome. The most the rest of us can hope for, as these scientists are spending our tax dollars, is that they will report their findings honestly, and many do. When a study on a major topic, say diet, has a quiet check on some other factor, say exercise, that is buried in the text of the paper and is not in the figures, or in the tables, or abstract or press release, it is buried treasure indeed. Such is the case from within reports on the two following diet studies.

The first observational study was from the Harvard School of Public Health and nearby institutions presented in Myth 2 on the bad effect of high *trans* fat intake on the RR of study subjects suffering CVD (Willett et al., 1993). Factors other than diet and vitamin supplements were checked for their influence on the RR of CVD in the Nurses Health Study. One of those factors was the amount of "vigorous physical activity", which was found to have *no* effect on the RR of CVD. Why was this finding buried?

The second observational study was also from the Harvard School of Public Health and nearby institutions and also presented in Myth 2 (Mozaffarian et al., 2004). In this case the actual progression of CVD in postmenopausal women was examined by accurate coronary angiography, so that the changes in the openings of several coronary arteries were followed for 3.1 years. Besides the striking effects of diet given in Myth 2, adjustments by the scientists for the amount of physical activity *had an insignificant effect* on the progression of CVD in these subjects.

As with diet and drugs, there are powerful economic interests who benefit from the sales of clothing, devices, facilities, stress testing, and other medical procedures associated with people who engage in strenuous exercise. Failure to exercise is also used to blame people who contribute to the current obesity epidemic. While there is some truth in this, more blame attaches to the low-cholesterol, low-fat, and bad-fat dietary advice that has been promoted as "heart-healthy" for the last 40 years (see Myth 2).

Recent books on exercise in general or on running will usually have testimonials, but rarely even a single citation to a controlled study that supports the author's claims for benefit (Hahn et al., 2003; Jackowski, 2004; Scott, 2000). There are exceptions (Gittleman, 2004). Most older and some very new books on exercise promote high-carbohydrate diets, even to the extent of recommending the USDA's ill-conceived Food Pyramid (see Myth 2), (Jackowski, 2004; Scott, 2000). Others have at least been enlightened partially but not sufficiently on diet issues (Hahn et al., 2003; Gittleman, 2004; Villepigue, 2004).


## Exercise Advice from Many Authors

Most authors caution that a medical examination should precede and may show that strenuous exercise would be unsafe. Some still think a stress test is valuable despite Solomon's evidence that it is not. All know that the level of exercise must start slowly and be appropriate to the individual. Most caution that bodily signs of stress should be heeded, but we all know how runners are encouraged to press past pain to obtain the vaunted "runner's high", and to succumb to the pressure from trainers, coaches, or co-workers to press on. Careful warming up and cooling down are stressed by some and minimized by others.

A glance at Table 6-3 will show that the range of views of what provides the most beneficial exercise is as varied as opinions on the amount and type of alcohol to drink; admittedly this advice has been oversimplified to fit on 1 page. Atkins and others had the most strenuous program for the youngest people. Barnard had less inflated claims for exercise later in his book, writing that only 10% of human bodies are really built for running with minimal damage, and that any physical activity was better than none. Jackowski, Scott and Whitaker provided no evidence from controlled trials, just testimonials, that strenuous exercise would benefit almost anyone by conferring longer life and weight loss; but like every one of these authors, they had diet and smoking cessation as part of their programs, thus obfuscating the contribution of each, along with the value of the testimonials. None gave the % who dropped out of their structured exercise programs. Atkins, Bernstein, Gittleman, Hahn and Solomon were most aware of the dangers of exercise, and that being more fit (which means being able to do even more exercise) may not make you healthier overall. Bernstein's whole chapter on exercise has the best distinction between aerobic and anaerobic exercise in this whole group of books, and explains the desirability of regressive anaerobic exercise to build muscle mass in order to reduce insulin resistance. This utilizes weight lifting during which one changes to lighter and lighter weights in order to keep going.

The range of advice is understandable considering that all the authors had access to the same peer-reviewed journals, because there is so little agreement among reports of studies, and because many studies were poorly conceived or poorly reported. Much of the advice was colored by the pervasive myths of exercise: (1) that stress tests reveal one's true tolerance for exercise; (2) that sedentary people simply lack will; (3) that athletes and runners live longer than the merely active; and (4) that strenuous exercise prevents CVD and CHF, thus preventing MI and sudden cardiac death.

In fact, there really is no placebo for exercise. Trial subjects in the low or no exercise groups in RCTs will believe they must do worse than people in the exercise group, and most trials are biased. Surveys by questionnaires were shown to be flawed in that the less healthy were less likely to respond.

Table 6-3. Types of Exercise Recommended by Various Experts and/or Authors.

| Source | Recommendations |
| --- | --- |
| Atkins, 2002, pp247-260* | for>35 years old: walking>slow bicycling, stretching, yoga, light swimming, machines, dancing, skating, tennis |
| Barnard, 2001, pp197-219 | sex>fast walking>golf=any physical activity>running |
| Bernstein, 2003, pp200-223* | for diabetics: decreasing anaerobic light weight lifting, exercycle, machines, walking, jogging with cooldown |
| Gittleman, 2004, p xvi ff | stretching, light weight lifting, low-impact aerobics |
| Hahn, Eades, Eades, 2003, pp12-17 | slow light weight lifting, machines, some calisthenics |
| Jackowski, 2004, pp50-63 | stress test, warm-up by aerobic walking, jogging, exercycling, machines, rowing for 5015 min; stretching, 2-30 min of aerobics or light weight lifting, cooldown, all individualized; anerobics for the thin |
| McCully & McCully, 2000, pp148-151* | walking>>swimming>yoga, stretching |
| Scott, 2000, pp18,228-249, 253-264 | running (less when pregnant), stretching, light weight lifting |
| Solomon, 1984, pp122-135 | walking>>swimmming>calisthenics=fastdancing>bicycling>limited jogging |
| Whitaker, 1987, pp74-77 | for diabetics: stress test, aerobic walking, bicycling, swimming, slow jogging, not yoga or weight lifting |

*See Myth #2 for complete citations to these books.

154

How many researchers would be likely to obtain a grant to show that strenuous exercise is *not* beneficial? Most sedentary people do not exercise or do much physical activity because they are sick and/or depressed. People who persist in strenuous exercise for long periods must have been in unusually good condition when they began.

## The Dangers of Strenuous Exercise

What a pity that the complete story is rarely told of the marathon run of Pheidippides, completed in 490 BCE to carry the news of the victory of the Greeks over the Persians. After his run of 26 miles (42 km) from Marathon to Athens, and delivering his message, he dropped dead (Solomon, 1984, p112).

James F. Fixx was addicted to running and wrote the famous jogger's book, *The Complete Book of Running*. He was a marathon runner and a vegetarian on a diet high in carbohydrates and low in protein (see Myth 2). He died on his daily run of a massive heart attack at age 52, proving to the world that neither a bad diet nor exercise will prevent CVD. Fixx admitted in his book that his own research showed that the athletes among his university alumni had a shorter life span than the "couch potato" students.

Dr. Richard K. Bernstein's overweight non-diabetic cousin began jogging with friends when he was about 50 years old. In his second month of jogging, minutes after stopping completely, as was his usual practice, he dropped dead. Bernstein attributed this to not doing a cooldown walk (Bernstein, 2003, pp221-222). Bernstein himself could not benefit from exercise until his serum glucose levels were controlled with a low-carbohydrate diet.

Brian Maxwell was ranked the number three marathon runner in the world in 1977. He and his nutritionist wife, Jennifer, came up with the PowerBar after he had to drop out of a 26-mile marathon race at the 21-mile mark, finally selling their PowerBar company to Nestle SA for $375 million. He collapsed and died of a heart attack at the age of 51 (AP Bulletin of 20 Mar 04), proving that neither strenuous exercise nor a bad diet prevent CVD. Maxwell and his wife were devotees of carbohydrate-loading (Bender, 2004), which was proven useless in trials conducted by Barry Sears and others (see Myth 2).

Harry A. Christensen finished a 5 km fun race, laughed at some jokes of his fraternity brother, and collapsed from a fatal heart attack. He was a controller for a company in Atlanta, GA, and had been a runner for much of his life (Anon., 2004).

Male compulsive runners resemble anorexic women in terms of family background, socioeconomic class, and such personality characteristics as inhibition of anger, extraordinarily high self-expectations, tolerance of physical discomfort, denial of potentially serious disability, and a tendency toward depression, especially when unable to be in motion. Anorexic women and other members of their families are often compulsively athletic. Compulsive runners may demonstrate a bizarre preoccupation with food and an unusual emphasis on lean body mass. It has been postulated that both phenomena represent partially successful attempts to establish an identity. All 3 individual case histories given by Yates et al. of ostensibly typical male runners revealed temporarily debilitating injuries from running. Incidentally, in the compulsive runners examined, all avoided carbohydrates in their diets except for ritual carb-loading before a run (Yates et al., 1983).

There is another common disconnect to confuse the issue: it is possible to be fit from exercise, yet sick with CVD and about to drop dead. Dr. Lionel Opie, Groote Schuur Hospital, Cape Town, Republic of South Africa, reported on some adverse effects of the 52 mile (84 km) Comrades' Marathon run from Durban to Pietermaritzburg, namely the deaths of 3 male runners. A 35-year-old died at home after the run, having reported chest pains during the run; he had 23 years experience as a marathoner. A 19.5-year-old who took part in the Marathon dropped dead in a later run. A third runner suffered sudden cardiac death after a 6-8 mile run, this after several 20-mile runs. His autopsy showed severe CVD with calcified plaques, but no recent clot (Opie, 1975).

In 1976 Dr. Per Björntorp et al., University of Gothenburg, Sweden, reported on normal and overweight subjects after 6 months of physical training. The normal weight subjects lost some weight, but the overweight ones did not. Two years later Dr. Martin Krotkiewski et al. reported on a similar study. Here mildly obese subjects lost some weight, while severely obese subjects gained weight (Groves, 1999, pp86-87).

In a Canadian study, 8 lean subjects, half male, age 30±6 (SD) years, 65±14 kg, and 12 very obese subjects, 42% male, age 36±10 years, 126±31 kg, were all exercised to exhaustion during 7±3 minutes on an exercise bicycle. A number of assays on components of their plasma were made. After an hour post-exercise, both glucose and insulin levels were back to baseline in the lean subjects, but remained elevated in the very obese subjects for the entire hour. Since insulin is the prime fat-building enzyme (see Myth 2) this may be a biochemical confirmation of fat synthesis in the very obese as actually found by Krotkiewski et al. (Yale et al., 1989). Strenuous exercise was certainly contraindicated for the very obese people in this study.

Endurance training, as in the military, allows people to do more and more strenuous exercise. Recruits who are initially able to walk 3-10 miles a day with no load can walk up to 20 miles a day with a heavy back pack after 3-6 months of training...except the ones who could not. They were medically discharged, and thus they were no longer visible on the parade ground. This fitness training did not prevent the high incidence of fatty streaks and plaques found in the arteries of young dead soldiers in the Korean and Viet Nam Wars (Solomon, 1984, p62).

While the benefits of the Peachtree Road Race were given in a previous section, there were adverse effects of running as well. Figure 6-1 shows the mounting damage of running increasing distances per week summarized for a year of running. From 22-70% of runners admitted to injuries during a single year! Taking mean values of injury frequency, fully 37% of men and 38% of women were injured in a single year of general running after the Peachtree Road Race (Figure 6-2). Knees were the most frequently damaged, 14% in a year. The frequencies add up to more than the totals for all sites because of multiple injuries to some runners (Koplan et al., 1982).

Delving into the body of the article on the University of Heidelberg study, whose minor benefits were given in a previous section, revealed that men with CVD of the left main coronary artery, previous angioplasty or bypass surgery, severe CHF, heart valve problems, arrhythmias, uncontrolled hypertension, diabetes (type not given), "hypercholesterolemia" (LDL > 210 mg/dL), or any condition precluding group exercise were excluded from the study. This means that the supposedly favorable results of this study apply only to men with stable angina and no other problems in the list. Moreover, poor randomization favored the intervention (exercise) group, since the controls had much more previous NFMI, more CHF, and were a year older. Even before the initial stress testing, 4 subjects from the strenuous exercise group vs 1 from the control group dropped out. From the strenuous exercise group, 3 more subjects were asked to stop exercise because of rapid heartbeat episodes. From the rapidly shrinking strenuous exercise group there were 4 more who dropped out and could not repeat stress testing at the end of the 1-year period against 3 dropouts and 1 cancer death in the control group. There were 2 cardiac arrests in the strenuous exercise group, 1 of whom was found dead in a street, vs 1 in the control group who was revived. This honest and complete description allows us to realize that there were 16 casualties in the strenuous exercise group of 45 (33%) vs. 10 in the control group of 43 (23%), counting all incidents reported. How could one believe that the strenuous exercise group as a whole became more healthy during the study? Only the survivors might have, and only for a single year. Note from Table 6-1 that the 2200 kcal/week supposedly found to reverse CVD can be expended by 1.3 hours/day of walking at 3 mph (5 km/hr) by a 154-lb (70 kg) person, and it does not necessarily have to be done on a treadmill.

From an editorial in the *European Heart Journal:*

"The general population has the perception that athletes are the healthiest members of society, since they are capable of such impressive physical performance. However, the cardiological community has been interested in the inherent risk of sport for many years. Although it is proven that moderate exercise is helpful in controlling risk factors for coronary artery disease and in decreasing its incidence, several studies have shown that acute myocardial infarction may be precipitated by exercise. On the other hand, athlete's heart is a well-known consequence of sport practice, and has been considered as a kind of physiological adaptation to extreme training. It was not until very recently that athlete's heart... was recognized as a possible risk factor for the development of atrial fibrillation [arrhythmias], establishing a link between excessive training and the presence of arrhythmias.

"Up until now, sudden death in athletes has been attributed to pre-existing cardiovascular diseases..." (Mont & Brugada, 2003)

The study by Heidbüchel et al. described above shows that strenuous exercise, in some individuals, may lead to arrhythmias that produce sudden death.

Uffe Ravnskov, MD, PhD, of Lund, Sweden, pointed out that some of the damage caused in people undergoing strenuous exercise is compounded by their use of performance-enhancing drugs, which have been found by post-mortem examinations by coroners. The use of steroid hormones and other drugs to enhance muscle mass is widespread in gyms in Sweden.

From an editorial in the Wall *Street Journal:*

"Just two years ago, the Institute of Medicine, a Washington-based independent adviser to the government on national health issues, announced its recommendations that people exercise at least an hour a day. That more than doubled recommendations from the Surgeon General and the American College of Sports Medicine, which had advised only moderate exercise at least three to five days a week. The hour-a-day exercise guidelines were widely criticized as being far too onerous and triggered fears that the report would end up setting back efforts to get more people to exercise.

" 'That report was really a disservice to so many people,' says Tim Church, medical director of the Cooper Institute in Dallas [TX], which has pioneered much of the research on exercise and health. 'I literally had participants in our studies who had been doing 30 minutes a day five days a week for the last six months almost crying in our office. They said, "If I have to do that, I'm just going to give up." '

"But much research shows it takes far less effort to reap the benefits of exercise. The most recent study from Sweden followed more than 3,200 men and women over the age of 65 [at baseline]. After accounting for differences in age, education, smoking habits, and illnesses such as diabetes or hypertension, researchers found that people who said they 'exercise only occasionally' still had a 28% lower risk of dying [RR = 0.72] during the 12-year study period than those who described themselves as inactive.

Occasional exercise was was described as exercising less than once a week and even as little as taking a ski trip twice a year. And those who said they exercised at least once a week had a 40% lower chance of dying [RR = 0.60]." (Parker-Pope, 2004).

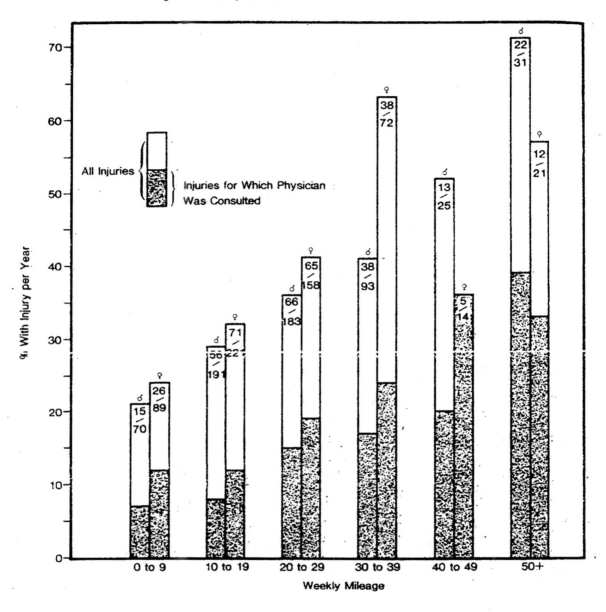

Figure 6-1: Percent of Runners with Injury during One Year according to Distance in Miles Run. Left column of each pair is men, right is women. From Koplan et al., 1982.

Long-term sport bicyclists who did it more than 3 hours per week had 3 times the incidence of erectile dysfunction as moderate bicyclists who did it less than 3 hours per week. The statistics in this epidemiological study could have been better (Marceau et al., 2001).

According to Alayne Yates, MD, former runner, stress fractures from running tend to occur in smaller bones, such as the ankle, and need to be treated to heal properly. Avulsed tendons usually do not protrude through the skin, but need repair. The most common injuries while running are the micro hemorrhages in the major muscles involved, and is the major source of the soreness and stiffness after extreme running.

**Figure 6-2: Incidence Rate of Injuries to Runners in a Single Year of Running. Exressed as Probability of Injury at Each Site. Totals at Any Site Higher than Individual Totals because of Multiple Injuries. Men left, women right. From Koplan et al., 1982.**

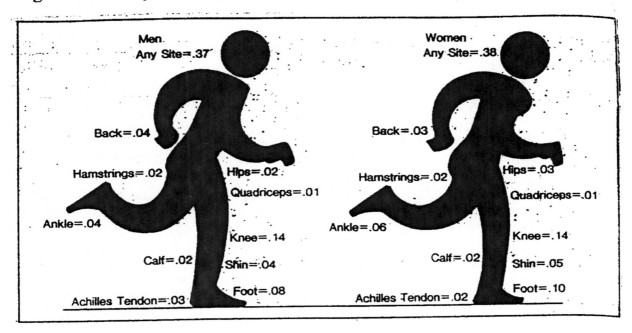

Men.
Any Site=.37

Back=.04

Hamstrings=.02

Hips=.02

Quadriceps=.01

Ankle=.04

Knee=.14

Calf=.02

Shin=.04

Foot=.08

Achilles Tendon=.03

Women
Any Site=.38

Back=.03

Hamstrings=.02

Hips=.03

Quadriceps=.01

Ankle=.06

Knee=.14

Calf=.02

Shin=.05

Foot=.10

Achilles Tendon=.02

## Summing Up

Of the many promises made for aerobics (strenuous exercise), only a few will be realized by most of the converts. Many will simply drop out. Doing aerobics makes one able to do more of them until the long-term damage ends the beneficial phase. One will have more endurance for other activities for a while, maybe even for decades. One may be better able to run away from some peril. The approval of one's spouse, friends, exercise group, or employer will provide a great psychological boost.

Since most exercise programs involve other lifestyle changes, it is uncertain which actually contribute which benefits claimed by the proponents of each program. Only some people will lose weight in these programs, which may be a result of a diet change, better sleeping patterns, smoking cessation, or a boost in self-esteem.

Henry A. Solomon, MD, Cardiologist, Cornell University Medical College, NY, may have overdone it only slightly when he wrote: "There is about the same relationship between activity and longevity as you might find if you were to compare the amount of chocolate pudding children eat with the likelihood of their coming down with chicken pox — that is, no relationship at all... By all indications, you must be truly sedentary — a slug who sits or lies about all day, or barely crawls from bed to breakfast, to car and desk, and back again — to be at any risk from inactivity."

Richard A. Friedman, MD, Cornell-Weill Medical School, and Fred Charatan, MD, retired geriatric physician, expressed the self-selection bias of exercisers as follows: "...I suspect that exercise is more often a marker of health than its cause — healthy people like to exercise more than unhealthy people to start with. And the real value of it is not in terms of abstract health benefits like longevity — an extra few hours or maybe months — but because it feels good when you do it or when it's over. To hell with Hygeia, the truth lies in the pleasure." (Friedman & Charatan, 2004)

Extreme aerobics such as running and marathon cycling not only do not prevent CVD and CHF, they appear to cause them. Knee problems, stress fractures of bones, and joint problems affect a majority of those doing strenuous exercise for years, not a small fraction. Warmup and cooldown phases can help somewhat. Athletes and runners do not live the longest. The mantra "No pain, no gain!" would better be: "More pain, more risk!"

Forced exercise in the very obese may cause cardiovascular problems and no weight loss.

Clinical studies on exercise measuring surrogate endpoints after short periods are about as useful as those employed to recommend cholesterol and blood pressure drugs — not of any use except in guiding researchers on how to perform better long-term studies.

When epidemiological results are reported, the use of relative risks and benefits rather than absolute ones can obfuscate the small size of either or both. Absence of statistical backup does not help either.

In general, people who are not too sick or depressed are active on their own volition. This self-selection process negates the reported results of most epidemiological studies. When RCTs are done, there can be no placebo for exercise as is supposed to be used in drug trials. For this and other reasons, results of such RCTs, in which there has been real randomization of the subjects, do not justify the pervasive exhortations to undertake strenuous exercise. Both types of study often fail to report all-cause death rates, which may include more falls, accidents, or collisions for those doing strenuous exercise.

On the other hand, it is clear that moderate activity such as fast walking, slow swimming, slow dancing, yoga, tai chee, light weight lifting, mild calisthenics, the use of exercise machines and maybe even moderate aerobics will make those who enjoy the activity feel better and possibly even live a little longer. If your body's stress messages are heeded, there will be no harm in such moderate exercises, and some benefits may accrue.

Acknowledgements for Myth 6

Frances E. H. Pane, MSLS, Prof. William Reinsmith, DA, Alice Ottoboni, PhD, Fred Ottoboni, PhD, MPH, and Alayne Yates, MD, critically reviewed this chapter. Duane Graveline, MD, MPH, provided the Synopsis.

References for Myth 6

Anon. (2004). Obituary of Harry A. Christansen. *The Trenton Times,* 22 Oct 2004, p B4.

Barnard C (2001). *50 Ways to a Healthy Heart.* London, England: Thorsons.

Bender K (2004). PowerBar founder was a visionary force. Brian Maxwell was remembered for his grace, charity and his incredible strength. *Oakland (CA) Tribune,* 3 Apr 2004.

Black HR, Backris GL, Elliott WJ (2001). Hypertension: Epidemiology, Pathophysiology, Diagnosis and Treatment in *Hurst's The Heart,* 10th ed., Fuster V et al., Eds., New York, NY: McGraw-Hill.

Carter JB, Banister EW, Balber AP (2003). Effects of endurance exercise on autonomic control of heart rate. *Sports Medicine* 33(1):33-46.

Colcombe SJ, Erickson KI, Raz N, et al. (2003). Aerobic fitness reduces brain tissue loss in aging humans. *Gerontology A, Biological Sciences, Medical Sciences* 58(2):176-180.

Dorn J, Naughton J, Imamura D Trevisan M (1999). Results of a Multicenter Randomized Clinical Trial of Exercise and Long-Term Survival in Myocardial Infarction Patients. *Circulation* 100:1764-1769.

Friedman RA, Charatan F (2004). The truth about exercise. *British Medical Journal* 328(7451):1315.

Gates PE, Tanaka H, Graves J, Seals, DR (2003). Left ventricular structure and diastolic function with human aging. *European Heart Journal* 24:2213-2220.

Gittleman AL (2004). *The Fat Flush Fitness Plan.* New York, NY: McGraw-Hill.

Groves B (1999). *Eat Fat, Get Thin!* London, England: Vermilion/Random House.

Hahn F, Eades MR, Eades MD (2003). *The Slow Burn Fitness Revolution.* New York, NY: Broadway Books, Random House.

Hambrecht R, Niebauer J, Marburger C, et al. (1993). Various Intensities of Leisure Time Physical Activity in Patients With Coronary Artery Disease: Effects on Cardiorespiratory Fitness and Progression of Coronary Atherosclerotic Lesions. *Journal of the American College of Cardiology* 22:468-477.

Hammond EC (1964). Some Preliminary Findings on Physical Complaints from a Prospective Study of 1,064,004 Men and Women. *American Journal of Public Health and the Nation's Health* 54:11-22.

Heidbüchel H, Hoogsteen J, Fagard R, et al. (2003). High prevalence of right ventricular involvement in endurance athletes with ventricular arrhythmias. *European Heart Journal* 24:1473-1480.

Jackowski E (2004). *Escape Your Weight*. New York, NY: St. Martin's Press.

Kaplan NM (2001). Hypertensive and Atherosclerotic Cardiovascular Disease in *Heart Disease: A Textbook of Cardiovascular Medicine,* 6th ed., Braunwald E et al., Eds., Philadelphia, PA: W. B. Saunders.

Koplan JP, Powell KE, Sikes RK et al. (1982). An Epidemiologic Study of the Benefits and Risks of Running. *Journal of the American Medical Association* 248:3118-3121.

Manson J-AE, Greenland P, LaCroix AZ, et al. (2002). Walking compared with vigorous exercise for the prevention of cardiovascular events in women. *New England Journal of Medicine* 347:716-725.

Marceau I, Kleinman K, Goldstein I, McKinlay J (2001). Does bicycling contribute to the risk of erectile dysfunction? Results from the Massachusetts Male Aging Study (MMAS). *International Journal of Impotence Research* 13:298-302.

Mont L, Brugada J (2003). Endurance athletes: exploring the limits and beyond. *European Heart Journal* 24:1469-1470.

Mozaffarian D, Rimm EB, Herrington DM (2004). Dietary fats, carbohydrate, and progression of coronary atherosclerosis in postmenopausal women. *American Journal of Clinical Nutrition* 80:1175-84.

Oguma Y, Sesso HD, Paffenberger Jr RS, Lee I-M (2002). Physical activity and all cause mortality in women: a review of the evidence. *British Journal of Sports Medicine* 36:162-172.

Parker-Pope T (2004). Health Matters. When it comes to exercise a little bit goes a long way. *Wall Street Journal* 9 Aug 2004, pR5.

Pauling L (1986). *How to Live Longer and Feel Better*. New York, NY: Freeman.

Rauramaa R, Halonen P, Väisänen SB, et al. (2004). Effects of Aerobic Physical Exercise on Inflammation and Atherosclerosis in Men: the DNASCO Study. *Annals of Internal Medicine* 140:1007-1014.

Robin ED (1984). *Matters of Life and Death: Risks and Benefits of Medical Care.* Stanford, CA: Stanford Alumni Association.

Rosenwinkel ET, Bloomfield, DM, Arwady MA, Goldsmith RL (2001). Exercise and autonomic function in health and cardiovascular disease. *Cardiology Clinics* 19(3):369-387.

Scott D (2000). *Runners World Complete Book of Women's Running*. Emmaus, PA: Rodale Press.

Solomon HA (1984). *The Exercise Myth*. Orlando, FL: Harcourt Brace Jovanovich.

Vedral JL (1993). *Bottoms Up! The Total-Body Workout from the Bottom Up, From Cellulite to Sexy - in 24 Workout Hours*. New York, NY: Warner Books.

Villepigue J (2004). *The Body Sculpting Bible for ABS. The Way to Physical Perfection. Men's Edition*. Long Island City, NY: Hatherleigh Press.

Walsh JH, Yong G, Cheetham C, et al. (2003). Effects of exercise training on conduit and resistance vessel function in treated and untreated hypercholesterolemic subjects. *European Heart Journal* 24:1681-1689.

Whitaker, JM (1987). *Reversing Diabetes,* New York, NY: Warner Books.

Willett WC, Stampfer MJ, Manson JE, et al. (1993). Intake of *trans* fatty acids and risk of coronary heart disease among women. *Lancet* 1993;341:581-585.

Yale J-F, Leiter LA, Marliss EB (1989). Metabolic Responses to Intense Exercise in Lean and Obese Subjects. *Journal of Clinical Endocrinology and Metabolism* 68:438-445.

Yates A, Leehey K, Shislak, CM (1983). Running — An Analog of Anorexia? *New England Journal of Medicine* 308:251-255.

# Myth 7:  EDTA chelation therapy for atherosclerosis is ineffective, dangerous and a fraud.

## Who Should Be Interested in This Topic?

• You or a loved one who has angina pain
• Non-fatal heart attack
• Any blocked blood vessel for which balloon angioplasty or bypass surgery has been recommended
• Anyone who has swollen ankles or wrists
• Severe edema not relieved by a diuretic
• Anyone who has been recommended to have an amputation
• Anyone who has sores that will not heal because of poor blood circulation
• You or a loved one who has lost the ability to walk more than a few yards or meters because of the pain caused by poor blood circulation

## Synopsis by Spacedoc

The use of EDTA chelation to reduce the risk of atherosclerotic cardiovascular disease has resulted in a 30-year battle between proponents and opponents. The opponents are organized medicine and the pharmaceutical industry. The firm stand of organized medicine is no doubt largely derived from the alternative medicine "flavor" of chelation combined with the extraordinary economic gain from such orthodox treatment options as by-pass surgery and angioplasties, whereas the pharmaceutical stand is basically an economic one of "no money to be made" on such a biochemically simple and therapeutically safe procedure. Imagine, of an estimated 20 million intravenous infusions of EDTA, no ill effects when properly done. This is an extraordinary safety record, far surpassing our safe household favorites, aspirin and Tylenol.

"Chelation doesn't work!" choruses the medical establishment, yet Kauffman's tabulation of some 50 clinical trials document an extra-ordinary 87% success rate based upon very reasonably objective indicators of benefit. His documentation of under-handed and deliberate manipulation of clinical data in support of medically orthodox views for journal presentation makes one cringe to be in the same professional group.

As to mechanism of action of this EDTA, the possibilities range from depriving nanobacteria of their calcium underpinnings to the decrement of LDL and cholesterol oxidation via excess iron store elimination, or perhaps some as yet unproven combination of the two. We all should feel deeply indebted to Doctor Kauffman for the immense effort he has expended in reviewing this difficult subject.

------Duane Graveline MD MPH

## What is EDTA and Chelation?

EDTA is ethylenediaminetetraacetic acid, a very simple synthetic compound first made commercially available in the 1930s. Acetic acid, $CH_3CO_2H$, is the pungent active ingredient of vinegar.  EDTA contains 4 of these attached on the left end thus:  $—CH_2CO_2H$. An amine is just a compound with a nitrogen atom bonded to 3 hydrogens or 3 carbon atoms, or any combination of hydrogens or carbons that adds up to 3. The simplest example is household ammonia, $NH_3$. A diamine has two such groups. An ethylene group (not ethylene gas) is $-CH_2-CH_2-$, so it follows that ethylenediamine is $H_2N-CH_2-CH_2-NH_2$. By removing the 4 outer hydrogen atoms and replacing them with 4 acetic acid groups, one obtains EDTA, which can be written compactly as $(HO_2CCH_2)_2N-CH_2-CH_2-N(CH_2CO_2H)_2$. It looks more formidable only when the structure is given some spreading out and a reasonable shape as in Figure 7-1A.

Figure 7-1A.  Structure of EDTA
ethylenediaminetetraacetic acid)

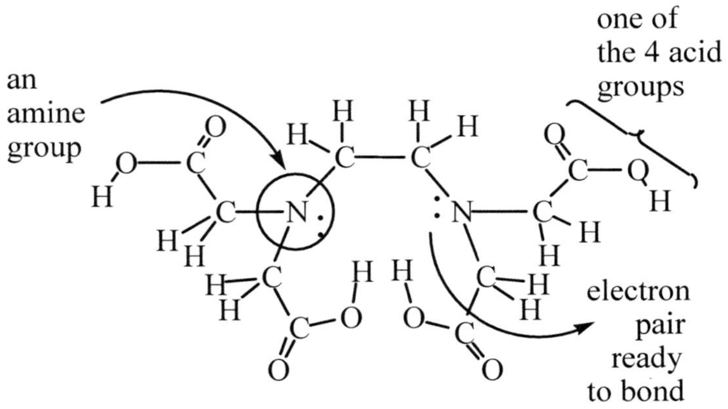

Acetic acid is a weak acid that can donate the hydrogen as an ion with a single positive charge to a base which can accept it. What is left behind is acetate ion with a single negative charge. Usually there is a common positive metal ion nearby such as Na+ to balance the negative charge (-) on the acetate ion. The main ingredient for the EDTA injection solution is purchased as disodium EDTA in which two of the acetic acid hydrogens have been replaced by sodium ions.

Chelation is derived from the Greek word for claw. Where ions of opposite charge are attracted to each other, each still can be interchanged for other ions of similar charge; the individual ions come and go easily in solution in water. But when a ring structure exists, especially a multiple ring structure as shown in Figure 7-1B, the metal ion is bound very strongly, as though held by a claw. This is what is called a chelate. Forming it is called chelation. In the mixture used for injections, magnesium chloride is an important component. The magnesium ion with its charge of 2+ is not only attracted to a pair of acetate ions, but is also attracted to both of the amine nitrogen atoms, each of which provides a pair of electrons for bonding. These electron pairs are negative in charge, as all electrons are. They are shown in Figure 7-1B as short straight arrows. The triple ring structure shown is one form of chelate, and is a very stable chelate.

Metal ions are bound very strongly by this type of EDTA chelate. The ions must have either a 2+ charge (magnesium, calcium, zinc, copper, manganese, mercury) or a 3+ charge (aluminum, iron). Iron is actually held the most strongly and magnesium the least in this listing. When the magnesium chelate is used, a more strongly held metal ion may change places with the magnesium to make a more stable chelate. Either chelate is excreted in urine with no other changes to the EDTA molecule; it is very stable in a human body. Chelates are not so strange. After all, iron is chelated in heme, the part of the red hemoglobin of blood that carries oxygen around. Magnesium is present as a chelate in the green chlorophyll of plants.

Figure 7-1B. EDTA Complex with Magnesium
(disodium magnesium EDTA)
Believed to be the active form that is injected

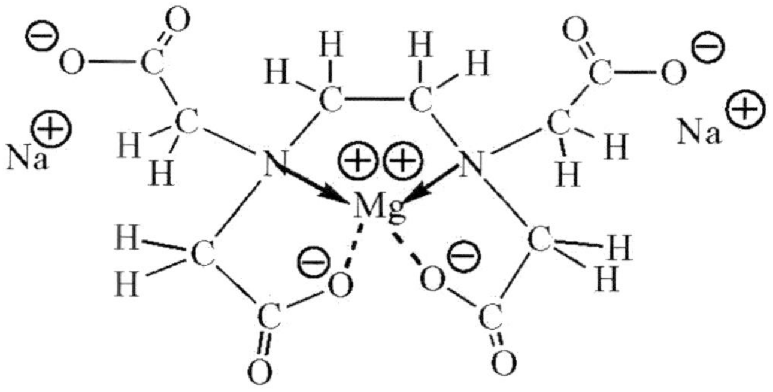

A safe and effective procedure first used to treat heavy metal poisoning, and then later to open up atherosclerotic blood vessels, EDTA chelation therapy has been attacked and vilified by mainstream medicine. The attacks extended to disbarment and delicensing of physicians who used EDTA chelation to treat patients by state medical boards. Randomized clinical trials (RCTs) were rigged to show no benefit from chelation, and the reports on those trials ended up in the most widely circulated peer-reviewed medical journals. The motives of the anti-chelation cliques have been described in detail (Cranton, 2001, pp329-342; Carter, 1992).

\*\*\*\*\*\*

The ingredients of the EDTA chelation solution for injection were optimized about 25 years ago (Cranton, 2001, 431-439). The amounts of each ingredient are usually customized for the weight and condition of the individual patient. Besides the usual 3 g of disodium EDTA in 500 mL of sterile water for a 70 kg patient there are:

Magnesium chloride, which reduces pain from the injection, and is therapeutic for many conditions that may benefit from chelation (see Myth 1);

Sodium bicarbonate, which holds the acidity (pH) of the solution within narrow bounds at the safest level for the body;

Local anesthetic, such as lidocaine or procaine, to prevent pain at the injection site;

Heparin to prevent clotting near the injection site;

Vitamin C as a synergistic chelating agent, antioxidant and free radical scavenger; and

B-complex vitamins, such as B1, B6, B12 and pantothenic acid, mostly as antioxidants. Now we know that some of the benefits of these may relate to lowering homocysteine levels (see Myth 2).

Some other vitamins and minerals are often given orally as supplements. Loss of the mineral manganese is the the most serious consequence of depletions by EDTA; zinc is the next most serious. Both are always given as a supplements by skilled providers of chelation.

The 250-500 mL of completed solution for chelation is usually injected through a small needle or butterfly (24-25 gauge) into a vein in an arm over the course of 1.5-4 hours. One or two injections, called infusions because they must be done slowly for safety and greatest benefit, are usually done at the rate of 1-2 per week for 10-30 weeks, average 20 times for a series. Sometimes the peak of patient response occurs after the end of the series. Often patients may not need additional treatments for

164

months, but the conditions that call for application of this treatment usually mean that more will be needed at intervals as long as the patient lives.

There is some choice among some chelators to give 1.5 g of EDTA in 250 mL of solution during 1.5 hours, if there are time constraints. Elmer M. Cranton, MD, estimated that this gives about 75% of the benefit of the normal 3 g given over 3 hours (his e-mail of 12 Mar 04). Only this lower dose is safe for kidneys if given in the shorter time. The 3 g dose that has been standard must be infused over 3-4 hours.

Pre-treatment examination, customization of the injection solution and injection rates, and careful monitoring of patients, including post-chelation, have helped patients with all kinds of ailments. It is expected that about 44% of patients will have substantial benefits, such as less angina pain, less edema, better and complete healing of sores, such as diabetic ulcers, and more walking distance. Another 44% will have more modest but still worthwhile benefits of the same types. Patients who were totally sedentary may expect to have more capacity for normal activity for household chores and traveling. And many who were supposed to have some potentially dangerous surgery may no longer need it.

Chelation is an excellent alternative to bypass surgery in 80-85% of cases, and should be tried first. The surgeon involved with former President Bill Clinton's bypass surgery quoted a death rate of 1% for bypass surgery. This figure is a generally used ploy to snare patients for bypass surgery. One large study actually found a 5.6% death rate, and another 5.7%. Loss of blood supply from where the replacement blood vessel was taken may cause gangrene and lead to an amputation of a leg. It has been recognized recently that use of a heart-lung machine leaves patients with an IQ loss of 10-12 points. Long term studies show almost no benefit from bypass surgery in mortality after 10 years. Balloon angioplasty may be somewhat safer, but its effects last only a few weeks to months (McGee, 2001, pp20-55).

*****

Oral chelation does not yet have the established record of intravenous chelation for treatment of atherosclerosis. For now it cannot be recommended, but this could change. For removal of certain heavy metals, oral administration of agents other than EDTA are valuable.

## Who Practices Chelation Therapy?

Very thorough training in chelation is necessary before it can be practiced with low risk and eventual benefit to people with atherosclerosis. An organization was set up to do this in 1973; it was re-named and is presently called the American College for Advancement in Medicine (www.ACAM.org). Physicians who have trained with ACAM may be found on the website. There are about 1,000 in the USA. These physicians are the brave ones who honestly try to do what will most benefit patients with atherosclerosis, which is so often preceded by NIDDM. You should expect that these physicians will prescribe fewer drugs and more supplements than a typical MD. Some try too hard to sell too many supplements from their offices, so one must be on guard. On the other hand, most of those willing to administer chelation are enlightened about the myths of mainstream medical practice.

The cost per infusion is usually $90-125. A typical course of 20 infusions runs $2000 and suffices for a year. Most of the time medical insurance will not pay for it, but it always makes sense to apply for reimbursement to show the insurers that there is a demand for chelation. Bear in mind that the co-payments for useless drugs for cholesterol lowering (see Myth 3) and a combination of drugs for blood pressure lowering (see Myth 4) would be about $960 per year. Refusing to take the useless drugs can cover about half the cost of chelation, and relieve you of most of the side-effects of these drug classes.

By 2002 the cost of multiple bypass surgery was about $50,000 (Leduc, 2002) to $65,000. Stenting cost $8,000 to $16,000 in 1998 (Goodwin et al.,1998); but has to be done over in 1-4 years. Naturally, medical insurers happily pay for these procedures, which have mainstream approval.

## Benefits of Chelation

The earliest benefit of chelation was for heavy metal poisoning. In the early 1950s disodium EDTA became an established treatment for serum calcium levels that are too high, a rare condition. Disodium calcium EDTA became the single most effective treatment for lead poisoning, and is so used to this day. The FDA approved it for this use. A recent study from Taiwan showed that too much environmental exposure to lead compounds accelerated kidney failure. Chelation improved kidney function with no toxicity at 1/20 the cost of dialysis (Lin et al., 2003). Other studies showed that some form of EDTA was valuable for removing heavy metals present accidentally in the body as radioactive isotopes.

Reasoning that atherosclerotic plaques that had accumulated calcium ion (Ca 2+), called calcified plaques, might be broken down by removal of the calcium, N. E. Clarke and associates tried disodium EDTA in patients who had actual plaques from CVD, noting an immediate improvement in many patients. Using too much EDTA too fast or without the additives listed above caused some toxicity in the early years; but no deaths have been reported since the early 1980s when the optimum protocol has been followed. The same cannot be said about bypass surgery.

Rather than go over trial after trial, the results of a meta-analysis will be given in Table 7-1 (Cranton, 2001, pp396-212). Of about 50 trials of EDTA for treatment of atherosclerosis, the ones included had to have data on humans, not test animals; data on whether subjects improved, not just survived; and data on some objective measure of improvement. The objective measure could be more normal EKGs, increased walking distance before pain, better circulation as shown by doppler ultrasound, or reduced plaque sizes as shown by arteriograms. EDTA chelation also improved blood circulation enough for patients to avoid bypass surgery or amputation, even when gangrene had been present. The mean benefit found in all of the trials was that about 87% of patients improved. The 2 very large trials had about the same overall result as small trials. Unpublished trial results solicited by the author of the meta-analysis, James P. Carter, MD, MPH, had the same % benefits as the trials published in peer-reviewed journals. Note that a medium-sized trial with negative results was included (Sloth-Nielsen). This is the Danish trial with misconduct discussed below.

Sharp readers will notice that there is no column in this table with all-cause death rates. This is regrettable. Part of the reason is that people who are candidates for chelation are really sick, unlike 90% of the people for whom antihypertensive drugs are prescribed (see Myth 4), and a majority of those for whom anticholesterol drugs are prescribed (see Myth 3). The endpoints of the chelation trials such as improved EKGs, much greater walking or treadmill distance, pulses in ankles where there were none before treatment, as shown by doppler ultrasound, and arteriograms showing regression of plaque, are much more meaningful endpoints than some endpoints of trials described in earlier chapters. Being able to walk 100 yards or meters rather than 5 is a dramatic improvement in the quality of life, as is avoiding amputation of feet, or the dangerous coronary bypass surgery. Another simple way to judge the benefits of chelation is the low dropout rate (the percent of those who quit). When patients get through the first few chelation treatments, most, the vast majority, return by choice week after week to complete the course of 10-30 treatments. One recent trial had a dropout rate of only 5% (Knudtson et al., 2002).

Table 7-1. Clinical Trial Benefits of EDTA Chelation for Treatment of Atherosclerotic Conditions such as Coronary or Peripheral Artery Disease and Gangrene (from Cranton, 2001, p301).

| Author(s) | Journal/Date 19__ | Benefit Test Type | Subjs. | Better (%) | | Same/Worse (%) | |
|---|---|---|---|---|---|---|---|
| Olszewer, Carter | Medical Hypotheses/88 | EKG, walk dist., DU* | 2482 | 2379 | (96) | 103 | (4) |
| Clarke | Am J Medical Science/56 | exercise ability | 20 | 19 | (95) | 1 | (5) |
| Kitchell et al. | Am J Cardiology/63 | exercise, lifespan | 38 | 23 | (61) | 15 | (39) |
| Sloth-Nielsen** | Am J Surgery/92 | arteriograms | 30 | 2 | (7) | 28 | (93) |
| Casdorph | J Holistic Medicine/81 | arteriograms | 15 | 14 | (93) | 1 | (7) |
| Casdorph, Farr | J Holistic Medicine/83 | avoid amputation from gangrene | 4 | 4 | (100) | 0 | |
| Casdorph | J Holistic Medicine/81 | arteriograms, heart ejection fraction | 18 | 17 | (94) | 1 | (6) |
| Olszewer, Carter | J Nat Medicine Assoc/91 | ankle/brachial BP | 10 | 10 | (100) | 0 | |
| Godfrey | New Zealand Medical J/90 | ankle/brachial BP, DU* | 27 | 25 | (93) | 2 | (7) |
| Morgan | J Advances in Medicine/91 | stress EKG | 2 | 2 | (100) | 0 | |
| Brucknerova | Cas Lekces/80 | arteriograms | 2 | 2 | (100) | 0 | |
| Hancke | ---/93 | avoid amputation or bypass | 92 | 82 | (89) | 10 | (11) |
| Hancke | ---/93 | EKG | 253 | 175 | (69) | 78 | (31) |
| Hancke | ---/93 | ankle/brachial BP | 262 | 217 | (83) | 45 | (17) |
| McGillem | New England J Medicine/88 | arteriograms | 1 | 0 | | 1 | (100) |
| Rudolph, McDonagh | J Advances Medicine/90 | DU* | 1 | 1 | (100) | 0 | |
| McDonagh et al. | J Advances Medicine/82 | eye blood vessel anal. | 57 | 50 | (88) | 7 | (12) |
| McDonagh et al. | J Advances Medicine/85 | ankle/brachial BP | 117 | 95 | (81) | 22 | (19) |
| Hoekstra et al. | ---/93 | thermography*** | 19147 | 16466 | (86) | 2681 | (14) |
| van der Schaar | J Advances Medicine/89 | exercise ability | 111 | 111 | (100) | 0 | |
| Rudolph et al. | J Advances Medicine/91 | carotid artery DU* | 30 | 30 | (100) | 0 | |

*blood flow by doppler ultrasound
**Danish Study subject to misconduct, see text
***blood flow by local measurement of heat

Patients who undergo chelation are really in such bad condition that administering a placebo in a double-blinded trial (RCT) would be unethical because the evidence for the safety and efficacy of chelation have been so strong since about 1985. Furthermore, the improvements among the treated patients in earlier blinded trials were so obvious as to break the blinding.

\*\*\*\*\*

There are anecdotal reports that EDTA chelation lowers systolic blood pressure (Cranton, 2001, pp266-268).

A 10-year follow-up of 59 patients treated with EDTA showed a 90% reduction in the incidence of cancer when compared with 172 control patients (Cranton, 2001, p130, 195-201). All were living in the same small Swiss city along a highway. The absolute number treated with EDTA who died of cancer was one (1.7% of 59) vs. 30 of the controls (17% of 172). As the observation period was 1959-1976, the interpretation was that lead compounds from gasoline may have caused the cancers, which were of many types. But patients in this study did not have toxic levels of lead at baseline by the standards of the time.

Interestingly, Elmer M. Cranton, MD, has pointed out that atherosclerotic plaques, also called atheromas, are a form of benign tumor (Cranton, 2001, p40).

## Dismissal of EDTA Chelation by Mainstream Medicine

The original motivation to discredit EDTA as a treatment for atherosclerosis may have stemmed from the turnabout of one of the early trial directors, J. R. Kitchell, from publishing on the benefit to later publishing that there was no benefit. This was about the time of the adoption of coronary bypass surgery and angioplasty, which, when they succeed, appear to do so in a short time span. These procedures are also much more costly and profitable, running 10-40 times the cost of chelation.

In recent years, mainstream medical journals have refused to publish the results of trials on chelation for atherosclerosis, while publishing a steady stream of frivolous letters to the editor and editorials criticizing chelation by selective citation of trials already shown to be flawed. Certain organizations oppose chelation violently, such as the American Council on Health Fraud, a bogus front for mainstream medicine that opposes all alternative methods, and which has lost lawsuits in California and several other states (http://www.vaccines.bizland.com/quackwatch.html).

Certain individuals take great pleasure in employing any methods of defamation against chelation. One such is Saul Green, PhD, Biochemistry, whose essay on chelation on the website www.Quackwatch.com reveals the depths to which opponents have gone, and the low quality of the criticism. Specific quotations from Green's essay and rebuttals to them are given below based on a recent critique of the Quackwatch website (Kauffman, 2002).

"Chelation Therapy: Unproven Claims and Unsound Theories
Saul Green, Ph. D.  Revised 14 Sep 00

"Chelation therapy...is a series of intravenous infusions containing disodium EDTA and various other substances.  Proponents claim that EDTA chelation therapy is effective against atherosclerosis and many other serious health problems.  Its use is widespread because patients have been led to believe that it is a valid alternative to established medical interventions such as coronary bypass surgery. However, there is no scientific evidence that this is so. It is also used to treat nonexistent 'lead poisoning', 'mercury poisoning', and other alleged toxic states..."

But later on p. 1: "After EDTA was found effective in chelating and removing toxic metals from the blood, some scientists postulated that hardened arteries could be softened if the calcium in their walls was removed." Note the inconsistency in the claim that lead and mercury poisoning are nonexistent followed by the statement that EDTA is effective for treatment of it! Green goes on to list 4 books he chose arbitrarily of the many that promote EDTA chelation. Then:

"The scientific jargon in these books may create the false impression that chelation therapy for atherosclerosis, and a host of other conditions, is scientifically sound. The authors allege that between 300,000 and 500,000 patients have safely benefited. However, their evidence consists of anecdotes, testimonials, and poorly designed experiments."

Green then gives an early history of 3 apparent successes with chelation, and dismisses them all. He then describes how the procedure is to be carried out according to the main proponent organization in the USA, the American College for Advancement in Medicine (ACAM), the cost, "$75-125 per treatment", and the fact that most medical insurance will not cover this cost. He continues with a critique of a 1989 study that will be detailed below, 15 reports of trials that found no benefit, and 2 trials in the 1980s that supposedly found no benefit. A page that warns about the lack of safety of the treatment follows, then a refutation of 4 theories of how the treatment works, and finally a report of a study in Denmark in 1992 that Green considered to be of the highest quality. Green does not cite a single study he thinks shows any success from this treatment. Note that 15 trials of some size in Table 7-1 show benefit; none were cited by Green. His summary reinforces this conclusion: "The few well-designed studies that have addressed the efficacy of chelation for atherosclerotic diseases have been carried out by 'establishment' medical scientists. Without exception, these found no evidence that chelation worked." He wrote:

> "The sources used for this review included position papers of professional societies, technical textbooks, research and review articles, newspaper articles, patient testimonials [which Green considered inadmissible in his previous paragraph], medical records, legal depositions, transcripts of court testimony, privately published books, clinic brochures and personal correspondence."

Rebuttal: Green's actual bibliography consisted of just 6 citations, all to papers in peer-reviewed journals, the most recent being from 1992. There were no reviews cited. Three of the citations lacked authors and titles, two of these lacked page numbers, and one of these had a misspelled journal title!

Green wrote of the success of the 1963 trial by Kitchell et al., citing it in his ref. 2, and then of Kitchell's later denial of success. Green wrote that the "improvement" (his quotes) was not significant because it was no better than than would be expected with proven methods, of which no examples were given, and that there was no control group for comparison.

Rebuttal: There was no description of the diagnosis of the patients in this 1963 trial, so one must assume that they suffered from atherosclerosis and one of its manifestations, such as intermittent claudication (blocked arteries). There were no "proven methods" at that time, no well-developed bypass surgery, no angioplasty. While the double-blind, placebo-controlled trial is the gold standard for treatment studies, it was not common before 1975. The patients were suffering from circulation conditions that would not be expected to improve without treatment, thus the patients served as their own controls. Even at present, since it is considered unethical not to treat a number of diseases, many trials do not utilize a placebo.

> Green: "In a retrospective study of 2,870 patients treated with NaMgEDTA [sic], Olszewer and Carter (1989) [sic] concluded that EDTA chelation therapy benefited patients with cardiac disease, peripheral vascular disease [this is blocked small arteries] and cerebrovascular disease [blocked carotid arteries]. These conclusions were not justified because the people who received the treatment were not compared to people who did not."

Rebuttal: No findable citation to this study was given by Green! The authors of the report on the study Green probably meant (Olszewer & Carter, 1988), which utilized $Na_2MgEDTA$, address the limitations of their study directly: "There was no placebo or control group and these studies are not double-blinded. It is a retrospective analysis of a large number of cases with standardized criteria for assessing improvement. Each patient served as his/her own control...the clinical response rates, especially for angina and intermittent claudication, are too high, i. e. from 77% to 91%, respectively, to be attributed to placebo-effect alone..."

Green then describes a study reported in 1990 by these same authors in which he ridiculed their description of double-blinding, while the actual results in exercise stress tests and blood pressure changes were not given by Green.

Rebuttal: Since there was no findable citation, this sarcastic description cannot be evaluated with certainty; but there is another description of this trial in which 10 patients with intermittent claudication were divided into 2 groups. The treatment group received 10 infusions of EDTA, with the usual additives, while the control group received all of the additives without the EDTA; this was double-blinded. The treatment group more than doubled their walking distance compared with no significant change in the placebo group. The differences were so striking that it was considered immoral to continue, and both groups received EDTA from then on, resulting in an equal improvement in what had been the control group, and further improvement in what had been the treatment group (Cranton, 2001, p285-293).

Green wrote that a randomized, controlled, double-blind clinical trial of chelation therapy conducted by Curt Diehm at the University of Heidelberg Medical Clinic with Bencyclan, a blood-thinning agent, as the control (no placebo) gave similar results in both groups, and both groups were said to have responded to the placebo effect.

Rebuttal: The citation for this was given as follows: "Zeit. Deutsch Herzstiftung. Vol 10, July 1986." An online search failed to locate this paper, thus this study could not be evaluated from the citation as given. Assuming that this was "The Heidelberg Study", others have interpreted the raw results to indicate that the EDTA-treated group enjoyed 5 times the increase of walking distance of the Bencyclan group (Cranton, 2001, pp xxiii-xxiv, 339-340). The raw results were smuggled out by researchers who saw how the official report for publication was to be altered. In contrast to the FDA's refusal to officially approve EDTA to alleviate the pain of walking due to poor blood circulation in the legs, there was a study in which pentoxifylline (Trental™) increased walking distance by just 1.25 times, yet this drug was given FDA approval (Cranton, 2001, pp340-341)! Even this small benefit has been disputed; moreover, pentoxifylline's fatal toxicity to bone marrow led the Public Citizen's Health Research Group to advise against using pentoxifylline for any purpose (Wolfe S, Sasich LD, 1999, pp166-167).

Green wrote that a randomized, controlled, double-blind clinical trial of chelation therapy conducted by R. Hopf at the University of Frankfurt, with normal saline as the placebo, gave similar results in both groups, with the conclusion that EDTA was of no benefit.

Rebuttal: The citation for this was given as follows: "Zeit. f. Kardiology, 76, #2, 1987". An online search of Zeitschrift für Kardiologie, Vol. 76, 1987, failed to produce this paper; thus, because of this possibly spurious citation, the work could not be evaluated.

Neither of the German studies was cited in any of the 3 major reviews in journals on EDTA chelation (Grier et al., 1993; Chappell et al., 1996; Ernst, 1997).

Green devotes a page to the supposed lack of safety of chelation, writing that there is no published scientific evidence that chelation will improve poor blood circulation, and that loss of zinc ion due to chelation is potentially serious. "People with coronary artery disease who need bypass surgery and choose chelation instead place themselves at great risk." This was in the context of attacking an advertisement for chelation therapy, which was reproduced on the web page.

Rebuttal: While it accepted the use of EDTA chelation for treatment of lead poisoning, the US Food & Drug Administration (FDA) has been quite hostile to its use for atherosclerosis. An official request was sent from the FDA to state health and regulatory agencies across the US asking that any information relating to untoward results, poor results, or patient complaints about EDTA chelation therapy be forwarded to the FDA; no such reports were received (Cranton, 2001, p xv). Despite the loss of zinc to EDTA chelation, the authors of the study to which Green referred recommended that zinc supplements be given, and that chelation be continued as both diagnosis and treatment for heavy metal poisoning (Allain et al., 1991). Bypass surgery has been shown in 3 major studies to have no significant effect on long-term survival rates, especially if function in the left main coronary artery had been adequate beforehand (McGee, 2001, pp24-28). A recent study from Canada is supportive in that bypass surgery improved 5-year survival rates only where dysfunction in the left main coronary artery was treated (Dzavik et al., 2001). The immediate death rate from bypass surgery is about 6% (McGee, 2001, p28), while the immediate death rate from properly applied and administered EDTA chelation is nonexistent, and chelation has been called one of the safest therapies available (Cranton, 2001, p345-351).

The attack on the advertisement for chelation reproduced on this web page of www.Quackwatch.com certainly exemplified one of the activities in the Mission Statement, "Investigating Questionable Claims", but the attack has been shown in this review to be groundless.

Green devotes 1/4 of the EDTA web page on www.Quackwatch.com to rebutting 4 theories of how chelation is supposed to work biochemically. His attempts to debunk these theories are supposed to show that chelation cannot have any beneficial effect because none of the theories stand up scientifically. With each of his debunkings is added a hypothetical scenario intended to scare the user into avoiding chelation.

Rebuttal: Green would appear to want to discourage the use of aspirin, morphine, codeine, general anesthetics, and antibiotics, since the biochemical explanation of these and other useful drugs were not understood when these drugs were adopted. For example, aspirin was used for more than 70 years before an explanation for its effects was found (see Myth 1). The clinical benefits of these medical treatments were so obvious that double-blind studies would have been superfluous. The sad corollary is that modern prescription drugs taken for life to treat chronic diseases often have such weak effects, yet they are accompanied by such profound side-effects, that any overall benefits can be proven only by large-scale controlled trials, and even these are often inadequate (Cohen, 2001). All of Green's scare scenarios ignore the fact that chelation has been very safe as well as effective.

As a specific example of Green's use of supposed chemical knowledge, the following quotation is given from one of his explanations of why chelation cannot work:

> "Ionic iron has two electrons in its outermost or N shell and 14 electrons in its M shell. This configuration gives ionic iron the distinct characteristic of being able to accept three pairs of electrons from other ions... When iron is dissolved in water at a pH of 7.0 or more, its three pairs of electrons will be bound to three OH groups of the water."

Rebuttal: Dear reader, this was a deliberate effort to feign knowledge of chemistry in order to discredit chelation by strewing non-facts of chemistry. In a transition metal such as iron the N shell is of lower energy than the M shell, so the N shell cannot be said to be outermost, especially since these two shells are combined to give hybrid orbitals of equal energy. In elemental iron the total number of electrons in these combined outer shells, said to be the valence shells where electron transfer or sharing takes place in chemical reactions, is 2 from the N shell and 6 from the M shell for a total of 8, not 14 or 16 (2 + 14). It follows that the unsolvated ion Fe 2+ would retain 6 of the 8, and that Fe 3+ would retain 5 of the 8 electrons. Iron ions are not unique either in their ability to form a trihydroxide or to share 3 pairs of electrons. While solvated iron ions may share up to 6 pairs of electrons provided by a donor; they do not provide a unique three pairs of their own (Holtzclaw et al., 1984). Thus it is unbonded pairs of electrons in water molecules or hydroxide ions (HO 1-) that are bound to the iron ion, not the other way around.

As the clinching argument, Green saved the Danish Study for last:

"In 1992, a group of cardiovascular surgeons in Denmark published results of a double-blinded, randomized, placebo-controlled study of EDTA treatment for severe intermittent claudication [Guldager B et al., *J Int Med* 1992:231:261-267]. A total of 153 patients in two groups received 20 infusions of EDTA or a placebo for 5 to 9 weeks, in a clinical protocol duplicating the conditions used by Olszewer and Carter in 1990. The changes seen in pain-free and maximal walking distances were similar for the EDTA-treated and the placebo group, and there were no long-term therapeutic effects noted in 3-month and 6-month follow-ups. These investigators concluded that chelation was not effective against intermittent claudication."

Rebuttal: The Danish Study is the darling of the opponents of chelation, which includes 2 of the 3 reviews cited above (Grier et al., 1993; Ernst, 1997). This Danish study was flawed by the fact that those conducting it were cardiovascular surgeons whose livelihood was threatened by EDTA. They even went so far as to pre-announce their expectation of a negative effect from their study! Instead of using the best cocktail for the purpose, which includes magnesium, they omitted it, thus they were *not* duplicating the cocktail used by Olszewer and Carter in 1990. The Danish surgeons used iron as part of the oral supplements, which predictably chelated more strongly with the EDTA than either magnesium or calcium, guaranteeing a lesser effect. Also, 70% of the patients were smokers despite the fact that it has been shown that smoking will neutralize the effect of chelation. The Danish surgeons were informed by telephone and in writing that there were errors and omissions which would invalidate the trial. Finally they were investigated very grudgingly by the Committee on Investigation into Scientific Dishonesty of the Danish Medical Association, which found that the correct cocktail was not used, that a mineral (iron) was used that was contraindicated, that the double-blinding was broken, and that the surgeons claimed they had used the correct cocktail even when informed they had not (Douglass, 1995). A more recent review (Chappell, 1996) agrees with Douglass, and cites 4 more critical reviews of the Danish study published in peer-reviewed journals. On top of this, the treatment group was pre-selected to be much sicker than the control group, with mean maximum walking distances of 119 meters before treatment for the EDTA group and 157 meters for the placebo group. When the raw data were examined the treatment group enjoyed an increase of 51% and the control group 24%, so this study actually had a slight positive result despite its denial by its own authors, who candidly admitted that they undertook the study to persuade the Danish government *not to pay* for chelation (Cranton, 2001, pp5-6)!

The PATCH Study on Chelation

The Program to Assess Alternative Treatment Strategies to Achieve Cardiac Health (PATCH) study was carried out in Alberta, Canada, from 1996-2000. Entry criteria included age at least 21 years with coronary artery disease proven by angiography or a documented myocardial infarction and stable angina while receiving "optimal medical therapy", which was not defined. Treadmill testing was done at baseline and at 15 and 27 weeks after randomization to EDTA or placebo. The placebo was normal saline, but with all the other chelation additives present in the solution to be infused, including magnesium, and there was double-blinding. An important endpoint was the time on the treadmill, as energy expenditure increased, to show a revealing change on an EKG recorded every 20 seconds. This was called "time to ischemia", which was puzzling since ischemia means clot formation. Quality of life scores were obtained at baseline and at 27 weeks. All patients were followed up for 1 year from randomization, recording all events of relevance. Of the 43 patients in the placebo group, 4 subjects dropped out vs. 2 chelation subjects of 41. Essentially no statistically important differences were found between the two groups of 39 subjects each at 27 weeks. The Conclusion of the Abstract of the article in the *Journal of the American Medical Association* said: "Based on exercise time to ischemia, exercise capacity, and quality of life measurements, there is no evidence to support a beneficial effect of chelation therapy in patients with ischemic heart disease, stable angina, and a positive treadmill test for ischemia" (Knudtson et al., 2002).

Stephen F. Olmstead, MD, Mount Ranier Clinic, Inc., Yelm, WA, found a number of inconsistencies in the trial and wrote to the Editor of the journal promptly with negative comments on the paper. He noticed that of 3140 patients screened, only a miniscule 171 or 5.45% were considered eligible for for treadmill screening. Of these only 2.68% of the original number passed the initial treadmill test and were randomized. This amounted to only 43 for placebo and 41 for chelation at baseline, not enough to detect with any certainty a 1 minute change in exercise time from the 10 minutes seen at baseline, and even worse for statistical validity after the dropouts occurred. The chelation group was sicker on some counts; for example, 49% had a previous heart attack vs. 28% of the placebo group, thus randomization was poor. Olmstead wrote that the exercise protocol was strange, incompletely described, and inconsistently applied. Another oddity was that the requirement for angina at baseline was ignored in 30% of the patients in both groups. His letter was not published.

L. Terry Chappell, MD, Bluffton, OH, noticed that there were 4 angioplasties and 1 bypass surgery in the placebo group vs. none in the chelation group. The chelation group gained twice the time on the treadmill to reach its anaerobic threshold (see Myth 6) as did the placebo group, and obtained twice the gain in oxygen utilization.

Neither Knudtson et al. or the two critics cared to speculate on whether infusion of magnesium alone, as in the placebo, might confer a significant portion of the benefits of chelation. The Danish Study was cited by Knudtson et al. without acknowledging any of the published refutations of it. Kitchell's study with negative findings was cited without citation of his positive study listed in Table 7-1. Olszewer and Carter's 10-subject study was cited, but not their 2482-subject study listed in Table 7-1. The whole picture is that of a deliberate effort to discredit EDTA chelation under the umbrella of the *Journal of the American Medical Association.*

*****

In 2000 the Harvard, UC Berkeley and Mayo Clinic newsletters showed their "independence of thought" by taking positions against EDTA chelation. According to Daniel Haley, Harvard graduate, successful businessman, New York State Assemblyman, then medical writer, the simultaneous attacks on EDTA after 50 years of its beneficial uses were probably coordinated (Haley, 2000, p406).

### Is Performing EDTA Chelation for Atherosclerosis Legal?

In 1978 Ray Evers, MD, won a precedent-setting case in Louisiana on the right of a physician to use an FDA drug approved for one condition, meaning that it was safe, for another condition not specifically mentioned by the FDA. This established the right for a physician to use EDTA chelation for atherosclerosis. Robert Rogers, MD, was restrained from using EDTA for atherosclerosis by the State Medical Licensing Board in Florida. This was overturned by the Florida Supreme Court, clearing the way for the use of chelation in that state. Both in 1979 and 1994-5 chelating physicians retained the right to use EDTA for atherosclerosis in California after court hearings for which ACAM prepared organized testimony. Other State Medical Licensing Boards have tried and failed to prevent usage.

Many other trials and harassments have been perpetrated with more or less open attacks from the FDA (Carter, 1992). The safety of EDTA chelation for atherosclerosis is not questioned by the FDA (Cranton, 2001, pp311-312). Using the excuse of the absence of double-blind studies the Federal Trade Commission cried fraud and tried to keep ACAM under scrutiny for 20 years based on "false advertising in ACAM's brochure". US Congressman Dan Burton was outraged and held hearings on the FTC's action (Haley, 2000, p406). Opposition by governmental bodies outside the USA has been countered with the obvious merits of the treatment, which has engendered considerable interest worldwide among patients and potential providers alike (Cranton, 2001, p393).

It is, therefore, lawful for you to receive EDTA chelation for atherosclerosis, but your provider may face harassment at any time.


## How Does EDTA Chelation Work?

You have been shown the structure of EDTA and how it is able to grab metal ions and hang on to them until the chelate is eliminated from the body. No one is really certain of exactly how it works.

Delivery of magnesium 2+ ion in slow-release chelated form may contribute. The most effective magnesium supplements for treating blood pressure, arrhythmias and cramps are chelates, especially the aspartate (see Myth 1). Elmer M. Cranton's clinical observations are that the anti-atherosclerotic effect of EDTA does not depend on the presence of magnesium, which is a fairly recent addition to the infusion cocktail.

Removal of calcium from calcified plaques as the major effect of EDTA was long thought to be the major mode of action. This seems less likely at present, but EDTA does lower the concentration of calcium 2+ ion in the blood and other extracellular fluids. This is the obverse of raising magnesium ion concentration, which prevents arrhythmias and may lower blood pressure (Cranton, 2001, pp31-33).

EDTA prevents clotting of blood.

Now it is thought that removal of iron 3+ ion (or even iron 2+ ion and/or copper 2+ ion) by EDTA prevents these ions from catalyzing oxidation of LDL or the cholesterol in it (Cranton, 2001, pp12-36). The hypothesis that oxidation of cholesterol is catalyzed by excess iron in the body was first published by Jerome L. Sullivan, MD, PhD, in 1981, and was elaborated upon at intervals since. His idea was that the resistance of pre-menopausal women to atherosclerosis and heart attacks compared with the far lower resistance of men of the same age was due to loss of iron in the menses. This was supported by the convergence of CVD rates in both sexes after menopause. He suggests that periodic blood donation is a good way to get rid of excess iron, and is safer than the internal blood loss caused by aspirin use (see Myth 1), (Sullivan, 1996). Newer evidence showed that a different iron chelator (not EDTA) prevented the oxidation of LDL in a lab experiment (de Valk & Marx, 1999). Most persuasive is a study in 31 humans who were said to be carbohydrate-intolerant (probably suffering from NIDDM), and who had iron stores at normal levels as measured by an assay for the iron-containing substance ferritin in serum. Bleeding was used to reduce the ferritin level to near-deficiency levels. This caused HDL to rise, but caused BP, LDL, TG and fibrinogen (a clotting promoter) to fall. All the changes were statistically significant, and all were in the direction expected for less inflammation in the blood vessels. Also, glucose and insulin responses to oral glucose loading were much lower (better), both being very statistically significant, while homocysteine levels were unchanged (see Myth 2). Thus individuals at high risk for CVD because of their NIDDM, who also had normal ferritin levels, did benefit, at least in the short term, as shown by the assays for serum ferritin, by having their iron levels lowered to those of pre-menopausal women. The effects were reversed by a 6-month period of restoration of iron levels (Facchini, Saylor, 2002). This is yet another piece of evidence that elevated LDL is a response, and a healthy one, to inflammation caused by oxidation, and is not a cause of atherosclerosis.

However, the discovery of nanobacteria in 1988 brings the chelation of calcium back into consideration. Nanobacteria are the smallest cell-walled bacteria, so small that they will pass through an 0.1 micron filter. They are visible only under extremely high magnification, as in scanning electron microscopy. Found in atherosclerotic plaques, kidney stones and other places in the body, nanobacteria produce calcium phosphate or other insoluble calcium compounds in their cell walls, and are thought to be the source of the calcium in calcified plaques (Kajander & Ciftcioglu, 1998). Perhaps removal of the plaque, a result of an evolutionary defense mechanism of the nanobacteria, by EDTA chelation allows better access by white blood cells to destroy the bacteria. A US Patent was issued for the treatment of atherosclerosis by EDTA chelation, which does remove these plaques, and co-administration of an antibiotic, with tetracycline being the most effective (Kajander & Ciftcioglu, 2004). If these observations are further confirmed, it may be that EDTA chelation will be carried out in the future with tetracycline in the injectable formulation.

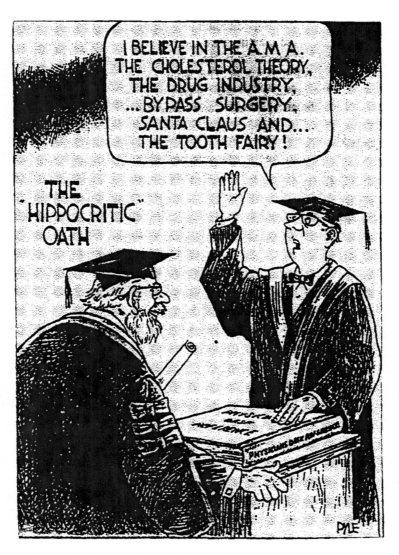

With permission from Charles T. McGee, MD, *Heart Frauds, HealthWise, Colorado Springs, CO, 2001.*

## Summing Up

While no one is certain of why EDTA chelation by intravenous drip works to reverse atherosclerosis, prevent cancer, lower BP, and increase walking distances by countering poor blood flow, there is little doubt that it does so when properly administered to appropriate patients. EDTA chelation also helps diabetic ulcers to heal and it delays or eliminates the need for the drastic mainstream treatments of angioplasty, coronary bypass operations, or amputation of limbs.

One has to be shocked that investigation of the procedure advanced only by means of low-cost studies, clinical observation, word-of-mouth communication, and publication of results in lesser-known journals. Lack of patent protection for the use of EDTA and the infusion process contributed, of course, but the lack of approval of EDTA by the FDA for atherosclerosis, despite evidence of far greater benefits than those of the toxic drug Trental, must leave one gasping at the iniquities of a treatment approval system so obviously biased toward Big Pharma, and against both patients who will benefit as well as physicians who want to provide this chelation treatment.

The low quality of the efforts to debunk EDTA chelation has been exposed. Officially sanctioned trials were rigged. Raw data had to be smuggled out by honest researchers in order to show some of the biases in the published articles on the trials that were debased. Chelation is one "alternative" treatment that works.

Discouraging sick people from undergoing an effective treatment such as EDTA chelation is despicable, even more so when dangerous procedures with limited applicability and no lasting benefit such as angioplasty or bypass surgery are recommended instead. Because of the bias in mainstream medicine against chelation, most patients who accept it do so as a last resort after all conventional treatments have failed, although a majority would have been better off using chelation as a first treatment. It is estimated that by the year 2000 more than a million patients had received more than 20 million intravenous infusions of EDTA. There were no ill effects when the procedure was correctly done. About 88% of the patients improved (Cranton, 2001, pp4, 324).

## Acknowledgments for Myth 7

This chapter was critically reviewed by Elmer M. Cranton, MD, Alayne Yates, MD, Frances E. Heckert Pane, MSLS, and William A. Reinsmith, DA.

## References for Myth 7

Allain P, Mauras Y, Premel-Cabic A, Islam S, Herve JP, Cledes J (1991). Effects of EDTA Infusion on the Urinary Elimination of Several Elements in Healthy Subjects. *British Journal of Clinical Pharmacology 31*, 347-349.

Carter JP (1992). *Racketeering in Medicine: The Suppression of Alternatives.* Norfolk, VA: Hampton Roads Press.

Chappell LT, Janson M (1996). EDTA Chelation Therapy in the Treatment of Vascular Disease. *Journal of Cardiovascular Nursing 10* (3), 78-86.

Cohen JS (2001). *Overdose: The Case Against the Drug Companies.* New York: Tarcher/Putnam.

Cranton EM (2001). *A Textbook on EDTA Chelation Therapy,* 2nd ed. Charlottesville, VA: Hampton Roads Publ. Co.

Douglass WC, Jr, (1995). Chelation Therapy — Better Than Ever! *Second Opinion,* Supplement, March, 1-4, and references therein.

Dzavik V, Ghali WA, Norris C, Mitchell LB, Koshal A, Saunders LD, Galbraith PD, Hui W, Faris P, Knudtson ML (2001). Long-Term Survival in 11,661 Patients with Multivessel Coronary Artery Disease in the Era of Stenting: A Report from the Alberta Provincial Project for Outcome Assessment in Coronary Heart Disease (APPROACH) Investigators. *American Heart Journal, 142,* 119-126.

Ernst E (1997). Chelation Therapy for Peripheral Arterial Occlusive Disease: A Systematic Review. *Circulation* 96, 1031-1033.

Facchini FS, Saylor KL (2002). Effect of iron depletion on cardiovascular risk factors: studies in carbohydrate-intolerant patients. *Annals of the New York Academy of Sciences* 967:342-351.

Goodwin S, Ovnic K, Korschun H (1998). http://www.whsc.emory.edu/_releases/1999january/010699stent.html Accessed 3 Oct 05.

Grier MT, Meyers D G (1993). So Much Writing, So Little Science: A Review of 37 Years of Literature on Edentate Sodium Chelation Therapy. *Annals of Pharmacotherapy 27* 1504-9.

Haley D (2000). *Politics in Healing: The Suppression and Manipulation of American Medicine.* Washington, DC: Potomac Valley Press.

Holtzclaw, Jr, HF, Robinson WR, Nebergall WH (1984). *College Chemistry with Qualitative Analysis,* 7th ed. (pp 102, 818-819), Lexington, MA: D. C. Heath.

Kajander EO, Ciftcioglu N (1998). Nanobacteria - An Alternative Mechanism for Pathogenic Intra- and Extra-cellular Calcification and Stone Formation. *Proceedings of the National Academy of Sciences (USA)* 95(14):8274-8279.

Kajander EO, Ciftcioglu N (2004). Methods for Eradication of Nanobacteria. U. S. 6,706,290 (16 Mar 04).

Kauffman JM (2002). Alternative Medicine: Watching the Watchdogs at Quackwatch, Website Review, *J. Scientific Exploration* 16(2):312-337.

Knudtson ML, Wyse DG, Galbraith PD, et al. (2002). Chelation Therapy for Ischemic Heart Disease, A Randomized Controlled Trial. *Journal of the American Medical Association,* 287:481-486.

Marc Leduc (2002). http://www.healingdaily.com/conditions/heart-disease-2.htm Accessed 3 Oct 05.

Lin J-L, Lin-Tan D-T, Hsu K-H, Yu C-C (2003). Environmental Lead Exposure and Progression of Chronic Renal Diseases in Patients without Diabetes. *New England Journal of Medicine* 348(4):277-286.

McGee CT (2001). *Heart Frauds: Uncovering the Biggest Health Scam in History,* Colorado Springs, CO: HealthWise Publishers.

Olszewer E, Carter JP (1988). EDTA Chelation Therapy in Chronic Degenerative Disease. *Medical Hypotheses,* 27:41-49.

Sullivan JL (1996). Iron versus Cholesterol—Perspectives on the Iron and Heart Disease Debate. *Journal of Clinical Epidemiology* 49(12):1345-1352.

Wolfe S, Sasich LD (1999). *Worst Pills Best Pills.* New York, N.Y.: Pocket Books.

de Valk B, Marx JM (1999). Iron, Atherosclerosis, and Ischemic Heart Disease. *Archives of Internal Medicine* 159:1542-1548.

# Myth 8: All Ionizing Radiation is Dangerous
# Except when an Oncologist Delivers It.

*A new scientific truth does not triumph by convincing its opponents and making them see the right, but rather because its opponents eventually die, and a new generation grows up that is familiar with it.* ---
*Max Planck, ≈ 1910*

### Spacedoc Speaks Out

It is easy to understand why ionizing radiation has such a bad reputation. Hiroshima, Nagasaki and Chernobyl have painted an indelible fear of radiation in the minds of all of us - physicians and lay persons alike. To even consider the possibility of health benefit from radiation is tantamount to swimming upstream against a very powerful current of opposition. Kauffman has done a remarkable job of reviewing relevant data and presenting a very compelling case for the amazing hormesis effect of ionizing radiation.

In support of NASA's efforts to return man to the moon and on to Mars, I have had the opportunity recently to participate in planning for the immense radiation challenge this will impose. Apollo took man beyond Earth's protective electromagnetic shield for short periods of time and now we know what to expect from the cosmic "heavies" to come in the future – those ions of common elements up to iron, stripped of their electrons and zipping through our spacecraft at nearly light speed.

Our focus on radiation as an enemy has been so narrow we have forgotten or have never been taught the reality that radiation is not all bad. The evidence for adverse health effects following large, acute doses of radiation is clear, and no one challenges it. But the compelling evidence of beneficial health effects following small doses (hormesis) is being ignored by the authorities, even though a biological explanation, based on measured stimulation of the body's natural defenses, has been provided. I am board certified in public health and preventive medicine. Why do I now find myself wondering why I have never heard of radiation hormesis?

Yes, I have been taught that the reason we can rationally discuss this as rational human beings is the result of eons of genetic mutations due primarily to the ionizing effects of cosmic radiation. Our Earth's protective electromagnetic shield allows just enough of this radiation to "get through". We now should know that this is beneficial. And the fact that we live in a sea of radiation cannot be denied. A background of 0.2 to 0.6 rads per year is natural, and it is thought provoking that fully one-tenth of this amount is emitted by the radiation from our internal stores of the potassium-40 isotope. Furthermore if you live at an altitude of 5-10 thousand feet, your background dose becomes three times that of your sea level colleagues.

My brainwashing in the past forty years has been that all radiation is bad, except for the undeniably beneficial effects of cosmic radiation on our mutation rates. As a young man I should have taken a much harder look at this zero-tolerance attitude. I admire those among us who, like Doctor Kauffman, have taken a harder look at this and proved, at least to my satisfaction, that low level amounts of radiation are not only tolerable but beneficial. They have critically examined those levels of radiation formerly thought to be harmful. Time and time again this effect has been proven to result in decreased malignancies of all kinds, improved general health, fewer congenital malformations and better recovery from gas gangrene and mastitis. People are now paying money to enter caves with radon-laced atmospheres for the purpose of helping their cancers and arthritis. Why? Because it works! This chapter should be required reading for every doctor. The positive effect of low levels of ionizing radiation on our immune systems is real.

----Duane Graveline MD MPH

## Overview

You already make a lot of decisions based on dose/response relationships. There may be foods you like such as spices, but you make the decision to eat a small amount at any one time because you know that ten times as much will give you a stomach ache or worse. Over-the-counter drugs such as cough medicines or Sudafed™ (pseudoephedrine hydrochloride) have instructions such as "Do not exceed 4 teaspoons (or tablets) in 24 hours". So you already know that many things that may be very good in moderation may not be better at higher doses.

In contrast to this common and correct knowledge we are told that ionizing radiation used in medical imaging, for example, from diagnostic Xrays for pictures, from CAT scans, or from isotopes used for bone scans, always has some acceptably small risk, usually of an increased cancer rate, at even the very lowest doses. This hypothetical dose/response relationship is called the linear no-threshold (LNT) model.

It has been found that some carcinogens do not cause cancers below a certain concentration. This is called the linear *with* threshold model, and it is not often observed.

The third typical model is the one first described for spices and drugs: a negligible amount of something has no effect, a little more of it is good, but much more of it is toxic. This is the hormetic dose/response relationship. The overall effect is called hormesis. Exercise is a perfect example of hormesis — some is better than none, and the optimum level is far from the maximum level (see Myth 6), (Calabrese & Baldwin, 2003).

Many substances, if not most, have a hormesis effect or a hormetic dose range, among them most prescription drugs, many heavy (and often essential) metals, the fat-soluble vitamins, and even water; all are toxic in high enough doses (Ottoboni, 1991; Calabrese et al., 1999; Calabrese & Baldwin, 2001; Gardner & Gutmann, 2002).

The prevailing view of regulatory agencies and advisory groups is that all high-energy (ionizing) radiation is bad for health, and exposure to any form of it should be minimized. The actual existence of a very measurable ambient or background level of radiation is ignored. A strong pretense is made or implied that the elimination of all background radiation would make us all healthier. In other words, the proclaimed official model for the health effects of ionizing radiation is the LNT model.

People took this seriously. A 1987 article in Newsline stated the following: "According to the IAEA, an estimated 100,000-200,000 ...[desired]... pregnancies were aborted in Western Europe because physicians mistakenly advised patients that the radiation from Chernobyl posed a significant health risk to unborn children."

Evidence opposing the LNT model is presented in this chapter showing that chronic (repeated) doses up to 100 times those of normal ambient (including medical) exposures are beneficial, mainly due to lower cancer rates. Further evidence is presented that single, acute doses of up to 50 rad are beneficial, including in the treatment of cancer and gangrene. Studies are cited to show that below-ambient radiation levels are unhealthful, and that some radiation may be essential for many life-forms.

Paradoxically, the use by radiation oncologists of gamma rays and other types of radiation from implanted "seeds" containing radioisotopes is seen as an overall benefit in the treatment of cancer. This includes delivery of acute doses of 6000 rad (10,000 to 30,000 times the typical ambient level), and delivery of several of these in a few weeks to give cumulative doses 40,000 to 120,000 times the typical ambient level. The inconsistency is obvious, and is ignored, minimized or explained away in a manner that would embarrass a used-car salesman.

Both parts of the paradox are promoted by the Nuclear Regulatory Commission (Kauffman, 2003a) and many other agencies. Is the pervasive advice from official and government agencies to minimize your exposure to ionizing radiation based on experimental science? Is radiation from any or all sources bad for you? Is advice to get rid of radon and limit medical exposures the best advice? Is high-dose irradiation with gamma rays for cancer treatment a good idea?

Evidence will be given that high-dose radiation, regardless of source or intention, is harmful to health, while low-dose radiation is beneficial. Radiation hormesis is real.

### What is Radiation Hormesis?

If increasing doses of radiation caused proportionally detrimental health effects, the relationship would be as shown in Fig. 8-1. That the higher doses produce a greater incidence of health problems has been determined experimentally, and this is shown by the solid right-hand part of the line. To estimate risks at lower doses in the absence of actual data, the line is extrapolated to a zero dose level of radiation. This hypothetical relationship is called the linear no-threshold (LNT) model and is used to set limits by all official and governmental associations such as the US Environmental Protection Agency (EPA), the International Commission on Radiation Protection (ICRP), the National Council on Radiation Protection and Measurements (NCRP) and the National Academy of Sciences-Nuclear Regulatory Commission (NAS-NRC) Board of Radiation Effects Research (BRER), (Cohen, 1997c). One justification claimed for using the LNT model is that too many test animals or too much time would be needed to evaluate chronic dose rates within 100 times background.

If the LNT model shown in Figure 8-1 were correct, then there is no "no observed adverse effect level" (NOAEL) for regulators to tell us to observe (Jonas, 2001), thus officials responsible for public health would be justified in calling for minimization of exposures to ionizing radiation. The LNT model was first considered in the 1940s on the theoretical grounds that a single hit by ionizing radiation on a single cell could cause chromosome damage which, in turn, could cause a mutation or cancer. After World War II a number of scientists promoted the LNT model in order to discourage nearly all uses of nuclear weapons and power; but other scientists disagreed with the LNT from the beginning (Calabrese & Baldwin, 2000). The polarization of opinions on whether radiation hormesis exists resembles that on low-carb diets (see Myth 2), where all government agencies are on one side, and a number of individual scientists and millions of people who have tried low-carb diets are on the

Figure 8-1: A Linear No-Threshold (LNT) Relationship

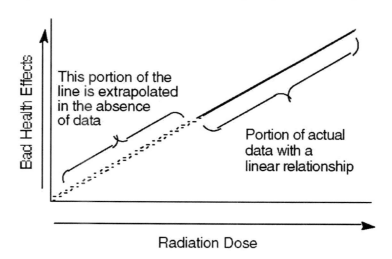

other. Yet the evidence to be presented shows that informed scientists and a small fraction of the public are ahead of the agencies in understanding the effects of low-level radiation exposure.

Evidence to be presented shows that the effect of radiation on the human body actually follows the relationship shown in Fig 8-2, whose curve shape should not be taken too literally. Below a certain level of exposure that does not differ in health effects from those of the normal background level,

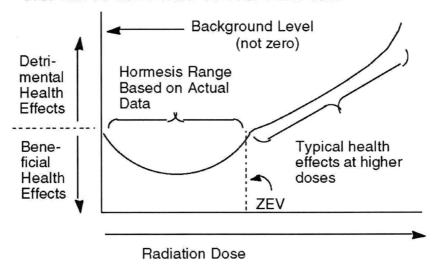

Figure 8-2. A typical real-life dose-response to radiation showing a hormesis range. ZEV = zero-equivalent value, the dose with the same health effect as a zero dose.

called the "zero equivalent value" (ZEV, also ZEP), there are beneficial health effects. This graphically represents the phenomenon called hormesis, and it does *not* follow from linear extrapolation of the rest of the curve. Adverse health effects at *higher* doses often follow a linear plus quadratic (curved) relationship as shown in eq. 1, where mortality from radiation exposure ($m_r$) is the sum of the death rate ($m_a$) in the total absence of the health factor of radiation (r), plus a linear term (br) plus a quadratic term ($cr^2$), (Luckey, 1991, pp148-158):

$$m_r = m_a + br + cr^2 \qquad (1)$$

This has no significance derived from theories of causation; it is just crude curve-fitting to the data.

By using the term "zero equivalent value" the radiation "experts" are trying to make us believe that the background levels of radiation do not exist, or may be ignored. The ZEV should have been called the background equivalent value.

<u>Units of Radiation Dose</u>

To understand some of the evidence and arguments, one must become familiar with several of the units used in measurements of radiation. The old unit of radiation dose, the roentgen (R) measures exposure in terms of how much ionization radiation produces in air. This has been replaced by the "radiation absorbed dose", the rad, which is the amount of radiation that deposits $10^{-2}$ J/kg of energy in any material. If animal tissue is placed at a point which is subjected to 1 R, it will absorb about 1 rad. With the move to SI units, the gray (Gy) was adopted, which equals 100 rad. So the centigray (cGy) equals 1 rad.

The amount of biological damage depends not only on the energy absorbed, but on the number of ions (or free radicals) formed. So the roentgen-equivalent-in-man (rem) was adopted to give a closer measure of the damage. The relation to the rad is shown in eq. 2, where the quality factor (QF) allows for the differences in types of radiation:

$$1 \text{ rem} = 1 \text{ rad} \times QF \qquad (2)$$

For low linear-energy-transfer (LET) electromagnetic radiation, such as Xrays and gamma rays, as well as beta particles, QF = 1. Beta particles are electrons. Electron beam tomography (EBT) was mentioned in Myth 3. It is an example of how we could be exposed to high-energy electrons. According to Jerry Cuttler, a radiation biology specialist, the QF (or "Q") is an arbitrary factor used in an attempt to model the supposed effects of different types of radiation, and has little scientific basis. For high LET radiation, alpha particles, neutrons and protons are said to have QF ≈ 5-20 (Luckey, 1991, p3). The SI unit now used for damage is the sievert (Sv) which equals 100 rem.  To compare units when QF = 1:  100 rad = 100 rem = 1 Gy = 1 Sv.

Units for the local level of radioactivity are used instead of dose in the special cases of radon gas and other airborne radionuclides. The older activity unit was the curie (Ci), which is $3.7 \times 10^{10}$ disintegrations per second. The newer SI unit is the becquerel (Bq), which is 1 disintegration per second: 1 pCi/L = 37 $Bq/m^3$, and these units are independent of the identity of the radionuclide (Tipler, 1987).

## Background Levels of Radiation

The background radiation at present is thought to be 0.25-4.0 mSv/year (mean worldwide value on land) with some locations 10x greater (Parsons, 2001). Others cite 0.2 rad/year, of which 10% is from decay of the $^{40}K$ (potassium-40, an unstable isotope with one more neutron than the common potassium-39) within the average human, which emits $4 \times 10^7$ gamma rays, $3 \times 10^8$ beta rays and $3 \times 10^8$ delta rays (weak ionizing electrons) each year (Luckey, 1999). The rest is from cosmic rays, the earth (including atmospheric) radiation, from buildings, industry, food and drink, explosions, fallout and medical sources (Luckey, 1991, pp6-31), as shown in Table 8-0. The background doses are given in cGy (rad) per year, while the medical imaging exposures are given in cGy per episode. According to Jerry Cuttler, a chronic background level as high as 70 rad/yr, as in Ramsar, Iran, does *not* produce symptomatic adverse health effects.

Typical levels of radon in living areas of homes vary, but ≈ 50 $Bq/m^3$ seems to be a median, and the major health effect is thought to be lung cancer, but only as a result of much higher levels of radon than the median one (Cohen, 1977b).

We live in a sea of radiation that we cannot detect directly using any of our senses. Plastic scintillators have been used for 50 years to detect ionizing radiation in addition to other devices, such as Geiger counters. Scintillators work by converting the energy of the particle hit into a flash of light, the scintillation. This is detected by a photomultiplier tube that can sense even a single photon, the minimum possible piece of light. When a block of plastic scintillator is used to detect ambient radiation, and the results are adjusted to the size of an adult human body, about 1,560,000 hits per minute are registered. This is 1,120,000,000 per day and about 409,000,000,000 per year! This information was  provided by Charles R. Hurlbut, Manager, Scintillation Products, Ludlum Measurements Corp. (e-mail of 16 Mar 04). According to Dixy Lee Ray, former nuclear engineer, chairperson of the Atomic Energy Commission, and governor of Washington, our bodies receive 900,000 hits per minute from radioactive particles; this is 648,000,000 per day, and is in reasonable agreement with the first estimate (Ray, 1990, p95).

All living things on Earth evolved while bathed in even higher levels of ionizing radiation, thought to be ten times as high.

## Destructive Effects of High Levels of Radiation

The destructive effects of cumulative doses of >250 rads of Xrays are unquestionable, although a latency period of 10 years after exposure to Xrays is recognized, and the peak response to Xrays may occur 30 years after the first exposure (Miller et al., 1989). A latency period of 5 years may apply after steady high-level exposure to radon (Cohen, 1977b).

Bone cancer mortality resulting from ingestion of radium by painters of luminous dials has a threshold of 1000 rad cumulative (Luckey, 1991, p51). There seems to be no hormesis range.

The use of single doses of 6,000 rads for cancer treatment are as high a dose as residents of Hiroshima received who were less than 1 mile from the atomic bomb explosion. Such doses are often

Table 8-0. Doses from Typical Radiation Sources in USA (adapted from Kauffman, 2003b)

| | |
|---|---|
| Background[a,b] | |
| AL, LA, MS | 0.22 cGy/yr |
| CO, ID, NM | 0.72 |
| $^{40}$K adult human | 0.026 |
| | |
| UK Radiologists[c] | 0.05-5 |
| | |
| Technological[b] | |
| nuclear power | 0.0003 |
| nuclear fallout | 0.004 |
| nuclear devices[f] | 0.005 |
| -------------- | |
| Medical Imaging | |
| mammograms[d,e] | 0.4 cGy |
| chest X-ray[g] | 0.025 |
| dental, full-mouth[g] | 0.017 |
| CT scan, head[g] | 2 |
| CT scan, body[g] | 6 |
| thyroid scan[e] | |
| $^{131}$I | 5-10 |
| $^{123}$I | 3-5 |
| $^{99}$Tc | 1 |

[a]Luckey, 1999
[b]Upton, 1982
[c]Sherwood, 2001
[d]Giuliano, 1996
[e]Lipman, 1995
[f]smoke alarms, pacemakers, guages
[g]see text

repeated (Elias, 2001, p137) and cannot possibly have a beneficial long-term effect. In fact, they do not, as shown by a recent report of a study with a 25-year follow-up, in which women irradiated as a breast cancer treatment had no significant change in rate of recurrence and no increase in lifespan compared with controls (Fisher et al., 2002). A meta-analysis of other studies on the same type of patients, with a mean follow-up time of 11 years, showed no or no significant decrease in all-cause mortality in 15 of 18 trials (Whelan et al., 2000). Earlier trials on the same type of patients showed increased all-cause mortality as a result of irradiation after 10 years of follow-up, with more heart deaths vitiating the effect of fewer cancer deaths (Cuzick et al., 1994).

The main effect of radiation in humans of the lower (but above hormetic) dose ranges is cancer of several types. Cancer incidence is said to rise linearly with acute doses of 30-50 rads of Xrays or gamma rays, and, depending on the irradiation mode, as a squared function of acute doses from 50-200 rad (eq. 1). At still higher acute doses (>400 rad is considered lethal to humans by some authorities) the probability of cell death becomes dominant; therefore, the cancer incidence declines because radiation sickness ensues, and is then considered to be the cause of death (Feinendegen & Pollycove, 2001; Luckey, 1991, p4).

## Examples of Hormesis from Low-Dose Radiation

In contrast to the destructive effects of high-dose radiation, there are many studies that not only showed no danger from low radiation levels — ones not too far from those of normal background levels — but actual health benefits. Some research articles on radiation hormesis in humans cite examples of:

(1) Decreased cancer mortality in government nuclear facility workers in Canada, the UK, and the US (Luckey, 1991, pp111-121). Whether exposed in uranium mines or processing plants, laboratories, or nuclear power plants; and whether the exposure was to uranium, plutonium, thorium or radium, so long as the dose was < 50 times background (chronic) or < 50 rad (acute, and QF = 1), nuclear facility workers were healthier than those in the general population, mainly due to lower cancer incidence. Any possible "healthy worker effect" (the opposite of the unhealthy, unemployed, overstressed, ex-worker) was eliminated in studies which showed that nuclear workers in a single large energy company had lower mortality than thermal-only workers or non-energy workers within the same company. All groups of workers had the same physical examinations and health care.

(2) Decreased cancer mortality, decreased leukemia rate, decreased infant mortality rate and increased lifespan in atomic bomb survivors from both Hiroshima and Nagasaki who received < 1.2 rad (Luckey, 1991, p148-158), and further discussed in detail below.

(3) A 20% lower cancer death rate in Idaho, Colorado and New Mexico, which have background radiation of 0.72 rad/year compared with Louisiana, Mississippi and Alabama with 0.22 rad per year (Luckey, 1999). However, a supposed inverse correlation of *all-cause* death with the level of background radiation in the southeastern states compared with the Rocky Mountain states (Luckey, 1991, p181-182) failed to exclude magnesium in drinking water as a confounder (see Myth 1 and Kauffman, 2000). But high background radiation in parts of China and in Kerala, India, confers longer lifespan, supporting the first USA data above (Luckey, 1991, p181).

(4) Slightly *lower* cancer mortality after a 1957 explosion that dispersed nuclear weapon wastes in the eastern Urals village of Chelyabinsk. About 1,000 people were exposed to about 0.5 Sv of strontium-90 over 1.5 years (Luckey, 1991, p26, 141).

(5) Lower incidence of breast cancer in women who received a cumulative 10-29 rad of Xrays during repeated fluoroscopy in Canada (discussed in detail below).

(6) Lower incidence of breast cancer in women who received a cumulative 10-19 rad of Xrays during repeated fluoroscopy for spinal curvature (discussed in detail below).

184

(7) Decreased cancer mortality and decreased total mortality in workers from the US Nuclear Shipyard Worker Study (Pollycove & Feinendegen, 2001).

(8) British male radiologists practicing after 1954, exposed to 0.05 - 5 rad annually of Xrays have a lower cancer and all-cause death rate than the most relevant peer group, other male medical practitioners (Sherwood, 2001).

(9) For half of all US counties, representing 90% of the US population, lung cancer rates *decrease* by about 35% as the mean radon level in homes (by county) *increases* from 0.5 - 3 pCi/L, and the cancer rate is still 25% below what was found at the ZEV, even at 3 - 6 pCi/L (Cohen, 1997a). Related smaller studies in England and France confirm these findings (Cohen, 1995). This effect was less pronounced in the results from a questionnaire study relating the ratio of lung cancer deaths to all cancer deaths vs individually measured radon levels, but the findings still did not follow the LNT relationship at all (discussed in detail below), (Cohen, 1997b).

(10) In the Holm Study in Sweden on about 35,000 normal subjects who received 50 rad of $^{131}I$ (a beta emitter) to the thyroid for diagnostic purposes, and who were followed for 20 years, the relative risk (RR) for thyroid cancer was 0.62 compared with that of controls (Yalow, 1995); in other words, this means that there were 62 cases of cancer in the treatment group for every 100 cases in the control group.

(11) An examination of older literature disclosed a 12-year study on the effect of 6 50-rad doses of Xrays in 364 patients with gas gangrene, a treatment which brought the death rate from 50% down to 5-12% without surgery or antibiotic (Cuttler, 2002).

(12) Dwellings in Taipei, Taiwan, contained rebar into which cobalt-60 was accidentally incorporated. About 10,000 people were exposed to gamma rays — about 3 rad per year for 9-20 years — and were much healthier than the surrounding population (discussed in detail below).

*****

The Canadian fluoroscopy study referred to above involved 31,710 Canadian women being examined and treated for tuberculosis with Xray doses to the chest beginning between 1930 and 1952, and followed for up to 50 years. The results from all provinces except Nova Scotia, for which too few low-dose data points were taken, are shown in Figure 8-3. These are age-adjusted, since first exposure at ages 10-14 was considered to be 4 times as damaging as exposure over age 35. The data are presented as breast cancer incidence (after a 10-year lag from the first Xray exposure of the patient) per million person-years of exposure to different Xray doses. The rate of breast cancer at 10-19 rad cumulative exposure is 34% lower than that at the lowest exposure, a clear hormetic effect. It was 15% lower at 20-29 rad, and not significantly higher at 30-69 rad. Nevertheless, the authors forced the data into a linear response based on the LNT theory, and thus estimated a positive risk of death from breast cancer per rad at all levels! I consider this study to be among the best evidence for radiation hormesis because the authors were not looking for it, and effectively denied that it existed. This differs from some of the other examples given above where the authors were *looking* for hormesis. This study is very typical of the literature in that biopositive effects at the lowest doses were discounted. Readers often have to ferret out the low-dose effects from the raw data.

Here is another case of hormesis denial: Lynn Ehrle, MEd, brought to my attention a paper in the journal *Spine* in which the authors investigated the effect of Xray exposure on future breast cancer mortality (Doody et al, 2000). This paper was said to illustrate that more cancer was found even at the lowest Xray doses, and, therefore, that the study did not show a hormesis range. This was a retrospective study on 5573 women with spinal curvature (scoliosis) who had been exposed to Xrays for diagnostic purposes. Their mean age at diagnosis was 10.6 years, and the mean follow-up time was 40.1 years. The cumulative Xray doses to the breasts were individually estimated, and arbitrarily

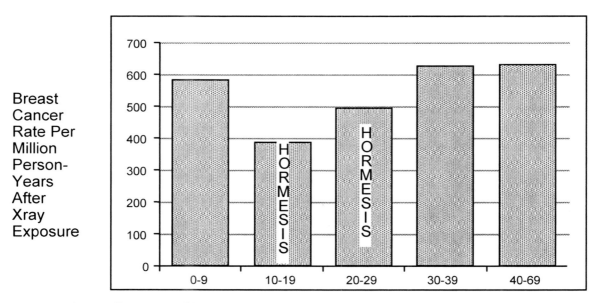

Fig. 8-3. Breast Cancer Rates vs. Cumulative Xray Doses in Canadian Fluoroscopy Study. Adjusted for age of first Xray exposure. Based on data from Miller et al., 1989

Dose Ranges of Xrays Used in Fluoroscopic Examinations in cGy or rad

divided into ranges as follows: 0 rad, mean dose 0 rad; 1-9, mean 4.4; 10-19, mean 14.5; and ≥20, mean 31.9. This means that the highest dose range contained all doses up to the highest amounts. The authors cited the article by Miller et al., 1989, without understanding that a hormesis range of 10-29 rad was demonstrated (see Figure 8-3). The articles by Boice et al, 1977, and of Shore et al., 1986, (see below) were cited with no understanding that hormesis probably was concealed because of the manner of data selection and presentation (see Tables 8-1 and 8-2). The Conclusions in the Abstract of the article by Doody et al. were: "...exposure to multiple diagnostic radiographic examinations during childhood and adolescence may increase the risk of breast cancer among women with scoliosis..."; hormesis was not even considered.

However, when the data in their Table 6 were charted as shown in Figure 8-4, made possible by their provision of both the numbers of patients and breast cancer deaths, it was clear that a hormesis range of 10-19 rad (mean 14.5 rad) was observed — quite similar to the range found by Miller et al. Because all cumulative exposures of 20 rads on up were lumped together, the chances are good that evidence of hormesis from 20-29 rads as found by Miller et al. was concealed. It was also clear that the typical death rate from breast cancer was quite low at under 1.5% overall (see Myth 9). This study by Doody et al. has been quoted by the authors of a popular book as "proof" that Xrays in any dose cause breast cancer (Lee et al., 2002, pp9-10,31-32).

An apartment complex in Taipei, Taiwan, built mainly of concrete, had the steel reinforcing rods (rebar) accidentally contaminated with discarded cobalt-60, a gamma emitter with a 5.3-year half life. About 10,000 residents were irradiated for 9-20 years. The mean cumulative dose was 40 rads, and 1,100 residents with the highest exposure received 400 rads. The mean annual dose was 3 rads, but the most exposed 1,100 residents received 20 rads per year. This incident was decried as a great disaster by the media in the late 1990s; some residents sued the government for compensation; but hospital workers in Taiwan did not find any signs of medical problems. The ICRP model predicted 232 natural cancer deaths in this population, plus 70 caused by the radiation; only 7 cancer deaths were observed, a 97% reduction. The number of congenital malformations (birth defects) expected in the

186

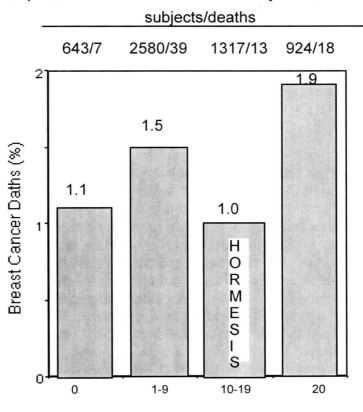

Figure 8-4.  Observed Breast Cancer Deaths Among Scoliosis Patients According Xray Exposure. Based on data from Doody et al., 2000.

surrounding population was 46, and the ICRP model predicted 67; only 3 were observed, a 95.5% reduction (Chen et al., 2004). Clearly, 400 rads of cobalt-60 gamma rays are not fatal, but beneficial, as a cumulative dose.

\*\*\*\*\*

In other animals, low-dose Xrays or gamma rays increase the lifespans of mice, rats, house flies, flour beetles, codling moths and house crickets, while higher doses usually decrease lifespans. Growth rates of *Paramecium* and *Synechococcus* strains are enhanced at dose rates of 2-5 rad/year of gamma rays, but reduced at higher doses. Antibody response to Staphylococcus in rabbits by prior whole-body Xray treatment is enhanced by 100 R, but inhibited by 1000 R. Antibody response to hemocyanin in mice was enhanced by 100-200 R per week, but inhibited by 300 R per week. Antibody response to sheep red blood cells by mouse spleen cells is enhanced by prior exposure of the spleen cells to 5-50 rad of Xrays, but inhibited by higher doses. Plaque formation and DNA synthesis in mouse spleen cells are enhanced by 2.5-7.5 rad of gamma rays in vivo, but inhibited at higher doses. The response of mouse splenic lymphocytes to antigen is enhanced by prior exposure to 2 rad of gamma rays in vivo, but inhibited by 200 rad (all from Upton, 2001).

In rats 25 rads of Xrays cut the breast cancer rate in half, but there was more breast cancer than in the controls above 200 rads. Also in rats 5 rads of neutrons cut breast cancer rate by two thirds, but there was more breast cancer than in the controls above 40 rads. In mice a type of desirable immune response peaked at 7.5 rads of Xrays, but dropped below that of controls at 9 rads (all from Calabrese & Baldwin, 1999b).

In mice bred to be tumor prone, a low dose of gamma rays significantly delays the development of bone tumors and lymphomas, according to Ron Mitchel of Atomic Energy of Canada, Ltd. (Mitchel et al., 2003; Kaiser, 2003).

In plants, the growth of tomato seeds is unchanged by an acute dose of 250 R, enhanced by 500-1000 R, and reduced by 2000 R. Pollen tube growth in Pinus sylvestris pollen grains was unchanged by 300 rad of Xrays or gamma rays, enhanced by 400-900 rad, but reduced at higher doses up to 10,000 rad (Upton, 2001).

*****

The major types of DNA damage, which are believed to be the most serious type of damage, are base changes, single-strand breaks, double-strand breaks and inter-strand crosslinks. About 60% of the total damage is indirectly caused by hydroxyl radicals. Most DNA damage is repaired rapidly. The probability of an oncogenic transformation with lethal consequences per stem cell in vivo at 0.1 rad (6 months of normal background) of Xrays or gamma rays is very low, on the order of $10^{-13}$ to $10^{-14}$, and is far lower than the "spontaneous" rate of cancer. Irradiated cells initiate protective responses within a few hours, including radical detoxification, DNA repair, cell removal by stimulated immune response, and apoptosis (normal programmed cell death). These responses are also used to repair endogenous DNA and other metabolic damage as well (Feinendegen & Pollycove, 2001; Luckey, 1991, p5).

Radiation damage caused by a low initial dose induces a DNA repair mechanism that allows efficient repair of a large number of breaks from a high later dose. This has been investigated by biochemical experimenters in great detail (Wolff, 1992). *Radiation hormesis, therefore, is a moderate overcompensation to a disruption in homeostasis caused by the radiation; it is a stimulus to the repair mechanisms that cope with non-radiation damage as well, so that the overall effect is a health benefit* (Cuttler, 2002). Acute doses of 1-50 rad are beneficial, and 10 rad/year appears to be the optimum hormetic dose for humans (Luckey, 1991, p228-230), but there is considerable individual variation, and more damage to children than to adults. These doses refer especially to external whole-body low-LET radiation.

Many experiments on isolated cells are known which appear to show that a single particle hit can damage not only a directly hit cell, but others nearby (Kaiser, 2003). However, isolated cells or even tissue cultures do not have an immune system to make repairs, so the old scare tale of the danger of a single hit does not apply. As noted above, we live in a sea of radiation all the time.

Much thought has been given to the idea that radiation is not merely beneficial at certain doses, but is essential to life. The radiation from the primordial radionuclides of potassium, thorium, uranium and others is thought to have been about 10 times more intense 4 billion years ago than now, based on simple back-calculation from known half-lives of these radioisotopes (Luckey, 1991, p220). Exposure of the protozoan *Euglena gracilis* to 5-10 rad/day causes *increased* growth rates, and 500 rad/day still engenders the same growth rate as ambient radiation, demonstrating the great radiation resistance of this ancient organism. The hatchability rate of the eggs of the brine shrimp, *Artemia,* is *reduced* from 60% at ambient radiation to 10% at am exposure level of about 1% of ambient radiation. This type of experiment is done by placing the test organism in a deep mine to shield it from radiation. There are more than a dozen additional examples given (Luckey, 1991, p211-223) which showed that the curve in Fig. 8-2 should be extended to the left and upwards to show that lower doses than ambient are less safe to life forms in general, and that above-ambient doses of radiation ($\approx$ 10 rad/year chronic, or $\approx$ 50 rad acute) are the optimum doses for mammals (Luckey, 1991, pp42,230).

## Radon Gas, the Awful Bugaboo

The supposed dangers of radon in causing lung cancer are based on extrapolation of high doses among afflicted miners to low doses using the LNT model; but the confounding factors in mining, such as inhaling toxic particulates, were not properly eliminated (Luckey, 1991, p13). Evidence presented below will negate the validity of such an extrapolation.

Volney Wallace of Dugway, Utah, made the following observations (Wallace, 1986):

"In the milling of uranium ore, the ore is ground finely and extracted with acid or alkali. Most of the radon in the ore is released in the process and surely ought to have given a lot of uranium mill workers a high-level exposure to radon. The normal incidence of lung cancer among them [or below normal, see Figures 8-5 and 8-6] raises considerable suspicion about the alleged carcinogenicity of radon. That suspicion is much strengthened when one considers mechanisms. A person breathing radon gets a whole-body exposure to radioactivity and only an incidental exposure to the lungs. On the other hand, a smoker breathing radioactive ore dust would have particles... lodge in his lungs... and those particles would repeatedly send... radiation into the same local region of lung tissue. The potential for radioactive dust to cause cumulative radiation damage to lungs is many orders of magnitude greater than that of radon. I would judge that the problem of lung cancer among uranium miners was due primarily to smoking, secondarily to radioactive dust, and not at all to radon.

"Salt Lake City had a uranium tailings pile that needed only to be covered with clay, but the fear of radon was hyped to the point that the state [of Utah] spent many millions of dollars that it could ill afford to move the tailings to a rural location. The Environmental Impact Statement [required by the US Environmental Protection Agency] justified the health hazard... [supposedly represented by] radon with nothing more than the statement that a high incidence of lung cancer had been found in workers in a mill 'in the uranium producing area of Eastern Europe'. The study turned out to be of machinists who worked with uncommon metals, including arsenic, but not uranium! It gives considerable cause for concern when our federal government can present no better case than this for the carcinogenicity of radon."

\*\*\*\*\*

Jay H. Lubin, National Cancer Institute, misrepresented some of the ecologic findings on radon exposure of Bernard L. Cohen, Department of Physics and Astronomy, University of Pittsburgh. As shown in Figure 8-8 (from Fig. 3 in Lubin & Boice, 1997), Lubin extrapolates Cohen's results out to 350 $Bq/m^3$, where, in fact, Cohen presented data only to 260 $Bq/m^3$. Lubin and Boice combined 8 case-control studies on radon exposure and found a RR = 1.14 for lung cancer at 150 $Bq/m^3$ using an LNT-based approach. However, in Lubin's Fig. 2 (not reproduced here), which showed the graphs with data points for each individual study, it is readily seen that the study called Finland-I showed decreased risk (= hormetic effect) at 300 $Bq/m^3$; that Finland-II showed a slight hormetic effect at 280 $Bq/m^3$; that Shenyang had a pronounced hormetic effect at all radon levels; that Winnipeg had a hormetic effect at 220 $Bq/m^3$; and that Missouri had a hormetic effect at 50-80 $Bq/m^3$. Only the high risks at higher levels of radon in the Stockholm and New Jersey studies made the combined RR positive. Cohen wrote that the disagreement of the 8 case-control studies with each other, and their poor statistical power invalidate Lubin's conclusions (Cohen, 1997c).

Lubin's results for miners as shown by the white squares in Figure 8-8 showed no obvious trend and could fit RR = 1 within the range of 95% CI bars. Sharp eyes will even see a hormetic effect at 400 Bq/m³.

Cohen's revised findings are shown in Figure 8-9 (from Fig. 1 in Cohen, 1997a), after he made allowances for a great number of potentially confounding factors. Typical radon levels in homes were around the value of 1. The dip at levels higher than 1 shown by the data points indicates a *decrease* in lung cancer rates as the radon levels *increased.* Lubin countered this presentation with a hypothetical example of how Cohen's results could have been due to bias, subject to the ecological fallacy (described in Milloy, 2001), and why these results should be rejected because they "are at odds with the overwhelming [sic] evidence from epidemiological...studies and are likely the result of confounding within county" (Lubin, 1998). In a final rejoinder, Cohen found faults in Lubin's treatment, and explained how the "ecologic fallacy" does not apply in testing the LNT. The results of a recent British study on radon levels were also presented by Cohen, showing no trend in toxicity below 120 Bq/m³ and no effects of high statistical significance even at 200 and 370 Bq/m³ (Cohen, 1999).

A recent case-control study found that, among children diagnosed with leukemia when under 2 years old, there was an *inverse* relation of home radon level with risk. There was no statistically significant relationship among children over 2 (Steinbuch et al., 1999). Both findings are at odds with the positions of Gofman and Lubin, and in agreement with those of Cohen.

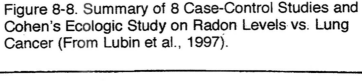

Figure 8-8. Summary of 8 Case-Control Studies and Cohen's Ecologic Study on Radon Levels vs. Lung Cancer (From Lubin et al., 1997).

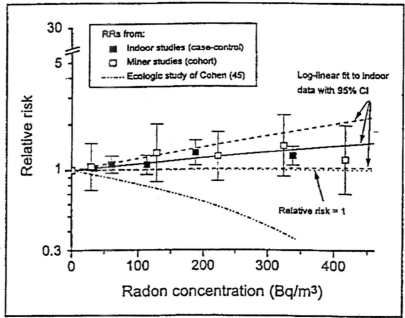

The EPA's estimate that radon exposure causes 20,000 of the 140,000 annual lung cancer deaths in the US is unreasonable (Yalow, 1995). Regarding radon levels, none of the 8 case-control studies cited above shows a statistically significant health detriment below 150 Bq/m³, and of the 5 with data in the 300-400 Bq/m³ range, only 1 shows a slight risk in this range (Lubin & Boice, 1997). If Cohen is correct about hormesis in this range, there is realizable benefit in achieving *lower* lung cancer rates by leaving *above*-average radon levels in homes undisturbed. Standards for radon levels could be relaxed from the current 150 Bq/m³ (4 pCi/L) to at least 250 Bq/m³ (7 pCi/L) with no increased risk and considerable health benefits. For example, the Commission of the European Communities (CEC, 1990) has recommended the following action levels for radon removal: 200 Bq/m³ for new homes and 400 Bq/m³ for existing homes. The World Health Organisation (WHO, 1988) on the other hand recommended a single value of 200 Bq/m³ for general application, with a maximum of 800 Bq/m³. (http://pachome1.pacific.net.sg/~sckmipil/radonpt2.htm). Most of the radon dispersal systems in US homes, which cost $800-1,500, have been valueless or worse, except to the vendors.

People are paying to be exposed to radon in caves or mines for treatment of cancer and arthritis. The benefits are now under study (http://www.radonmine.com/letter.shtml#N_8_).
The radon levels in one Montana mine are 1600 pCi/L! Many people inhaling the radon in the mine to treat arthritis can stop taking medication and remain pain-free for a year, at least this is claimed. At least 83 of the people have been using the mine for over 20 years, and 173 for over 10 years, all with repeat visits and all with complete satisfaction. The American Medical Association declined to send a qualified person to assess the radon treatment. In Austria and Germany the national health insurance pays for visits to radon mines or spas (Erickson, 2004).

Fig. 8-9. Recent Presentation of Cohen's Ecologic Study on Radon Levels vs. Lung Cancer, where $m_0$ is mortality from lung cancer at $r_0$, a mean radon level of 1 pCi/L or 37 Bq/m³ (from Cohen, 1997a). Shows $m/m_0$ vs. $r/r_0$ for all 1,601 counties. Males left, females right graph.

Each data point represents all counties within a range of $r/r_0$ values: <0.5, 0.5-0.75, 0.75-1, 1-1.25, 1.25-1.5, 1.5-1.75, 1.72-2, 2-2.25, 2.25-2.5, 2.5-2.75, 2.75-3, 3-3.5, 3.5-4, 4-5 and >5. Each datum point is the mean value of $m/m_0$ for these, and the error bar is the std. dev. of the mean.

The dotted line represents the best fit for the 1,601 underlying data points to $m/m_0 = A + Br$. The dashed line represents the best fit to $m/m_0 = A + Br + Cr^2$.

The solid straight line at the upper left going up to the right is the prediction of the LNT model.

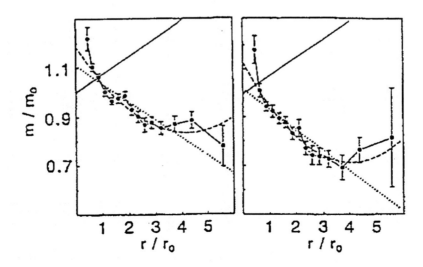

<u>Existence of Radiation Hormesis Challenged</u>

The evidence for hormesis is not viewed as reliable by key members of the radiation protection community for the following putative reasons: (1) Data in support of radiation hormesis in human populations is limited, and much of it is based on reevaluation of selected epidemiological data that has been used to test a different hypothesis; (2) hormetic effects are weak and inconsistent, and are subject to large statistical uncertainties; (3) a consensus is lacking on how hormesis should be defined and quantified; and (4) it is unclear to some administrators how hormesis can be incorporated into the regulatory framework when beneficial health effects occur just below the doses that cause health problems (Mossman, 2001).

Regarding (1), the supposed paucity of data: more than 30,000 Canadian women and almost 6,000 American women were in the fluoroscopy studies that showed hormesis; Cohen's ecological study related radon levels in 1,600 US counties to lung cancer deaths in 90% of the population, and some of the results were 20 standard deviations from the LNT relationship; see below (Cohen, 1995); and more than 7,000,000 government nuclear facility workers were included in 9 studies (Luckey, 1999). One is reminded of the tobacco industry's response to research findings that smoking is a cause of lung cancer by invariably calling for more research.

Regarding (2), weak data: charts depict the cumulative radiation exposure vs. the death rate in the UK Atomic Energy Authority work force, Figure 8-5 being death from all cancers and Figure 8-6 death from leukemia. First, it can be seen that there is no trend; second, the highest doses were still very low and might have marked the *onset* of a hormetic effect; and third, *both* death rates were below expectations compared with those for all UK workers. This kind of finding is not equivocal even though it neither proves nor disproves hormesis because the *maximum* doses, from film badges, were too low (Beral et al., 1987).

Fig. 8-5. Mortality from all malignant neoplasms vs. cumulative whole-body radiation exposure in the UKAEA workforce of - 50,000 from 1946-1979 (from Fig. 3 in Beral et al. 1987). Actual deaths are shown above columns. Chart shows neither a trend nor an LNT relationship.

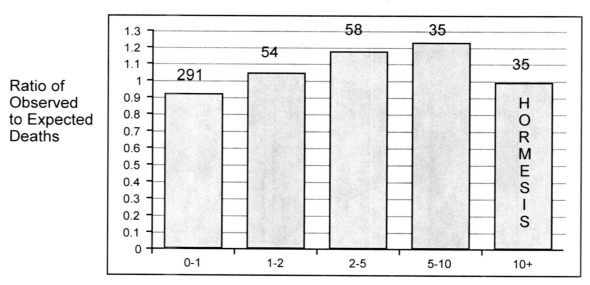

Cumulative Radiation Exposure in Rads

A US study of breast cancer incidence vs. Xray exposure of women being checked for tuberculosis seemingly did not show the hormesis effect of the Canadian study (Table 8-1). The authors here gave the mean Xray exposure for the second datum as 50 rads. In fact the range was 2-98 rads, which could have concealed a hormetic effect between 2 and 50 rads. The authors wrote that the

Fig. 8-6. Mortality from all leukemia vs. cumulative whole-body radiation exposure in the UKAEA workforce of - 50,000 from 1946-1979 (from Fig. 4 in Beral et al. 1987). Actual deaths are shown above columns. Shows neither a trend nor an LNT relationship.

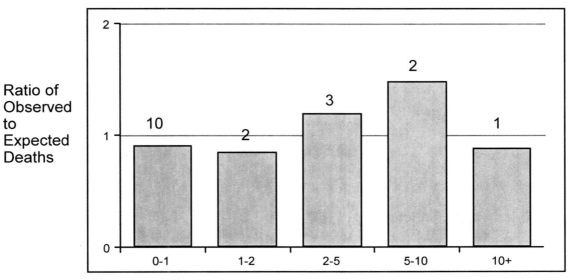

Cumulative Radiation Exposure in Rads

data supported the LNT hypothesis (Boice & Monson, 1977), which, of course, is nonsense, because the % of women with no breast cancer at death was the same for both zero rads and 2-98 rads. The LNT hypothesis requires that more breast cancer be found at 2-98 rads.

Table 8-1. Xray exposure vs. breast cancer incidence for which LNT was reported. Women subjected to fluoroscopic examinations and followed for 28 years (mean) after first exposure. (Based on data in Fig. 2 and Table 6 in Boice et al. 1977).

| No. of Exams Using Xrays | 0 | 1-49 | 50-99 | 100-149 | 150-199 | 200+ |
|---|---|---|---|---|---|---|
| Est. Exposure in rads | 0 | 2-98 | 100-198 | 200-298 | 300-398 | 400+ |
| % Treated Who Had No Breast Cancer at Death | 98 | 98 | 96 | 93 | 95 | 96 |

Another study, in which women were treated with Xrays for acute postpartum mastitis (Table 8-2) shows the RR of cancer steadily rising from that of the controls. However, the second datum, in which only 2 breast cancers appear, has a 90% (not 95%) lower CI value of 0.4, which is far below 1.0 for the controls. These authors also reported an LNT relationship (Shore et al., 1986). Again I calculated the % breasts with no cancer after a mean period of 29 years of follow-up, and again one can see that a hormetic effect could be concealed in the lower doses of the second datum (60-149 rad) or, more likely, missed in the unexamined range below 60 rad. Was the 1-59 rad range left out deliberately? So neither of these studies *disproved* the existence of a hormetic effect of Xrays on breast cancer because of the choices of dose ranges to report.

Table 8-2.  Xray exposure vs. breast cancer incidence for Which LNT was reported.  Women treated with Xrays for acute postpartum mastitis and followed for 29 years (mean) after first exposure.  (Based on data in Table 5 of Shore et al. 1986.)

| Xray Dose Range | Control | 60-149 | 150-249 | 250-349 |
|---|---|---|---|---|
| Mean Dose (rad) | 0 | 109 | 199 | 295 |
| No. of Breasts | 2,891 | 48 | 149 | 203 |
| No. of Breast Cancers | 64 | 2 | 12 | 15 |
| RR of Breast Cancers (90% CI) | 1.00 | 1.37 (0.4-4.2) | 3.26 (1.9-5.5) | 4.10 (2.5-6.6) |
| % Breasts With No Cancer | 0.98 | 0.96 | 0.92 | 0.93 |

Regarding (3), consensus: such cannot be imagined until the regulators stop denying the very existence of hormesis, nor should more than the acquiescence of a majority be required; see below.

Regarding (4), difficult implementation of hormesis: it should be possible (and it is certainly desirable) to keep a tally of all the radiation exposure of each citizen, including background, incidental, medical, and employment sources of radiation. With actual knowledge of dose levels, some health-enhancing decisions could be made and refined with confidence. Measuring only external low-LET radiation, a potentially easier task, would be better than no measurements at all.  An identification tag worn around the neck, and placed to receive medical Xrays, and readable in an instrument, seems an achievable goal.

Radiation Hormesis Denied and Dismissed

An entire book was written by John William Gofman, MD, PhD, Professor Emeritus of Medical Physics at UC Berkeley whose sole purpose was given on the fly leaf: "...an expert who is independent [sic] of the radiation community provides the human and physical evidence proving that carcinogenesis from ionizing radiation does occur at the lowest conceivable doses and dose-rates (Gofman, 1990). This finding refutes claims by parts of the radiation community that very low doses or dose-rates may be safe." In charting data on radiation dose vs. all-cancer death rates for atomic bomb victims from his Table 11-F, a hormetic effect is seen despite Gofman's denials (Figure 8-7). This effect is now accepted by some scientists, despite Gofman's determined efforts (Kaiser, 2003). In discussing the Canadian Study ex Nova Scotia (Figure 8- 3) on his pp18-8 and 21-4, Gofman does not address the actual observations. In discussing the Massachusetts Study (Table 8-1) on his pp 18-8 and 21-5, Gofman does not address the lack of separate data in the 2-50 rad range. Gofman wrote (pp 22-

15 - 22-25) that the Holm Study in Sweden of [131]I cited above was fatally flawed due to an improperly chosen control group, and that there was 4 times as much thyroid cancer in the diagnostic group as in the controls, disagreeing with evidence published by other workers (Luckey, 1991, pp139-141; Yalow,1995).

Figure 8-7. Hiroshima and Nagasaki Victims, Radiation Dose vs. all Cancer Deaths. (From Table 11-F in Gofman, 1990.)

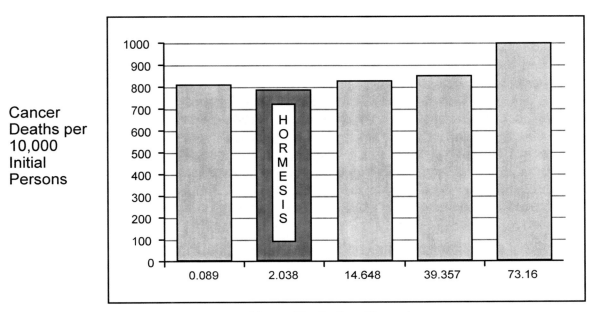

Mean Radiation Dose in rem

Carl J. Paperiello, US Nuclear Regulatory Commission (NRC), wrote an essay in which no single example of hormesis was cited, and he wrote as though the possibility of it was hypothetical. "The arguments in support of the LNT model are based on plausibility [sic]." That there might be a "threshold" for damage (a NOAEL) in the 0.1 rad dose range was admitted, but not hormesis. "Loss of the LNT model would result in 20 years' worth of of calculational work being discarded as well as every environmental analysis being dependent upon this dosimetry." How could this imagined "catastrophe" be true if only regulation below 5-10 rad/year or 50-100 rad acute were dropped? Paperiello also wrote as though neither the dose-rate nor the additivity of radiation had ever been investigated, and that the existence of occupational and medical exposure would throw all regulators into a tizzy if the LNT model were dropped. "In addition, because hormetic effects [the ones he does not admit to exist at all] are based on repair stimulation by many small doses, the trend in the past 50 years to base occupational standards on annual limits rather than weekly or monthly limits might be reversed." I am underwhelmed by this. And as a final warning shot: "The current LNT model evolved over a period of 50 years [sic]. If past history is predictive of the future, change could be comparably slow." (Papariello, 2000)

As the historian of the US Nuclear Regulatory Commission (NRC), J. Samuel Walker probably wrote an accurate record of what the NRC, its peers and its antecedents did to protect us from excess radiation in his book: *Permissible Dose: A History of Radiation Protection in the Twentieth Century*. Moreover, the writing is outstandingly clear, perfectly edited, and well-organized, mainly chronologically, and has footnotes to sources that appear to be in the best academic tradition. The NRC is to be congratulated on its successful protection of the public except for accidental individual blunders in industrial or medical practice for which the NRC could not be blamed. It may feel proud of

195

resisting the excessive demands of the EPA, John W. Gofman, MD, PhD, and self-styled environmental groups, and it certainly did not cave into the opposing demands of industry and medicine by allowing exposures to dangerous levels of ionizing radiation. However, Walker does not think the NRC bears any responsibility for the myth that all radiation exposures are risky, and thus has contributed to unfounded fears, because the level of emissions, as nuclear waste decays, eventually would be in the beneficial (hormetic) range until it dropped below even that. The linear no-threshold (LNT) extrapolation from high doses is "justified" throughout the book despite overwhelming evidence for its failure to account for the observations set out in this chapter. Of the hundreds of journal articles and books reporting or reviewing radiation hormesis (Luckey, 1991), not one is cited. Of the 4500 individual examples of hormesis (Hively, 2002), not one is cited. Of the dozens of reviews in peer-reviewed journals by respected scientists, specifically T. D. Luckey, E. J. Calabrese, B. L. Cohen, J. M. Cuttler, M. Pollycove, L. E. Feinendegen, K. L. Mossman, A. C. Upton and S. Wolff, among others, not one is cited. After admitting only that "controversy" exists over the biological effects of low doses, Walker gives one token quotation based on newspaper and magazine articles by Myron Pollycove, and even this was probably chosen because Pollycove was a consultant to the NRC. This was presented so as to marginalize it. Walker did not cite a single piece of evidence for hormesis (benefit), or even use either word, maintaining the fiction that the choices were between minor risk or no risk, never benefit. Nor does Walker believe that the NRC should be censured for the very high costs of implementing its unnecessarily excessive requirements (Kauffman, 2003).

## Public Policy Implications of Radiation Hormesis

The supposed increased risk of breast cancer from Xrays in annual mammograms has led to recommendations for women to avoid them altogether (Lee et al., 2002, pp9-10,31-32). Gofman estimated that 75% of breast cancers are *caused* by mammograms combined with other medical sources (as quoted in Diamond et al., 1997, p721). The data presented above in Figures 8-3 and 8-4 as well as Tables 8-1 and 8-2 all refute this. Gofman estimated that the entrance dose of Xrays in a typical examination was about 2 rads (Gofman & O'Connor, 1985, p221). In an updated review of the 5 Swedish mammography studies, the RR = 0.79 for breast cancer mortality, and, one must note, RR = 0.98 for all-cause mortality (Nystrom, et al. 2002). The total dose was calculated by me for each individual study based on the number of examinations (2-7), the number of views (1-2), and the attendance rate. The mean value was 12 rads of cumulative Xray dose. From the Canadian fluoroscopy study in Fig. 8-3 it can be seen that the RR = 0.66 for breast cancer at the closest cumulative dose range (10-19 rads). Even if the Swedish women continued to receive mammograms at the same rate until the end of the study, and doubled their cumulative dose to 24 rads, their RR = 0.85 for breast cancer based on the Canadian fluoroscopy study. A very critical review of the results of the 5 Swedish trials along with 3 others found RR = 0.76, 0.79 and 0.87 for death from breast cancer in those 3 others, which were considered to be of poor quality (Gøtzsche & Olsen, 2000). It must be added that these latter reviewers found RR = 1.00 for all-cause mortality in all the trials (Gotzsche & Olsen, 2000; Olsen & Gotzsche, 2001). The main criticism of the trials was poor randomization. Neither the Danish nor the Swedish reviewers allowed for any possible hormesis effect, or even considered the effects of different cumulative Xray doses; thus all trials of mammography are confounded by the failure to have control groups, whose subjects' breasts should have been squashed and pretended to be Xrayed without using film! (Or better yet, appearing to use film as part of a placebo effect. Obviously there would be ethical issues in attempting any such effort.)

Even a *recent* oncology text presents the results of the same 8 mammography trials *without* all-cause mortality, and as though there had been no criticism of mammography (Rimer et al., 2001). This despite the fact that there *was* serious criticism from mainstream physicians 12 years before

(Skrabanek & McCormick, 1989) and 17 years before (Robin, 1984). A recent gynecology text presents extensive tables of risk/benefit ratio, obviously based on the LNT theory for the supposed radiation risk, without specifically noting what basis was used, and thus is misleading by not allowing for hormesis. The supposed benefits from screening, reductions in breast cancer mortality of up to 25%, are also misleading, because *all-cause* mortality is not given (Mishell et al., 1997).

Modern mammography routines in the 1990s are now claimed to deliver as little as 0.2 rad, apparently for each pair of views of each breast, thus totaling 0.4 rad per total examination (Giuliano, 1996; Lipman, 1995). If a woman of 50 began in 1990 to have annual mammograms until age 75, the cumulative dose would be 10 rads, seemingly the low end of the optimum hormetic dose, so avoiding mammography because of the radiation "hazard" is not the best reason. (The unchanged all-cause mortality rate, as noted above, due to aggressive treatment of the many false positives, is a better reason. See Myth 9.)

In the 1970s the mean exposure to a single dental Xray was supposedly about 0.6 rad per shot (that is, the entrance dose, which is comparable with the doses of chest or breast Xrays), (Gofman & O'Connor, 1985, p235). Faster film had cut the dose considerably by the year 2002. According to an e-mail from Sarah Acker, Eastman Kodak Co., in 2002, a single dental shot now requires only 0.0009 rad, rem, cGy or cSv, and a full-mouth series of 19 shots requires only 0.017 rad. A lifetime annual dose at this low level, from age 20-80, would be 1 rad, which is in the hormetic range.

Low-dose total-body (or half-body) radiation for treatment of certain types of cancer, typically with 150 rad in divided doses, leading to up to a doubling of survival rates at up to 12 years, has been reported at least 5 times. This is not to be confused with the 4,000 to 6,000 rads used in conventional cancer treatments given by radiation oncologists, which are debilitating and deadly. Ironically, many radiation oncologists refuse to perform the low-dose procedure despite the evidence for its effectiveness and its almost total lack of side-effects (Cuttler et al., 2000). More specifically, several medical groups have used this low-dose treatment successfully for ovarian, colon, blood and lung cancers and for non-Hodgkin's lymphoma (Cuttler & Pollycove, 2003).

The radiation community should work out methods for determining the total radiation exposure, including background, for all our citizens. Perhaps simple dosimeters could be provided to be carried on key rings, built into licenses or social security cards, or carried on identification tags, at least for infants. Ideally, extremely high readings would generate an audible or visual signal. Since the actual output of medical Xray devices for dental work varies by a factor of as much as 40 (Gofman, 1985, p235), the dosimeter should be placed in the beam, or each instrument needs to have its output measured, at least annually, and the entrance dose entered into each patient's medical record. At the least, this will give some basis for determining total death rates (and causes) vs. radiation dose from cosmic, gamma and Xrays; but with the caveat that alpha and beta particles and neutrons would not be counted. This could lead to great cost savings by not overcompensating for low-level radiation from any external source, and to better health by eliminating fear of *low-dose* radiation from radon and the beneficial medical procedures. Such dosimeters would give the U. S. Department of Homeland Security early warning of any radiation contamination by terrorists.

Such a dosimeter that measures higher doses, 1 roentgen (R) per hour on up, was introduced in January, 2003. With a 10-year-life battery as its power source, this tiny device is to be carried on a key chain. The NukAlert™ sensor is composed of a cadmium sulfide photocell exposed to light emitted by a radioluminescent rare earth phosphor (scintillator) that emits light pulses when struck by Xrays or gamma rays. The NukAlert™ is always on, continuously monitoring and sampling its immediate environment. The number of chirps it emits is proportional to the number of light pulses detected, and thus indicates the dose level of the radiation. It costs $160. (http://www.nukalert.com/)

Those who are certain of the hormesis effect have taken the implications to the logical extreme: people who are not receiving the optimum dose of radiation should take it as supplements! It is suggested that 0.4 rad/month above background for people not located in high-background regions would be optimal, with a maximum of 5 rad/year from all non-background sources. A number of radioisotopes that might be taken as nutritional supplements have been listed. Since the potassium-40 in $^{40}$KCl already provides 2/3 of our endogenous radiation, this would seem the most logical supplement to "...alleviate our radiation deficiency" (Luckey, 1999); but Luckey made no allowance for age or sex. Your author notes that medical Xrays may contribute about 2 rads per year, not counting worthless (except for radiation hormesis) mammograms (see Myth 9), so less supplementation is indicated, another reason for measuring the total exposure of every person. It also might make more sense to have a 5-rad CAT scan for cause, such as a positive blood test for cancer (<www.amascancertest.com>) rather than ingest radioactive supplements, so that some worthwhile information can be obtained from the radiation in addition to hormesis. Conversely, people who have already had the optimum radiation dose (or more) should be directed to MRI scans instead.

## Summing Up

Small doses of ionizing radiation, say 5-20 rad per year, or an acute dose of 50 rad, from Xrays or gamma rays, are not harmful. In fact, they are probably beneficial to humans and other animals by lowering cancer rates. This feature of benefit at low dose and harm at much higher doses is called a hormetic effect or radiation hormesis in this case.

Regulators and pseudo environmentalists deliberately generate public fear by opposing the very concept of radiation hormesis, ignoring the overwhelming evidence for it. This has led to needless expense both in dwellings and workplaces, resistance to nuclear power plants, as well as avoidance of exposure to beneficial medical procedures utilizing low-dose radiation. This opposition has been shown to be unwarranted by the many examples of radiation hormesis presented.

According to T. D. Luckey, the benefit of radiation hormesis is such that: "...for every thousand cancer mortalities predicted by linear models [the LNT], there will be a thousand decreased cancer mortalities and ten thousand persons with improved quality of life." (Luckey, 1991, p177) Efforts to minimize exposures to the "lowest achievable level", or to the "no observed adverse effect level" (NOAEL) or to "below regulatory concern" (BRC) are all counterproductive to health, diverting resources from more worthy endeavors.

The scare over low radon levels, combined with the lawfully mandated remediation cost is one of the most arrant frauds ever perpetrated on an innocent public in the radiation protection field by self-serving "health-scare professionals".

Fear of medical Xrays is unfounded except possibly for the cumulative effect of more than two CAT scans in a single year. Bone scans and other scans with short-lived radioisotopes in your body are usually not to be feared. Far from being a "low but acceptable risk", low doses of ionizing radiation are a benefit, mainly by lowering cancer rates.

### Acknowledgment for Myth 8

Editorial aid and key source materials were provided by Leslie Ann Bowman. Other references and valuable advice were given by Frances E. H. Pane, MSLS, Jerry Cuttler, PhD and Charles T. McGee, MD.

### References for Myth 8

Beral V, Fraser P, Booth M, Carpenter L (1987). Epidemiological Studies of Workers in the Nuclear Industry. In Radiation & Health, Jones, R. R. & Southwood, R., Eds., New York, NY:Wiley, pp97-106.

Boice JD, Jr, Monson RR (1977). Breast Cancer in Women after Repeated Fluoroscopy of the Chest. *Journal of the National Cancer Institute, 59*(3):823-832.

Calabrese EJ, Baldwin LA, Holland CD (1999a). Hormesis: A Highly Generalizable and Reproducible Phenomenon with Important Implications for Risk Assessment. *Risk Analysis* 19(2): 262-281.

Calabrese EJ, Baldwin, LA (1999b). Reevaluation of the Fundamental Dose-Response Relationship. *BioScience* 49(9):725-732.

Calabrese EJ, Baldwin LA (2000). Radiation hormesis: the demise of a legitimate hypothesis. *Human & Experimental Toxicology* 19:76-84.

Calabrese EJ, Baldwin LA (2001). U-Shaped Dose-Responses in Biology, Toxicology, and Public Health. *Annual Reviews of Public Health* 22:15-33.

Calabrese EJ, Baldwin LA (2003). Toxicology rethinks its central belief. Hormesis demands a reappraisal of the way risks are assessed. *Nature* 421:691-692.

Chen WL, Luan YC, Shieh MC, et al. (2004). Is Chronic Radiation an Effective Prophylaxis Against Cancer? *Journal of American Physicians and Surgeons* 9(1):6-10.

Cohen BL (1995). Test of the Linear-No Threshold Theory of Radiation Carcinogenesis for Inhaled Radon Decay Products. *Health Physics* 68(2):157-174.

Cohen BL (1997a). Lung Cancer Rate vs. Mean Radon Level in U. S. Counties of Various Characteristics. *Health Physics* 72(1):114-119.

Cohen BL (1997b). Questionnaire Study of the Lung Cancer Risk from Radon in Homes. *Health Physics* 72(4):615-622.

Cohen BL (1997c). Problems in the Radon vs. Lung Cancer Test of the Linear No-Threshold Theory and a Procedure for Resolving Them. *Health Physics* 72(4):623-628.

Cohen BL (1999). Response to the Lubin Rejoinder. *Health Physics* 76(4):437-439.

Cuttler JM, Pollycove M, Welsh JS (2000). Application of Low Doses of Radiation for Curing Cancer. *Canadian Nuclear Society Bulletin* 21(2):45-50.

Cuttler JM (2002). Low-Dose Irradiation Therapy to Cure Gas Gangrene Infections. *American Nuclear Society Winter Meeting* Washington, DC, 17-21 Nov 2002.

Cuttler JM, Pollycove M (2003). Controlling Prostate Cancer with Low-Dose Radiation. Abstract, American Nuclear Society, Winter Meeting, New Orleans, USA, 16-20 Nov 2003.

Cuzick J, Stewart H, Rutqvist L, et al. (1994). Cause-Specific Mortality in Long-Term Survivors of Breast Cancer Who Participated in Trials of Radiotherapy. *Journal of Clinical Oncology* 12(3):447-453.

Diamond WJ, Cowden WL, Goldberg, B (1997). *An Alternative Medicine Definitive Guide to Cancer.* Tiburon, CA: Future Medicine Publishing.

Elias TD (2001). The Burzynski Breakthrough, Rev. Ed., 40% New Content with Clinical Trial Statistics. Nevada City, CA: Lexikos.

Erickson BE (2004). The Therapeutic Use of Radon: A Biomedical Treatment in Europe; An "Alternative" Remedy in the United States. *Proceedings of the 14th Pacific Basin Nuclear Conference, New Technologies for a New ERA,* 21-25 Mar 2004, Honolulu, Hawaii.

Feinendegen LE, Pollycove M (2001). Biologic Responses to Low Doses of Ionizing Radiation: Detriment Versus Hormesis: Part 1. Dose Responses of Cells and Tissues. *The Journal of Nuclear Medicine* 42(7):17N-27N.

Fisher B, Jeong J-H, Anderson S, Bryant J, Fisher ER, Wolmark N (2002). Twenty-Five-Year Follow-Up of a Randomized Trial Comparing Radical Mastectomy, Total Mastectomy, and Total Mastectomy Followed by Irradiation. *New England Journal of Medicine* 347(8):567-575.

Gardner JW, Gutmann FD (2002). Fatal water intoxication of an Army trainee during urine drug testing. *Military Medicine* 167(5):435-437.

Giuliano AE (1996). Benign Breast Disease in *Gynecology,* Mitchell, C. W., Ed., Baltimore, MD: Williams & Wilkins, pp525-529.

Gofman JW, O'Connor E (1985). *X-rays: Health Effects of Common Exams,* San Franciso, CA: Sierra Club Books.

Gofman JW (1990). *Radiation-Induced Cancer from Low-Dose Exposure: An Independent Analysis,* San Franciso, CA: Committee for Nuclear Responsibility, Inc.

Gøtzsche PC Olsen O (2000). Is screening for breast cancer with mammography justifiable? *Lancet* 355(9198):129-134.

Hively W (2002). Is Radiation Good for You? *Discover,* Dec., 74-80.

Jonas WB (2001). The Future of Hormesis: What is the Clinical Relevance to Hormesis? *Critical Reviews in Toxicology* 31(4&5):655-658.

Kaiser J (2003). A Healthful Dab of Radiation? *Science* 302:378.

Kauffman JM (2000). Should You Take Aspirin to Prevent Heart Attack? *J. Scientific Exploration* 14(4):623-41.

Kauffman JM (2002). Alternative Medicine: Watching the Watchdogs at Quackwatch, *Journal of Scientific Exploration* 16(2), 312-337.

Kauffman JM (2003a). Book Review of "Permissible Dose: A History of Radiation Protection in the Twentieth Century", by J. Samuel Walker. Berkeley, CA: University of CA Press, 2000, in *J. Scientific Exploration* 17(3):563-564.

Kauffman JM (2003b). Diagnostic Radiation: Are the Risks Exaggerated? *Journal of American Physicians and Surgeons* 8(2), 54-5.

Lee JR, Zava D, Hopkins V (2002). *What Your Doctor May* Not *Tell You About Breast Cancer — How Hormone Balance Can Save Your Life,* New York, NY: Warner Books, p9.

Lipman JC, Ed. (1995). *Quick reference to radiology,* East Norwalk, CT: Appleton & Lange, p251.

Lubin JH, Boice JD, Jr. (1997). Lung Cancer Risk from Residential Radon: Meta-Analysis of Eight Epidemiologic Studies. *Journal of the National Cancer Institute* 89(1), 49-57.

Lubin JH (1998). On the Discrepancy between Epidemiologic Studies in Individuals of Lung Cancer and Residential Radon and Cohen's Ecologic Regression. *Health Physics* 75(1), 4-10.

Luckey TD (1999). Nurture with Ionizing Radiation: A Provocative Hypothesis. *Nutrition and Cancer* 34(1), 1-11.

Luckey TD (1991). *Radiation Hormesis,* Boca Raton, FL: CRC Press.

Miller AB, Howe GR, Sherman GJ, Lindsay JP, Yaffe MJ, Dinner PJ, Risch, HA, Preston DL (1989). Mortality from Breast Cancer after Irradiation during Fluoroscopic Examinations in Patients being Treated for Tuberculosis. *New England Journal of Medicine,* 321(19):1285-1289.

Milloy SJ (2001). *Junk Science Judo.* Washington, DC: Cato Institute, 92-95.

Mishell DR, Jr, Stenchever MA, Droegemueller W, Herbst AL (1997). *Comprehensive Gynecology,* St. Louis, MO: Mosby, pp366-372.

Mitchel RE, Jackson JS, Morrison DP, Carlisle SM (2003). Low Doses of Radiation Increase the Latency of Spontaneous Lymphomas and Spinal Osteosarcomas in Cancer-Prone, Radiation-Sensitive Trp53 Heterozygous Mice. *Radiation Research* 159(3):320-327.

Mossman JL (2001). Deconstructing Radiation Hormesis. *Health Physics* 80(3), 263-269.

Nystrom L, Andersson I, Bjurstam N, Frisell J, Nordenskjold B, Rutqvist ER (2002). Long-term effects of mammography screening: updated overview of the Swedish randomised trials. *Lancet* 359(9310):909-919.

Olsen O, Gøtzsche PC (2001). Cochrane review on screening for breast cancer with mammography. *Lancet* 358:1340-1342.

Ottoboni MA (1991). *The Dose Makes the Poison,* 2nd ed., New York, NY:Van Nostrand Reinhold.

Papariello CJ (2000). Risk Assessment and Risk Management Implications of Hormesis. *Journal of Applied Toxicology* 20:147-148.

Parsons PA (2001). Radiation hormesis: an ecological and energetic perspective. *Medical Hypotheses* 57(3):277-279.

Pollycove M, Feinendegen LE (2001). Biologic Responses to Low Doses of Ionizing Radiation: Detriment Versus Hormesis: Part 1. Dose Responses of Organisms. *The Journal of Nuclear Medicine* 42(9):26N-32N, 37N.

Ray DL, Guzzo L (1990). *Trashing the Planet,* Washington, DC: Regnery Gateway.

Rimer BK, Schildkraut J, Hiatt RA (2001). Cancer Screening in *Cancer Principles & Practice of Oncology,* DeVita, V. T., Jr., Hellman, S. & Rosenberg, S. A., Eds., Philadelphia, PA: Lippincott Williams & Wilkins, pp627-632.

Robin ED (1984). *Matters of Life & Death: Risks and Benefits of Medical Care,* Stanford, CA: Stanford Alumni Assoc., pp140-143.

Sherwood T (2001). 100 years' observation of risks from radiation for British (male) radiologists. *Lancet* 358:604.

Shore RE, Hildreth N, Woodard E, Dvoretsky P, Hempelmann L, Pasternack B (1986). Breast Cancer Among Women Given X-Ray Therapy for Acute Post-Partum Mastitis. *Journal of the National Cancer Institute* 77:689-696.

Skrabanek P, McCormick J (1989). *Follies and Fallacies in Medicine,* Glasgow, Scotland, UK: Tarragon Press, pp98-107.

Steinbuch M, Weinberg CR, Buckley JD, Robison LL, Sandler DP (1999). Indoor residential radon exposure and risk of childhood acute myeloid leukaemia. *British Journal of Cancer* 81(5):900-906.

Tipler PA (1987). *College Physics,* New York, NY: Worth Publishers, pp856-858.

Upton AC (1982). Biological effects of low-level ionizing radiation. *Scientific American* 246(2):41-49.

Upton AC (2001). Radiation Hormesis: Data and Interpretations. *Critical Reviews in Toxicology* 31(4&5):681-695.

Wallace V (1986). Fear of Radon. *Chemical & Engineering News,* 7 July, 64(27):4.

Whelan TJ, Julian J, Wright, J, Jadad AR, Levine ML (2000). Does Locoregional Radiation Therapy Improve Survival in Breast Cancer? A Meta-Analysis. *Journal of Clinical Oncology* 18(6):1220-1229.

Wolff S (1992). Is Radiation All Bad? The Search for Adaptation. *Radiation Research,* 131:117-123.

Yalow R.S (1995). Radiation and Public Perception, in *Radiation and Public Perception, Benefits and Risks,* Young, JP, Yalow RS, Eds., Washington, DC: American Chemical Society, pp13-22.

# Myth 9:  Annual mammograms and follow-up treatment prolong life.

## Synopsis by Spacedoc

There is no doubt that in our country today the present climate regarding routine mammography is that both patients and physicians demand them or feel guilty if, for whatever reason, they are not riding the periodic mammogram bandwagon. Once mammography received FDA approval and support of both our American Cancer Society and National Cancer Institute, the average primary care physician became a pawn for our burgeoning cancer industry under the assumption that our very best scientific minds had come up with the very best recommendations. Who were we to argue? The truth is that mass cancer screening with follow-up and treatment is big business. It is the old story — how much can we trust those who stand to gain economically from their own recommendations?  Kauffman says look at the figures, and he has done a superb job of telling it like it is. Despite my 25 years of clinical practice as a family doctor with Board certification in both family practice and preventive medicine, I didn't know these figures. Once you read them and look at his resources and documentation there can be no argument. Now my only question is how can one put the brakes on this rapidly rolling juggernaut?

You may recall my aphorism from another chapter, "Figures don't lie but liars figure". Think about this when you read the following statement: "1 in 9 women will get breast cancer". Innocent enough – right? In what way could this be a lie? The media says it repeatedly, the mammography industry quotes it almost daily and even medical articles refer to it as the lifetime risk for women. I cannot think of a better scare tactic to drive women into mammography screening centers.

The reality is that this simple statement is grossly misleading – not technically a lie but far, far removed from the truth. This is like questioning a child on his way to become a lawyer about the empty cookie jar. "Did you steal the cookies? The child says, "No", then afterwards explains, "I just borrowed them."

When we look at our national disease incidence rates we find that the chance of a woman under 50 years of age contracting breast cancer is under 2% and the chance of that same woman dying from it is 0.3%. And to look at it another way, of the women who do contract breast cancer, fully half will be over 65 years of age and will be very likely to die from another cause. We are talking the same 1 in 9 women here as mentioned earlier but looking at the figures from a different perspective, one far less inclined to drive women into mammography screening centers and much closer to reality.

Now let us examine figure 9.1, the true picture of Doctor Kauffman's presentation, a must reading for every doctor and a sobering education. If 1,000 women of ages 40-50 had periodic mammograms what would be the impact, the true effect on public health, the real results? We know from years of observation and statistics that 8 of these women will actually have breast cancer. Seven of these positives will be found by mammography. The other will be missed. Of the 992 women who do not have breast cancer, 70 will be identified as falsely positive. Of our total of 77 "positives" discovered by our much touted, periodic mammography program, only 7 will be correct. Applying the legal term of "Res ipso loquitor", if one but just looks at the figures "the thing speaks for itself". This is the test now firmly entrenched in American society. It is truly mind-boggling to try to fathom how this has come about. Read on. Kauffman's story is a true public service.

## A True Picture of Mammogram Accuracy

For a hypothetical group of 1000 American women of ages 40-50 who have mammograms, the true picture, literally, may be seen in Figure 9-1. In such a group, 8 women will actually have breast cancer, which is usually determined by examination of cells obtained by biopsy. This is called a prevalence rate of 0.8%. There will be 7 positive tests with correct results. Mammography is therefore said to have a sensitivity of 87%. There will be 1 negative and incorrect test result, a 13% false negative rate. If mammography is actually repeated annually, the false negative probably would not be repeated.

In the 992 women who do *not* have breast cancer, there will be 922 negative and correct test results. Mammography is therefore said to have a specificity of 93%. This may seem to be pretty good until the rest of the results are considered. The other 70 mammograms on the non-cancerous 992 women are false positives. In every case, there will be anguish, repeat mammograms or other imaging procedures, and biopsies, and all of these are error-prone as well. At the very least, quality of life will be lowered, and will never recover, because there will always be the dread that the next mammogram will be positive, even if the biopsy is not.

Now remembering that the 1000 women aged 40-50 do not know beforehand which ones have breast cancer, the total of 77 positive tests must be looked at as follows: 91% are incorrect, and 9% are correct! How such a poor test could have achieved such entrenched status, engender such blind faith among some women, and have its costs be accepted by health insurers is almost beyond belief.

## Mammography Procedure

The process of mammography is the preparation of an Xray of the breasts recorded on black and white film to give pictures, negatives, called mammograms. A digitized image stored in a computer is called a digital mammogram. As noted in Myth 8, the Xrays used were and are too weak to be a danger, and may be a benefit in reducing cancer rates by radiation hormesis. Mechanical squashing of the breasts in each of two planes is done to obtain a clearer picture. This can be quite painful, in some cases intensely painful, and is a major cause of "noncompliance" not only with mammography, but with self-examination or palpation by a physician (Porter-Steele, 1996). Of 125 women over age 50 undergoing mammography, 93% reported pain. Patient-controlled breast compression alleviated the pain or fear of it somewhat (Kashikar-Zuck et al., 1997). Mammography costs $100-150 and takes 10-15 minutes.

The pictures obtained are blurry and lack contrast. Any denser tissue seen in the mammogram might be used to justify a positive diagnosis, because mammography cannot distinguish malignant tumors from denser tissue of any other type. The decision of the technician is very subjective, which is another reason why there are so many false positives and negatives.

Mammography was approved by the FDA in the 1970s as a mass screening procedure for detection of breast tumors. As shown in Myths 2-4, approvals or recommendations from the FDA are sometimes not worth much. They often appear capricious, rather than being based on findings that include contradictions to the claims of the seeker of FDA approval. So, as will be seen, there is no benefit to be gained from the repeated assaults of mammography in terms of lowered all-cause mortality.

## The Cancer Industry Overpromotes Mammography

The media says it: 1 in 9 women will get breast cancer. The profitable mammography industry quotes the same risk in its handouts. Medical articles quote the same lifetime risk. Young women think this risk applies to them. The scare tends to imply that the 1 in 9 women who contract breast cancer will die of it unless it is treated, and treated early. In the 1970s the American Cancer Society actually used the more alarming statistic that 1 in 8 women would get breast cancer (Lomborg, 2001, pp223-224).

The USA and Canada have the highest incidence of breast cancer in the world (Table 9-1). Even so, the lifetime risk of contracting breast cancer is 10.4%, 1 in 10. The chance of dying from breast cancer is 4%, 1 in 25. The chance of dying from lung cancer is the same (Phillips et al., 1999), but women seem much more worried about breast cancer. The chance of a woman under 50 years old contracting breast cancer is under 2%, and of dying of it when under 50 is 0.3%. For this reason alone, it was always predictable that mass screening of women under 50 for breast cancer would not achieve much beyond profit for the cancer industry and plenty of anguish for the women.

What is not shown in Table 9-1 is how many women who were diagnosed with breast cancer received treatment for it. As will be shown later and in Myth 10, the past and present treatments for breast cancer can remove tumors, sometimes minimize future tumor growth, and occasionally prevent the spread of cancer cells (metastasis), but they do not prolong life. High-dose radiation, for example, does a good job of preventing recurrence of breast cancer, but it causes fatal heart disease (Lee et al., 2002, pp5-6; Cuzick J, et al., 1994). So it is not clear how many of the 10.4% of women who contract breast cancer are treated for it, and die of other causes as in the two right-hand columns of Table 9-1.

But of the 10% of women who will contract breast cancer, there is a 50% chance that a woman will receive the diagnosis after the age of 65, and she will have a 60% chance of dying from another cause, including treatment. The "1 in 9" dramatics was a scare tactic used by the American Cancer Society to coerce women to submit to mammographic screening programs (Phillips et al., 1999).

<u>Warnings About the Futility of Mammography</u>

Eugene D. Robin, MD, held faculty posts at the University of Pittsburgh and Harvard Medical Schools before settling at Stanford University Medical School. He observed and analyzed in his book the period of the beginnings of mammography in 1973 when it was recommended annually for women aged 35-70.

Robin examined the results of the Health Insurance Plan trial in New York City on 62,000 women aged 40-70. Half were offered annual mammography *and* physical examination, while the control group, the other half, was observed. The trial results seemed impressive at first. But of the 299 breast cancers found in the mammography group, *only 132 were detected by mammography alone.* After 10 years of follow-up, cancer deaths were slightly, but statistically significantly, lower in the mammography group. (Even Robin did not cite any *all-cause* mortality!) There were 93 deaths in the mammography group vs. 133 deaths in the control group. This difference, which would have been called "a 30% reduction in deaths" was extrapolated to indicate a great benefit to millions of women.

Using the "survivor" method as is so often done in earlier chapters of this book, one may calculate that 99.7% of the mammography group did not die of cancer after 10 years, and that 99.6% of the controls did not die of cancer, not a big difference. Moreover, there was evidence that women at high risk for breast cancer based on heredity tended to self-select for screening, meaning that there was poor randomization, thus possibly there was no real difference in outcome at all! (Robin, 1984, p140).

Careful re-examination of the data by an "expert" committee showed no difference in outcome for women under 50. This did not stop the original recommendation for all women aged 35 or older to have mammograms. In 1976 the recommendation was modified to say that a woman aged 35-40 should have a baseline mammogram, and then annual ones beginning at 50. In 1983, in the total absence of new data, an annual mammogram was recommended for women 40 or older. The earlier

Table 9-1:  Incidence of Breast Cancer and Causes of Death for a Birth Cohort of 1000 Women According to Five-Year Age Intervals (based on the 1995 incidence and mortality rates in the Ontario Cancer Registry in Phillips et al., 1999).

| Age Group (yr) | Number Alive at Beginning | Incident Breast Cancers | Breast Cancer Deaths | Cardio- and Cerebrovas-cular Deaths | Other Causes of Death |
|---|---|---|---|---|---|
| 0-4 | 1000 | 0 | 0 | 0 | 6 |
| 5-9 | 994 | 0 | 0 | 0 | 1 |
| 10-14 | 993 | 0 | 0 | 0 | 1 |
| 15-19 | 992 | 0 | 0 | 0 | 1 |
| 20-24 | 991 | 0 | 0 | 0 | 1 |
| 25-29 | 990 | 0 | 0 | 0 | 2 |
| 30-34 | 988 | 1 | 0 | 0 | 2 |
| 35-39 | 986 | 3 | 0 | 0 | 3 |
| 40-44 | 983 | 5 | 1 | 1 | 4 |
| 45-49 | 977 | 8 | 2 | 1 | 6 |
| 50-54 | 968 | 11 | 3 | 2 | 11 |
| 55-59 | 952 | 12 | 3 | 5 | 15 |
| 60-64 | 929 | 12 | 3 | 9 | 25 |
| 65-69 | 892 | 14 | 4 | 16 | 36 |
| 70-74 | 836 | 13 | 5 | 28 | 51 |
| 75-79 | 752 | 11 | 6 | 52 | 70 |
| 80-84 | 624 | 9 | 6 | 89 | 95 |
| ≥85 | 434 | 5 | 7 | 224 | 203 |
| Totals ——> | | 104 | 40 | 427 | 533 |
| | | 10.4% | 4% | 43% | 53% |
| | | 1 in 10.4 | 1 in 25 | 1 in 2.3 | 1 in 1.9 |

recommendation by an expert committee was based on a very close vote. A few months later, with minor changes in the people in the committee, the vote was equally close, but for beginning at age 40. The new policy was announced with great public hoopla and devoid of the doubts and close vote (Robin, 1984, pp141-143). In those days before the needle biopsy, this meant 77 surgical biopsies were performed to find 7 actual cancers (Figure 9-1). This means that full compliance with annual mammograms in the USA in women 40 or older would yield about 5,000,000 false positives per year — every year, a very nice source of income indeed.

Around 1987 John C. Bailar III, MD, observed that mammography detects breast tumors only about a year before they would have been found by palpation. When this year is subtracted from the survival time of women who were treated after a mammographic finding, there was no difference in life expectancy compared with women who did not have mammograms. Long-term survival time is about the same. This year is the "lead-time" bias observed in trials of mammograms, and even includes treatment beginning a year earlier (Lee et al., 2002, pp10-11).

In 1989 in a book called *Follies and Fallacies in Medicine,* the authors had the advantage of 3 more trials of mammography to form an opinion on its value. Based on the Number Needed to Treat (NNT) to obtain 1 benefit, that is, 1 woman not dying of breast cancer thanks to mammography, the NY Health Insurance Plan trial had an NNT of 5061. The Two-Counties trial in Sweden had an NNT of 12,755; the Edinburgh and Guildhall trial in the UK had an NNT of 18,315; and the Malmö trial in Sweden had an NNT of 67,568. These figures do not even count all-cause mortality! Obviously, mammography is not worth doing; but since so many women treat it as a religious belief, this chapter will continue with the hope that overwhelming evidence can unglue even a religious belief. The authors, Skrabanek and McCormick, think that the theory behind breast cancer screening is flawed because a tumor that can be felt (become palpable) has been growing for a mean time of 8 years. Earlier detection by mammography by two years at most can only be valuable if metastasis is confined to years 6 through 8. There is no reason to think this is the case. They also note that wounds to the psyche heal more slowly than the wounds of the many biopsies.

These authors also noted that women with breast cancer who are followed up for 30 years or more after the diagnosis are still dying of metastatic cancer. They think that most breast cancer is incurable at the time of diagnosis. Survival is determined by the nature of the growth, which varies greatly, rather than by the type of treatment. In the 1980s rates of mastectomy increased dramatically in the USA and were much higher than in the UK, although the incidence of breast cancer and mortality from it remained about the same (Skrabanek & McCormick, 1989, pp100-103).

Note that both these authors and Robin made an error so often exposed in other chapters of this book: they used mortality from breast cancer without including the more valuable all-cause mortality.

Shortly before dying of breast cancer, the clinical director of the Edinburgh Breast Cancer Screening Project, Maureen Roberts, wrote of mammography in 1989: "We can no longer ignore the possibility that screening may not reduce the mortality in women of any age, however disappointing that may be...I hope that pressure is not put on women to attend [mammographic breast cancer screening]. The decision must be theirs, and a truthful account of the facts must be available to the public and the individual patient. It will not be what they want to hear." She went on to remark on what she called the "brainwashing of physicians and the public: There is also an air of evangelism [in the national screening programs, with] few people questioning what is actually being done." (Gigerenzer, 2002, p55).

The complete failure of the Canadian National Breast Screening Study to demonstrate lower rates of death from breast cancer, not to mention lower all-cause mortality, led to charges that there had been subversion that led to poor randomization or other aberrations. An investigation was done under the direction of John C. Bailar III, MD, in which KPMG Investigation and Securities, Inc., of Toronto, Ontario, reviewed the records of the study. KPMG found only 467 records among 30,182 which warranted investigation. Half had clerical errors and the other half showed erasures and substitution of names. This was too small a set of flaws to influence the outcome (Bailar & MacMahon, 1997). The charges were proved false. This trial of mammography showed no benefit.

Mass screening for breast cancer was first introduced in Germany in the 1930s. Physicians were exhorted to recognize the value of early detection, and those who did not perform mammography screening were accused of contributing to the deaths of thousands of women each year. In the USA 60 years later, both the National Cancer Institute and the American Cancer Society recommend annual mammograms and clinical breast examinations beginning at age 40. The American Cancer Society also recommends self-examination from the age of 20. These organizations are not to be swayed by the facts (Gigerenzer, 2002, p56-58).

Gigerenzer also noted that early detection of breast cancer is not prevention. And if there is no effective therapy, early detection does not increase life expectancy, but only the time the patient is worried about the cancer, many of which will progress so slowly that they will not be fatal. Most

# Figure 9-1:  Mammogram Accuracy Exposed and Clarified

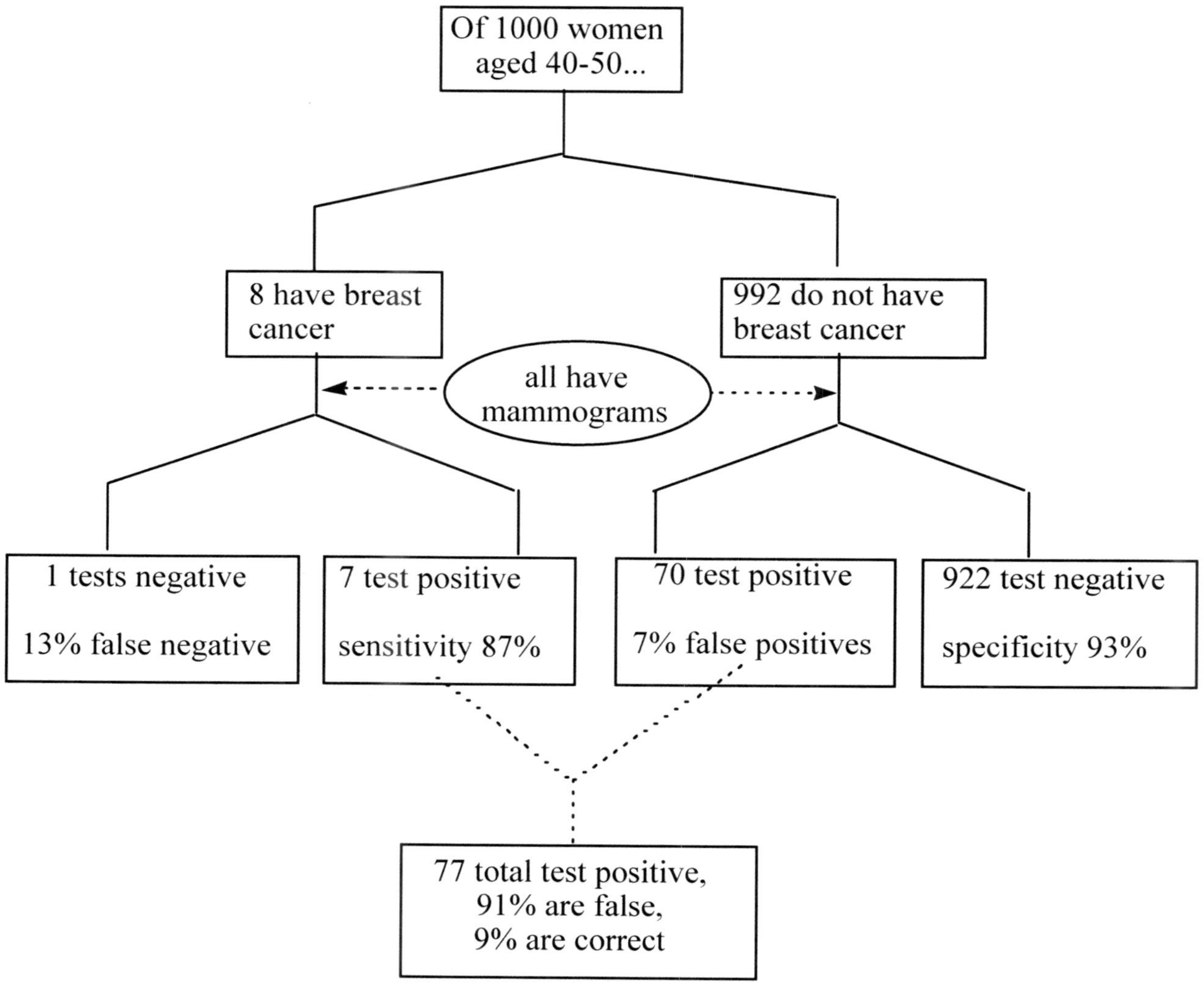

```
                    ┌─────────────────┐
                    │ Of 1000 women   │
                    │ aged 40-50...   │
                    └─────────────────┘

        ┌──────────────────┐              ┌──────────────────┐
        │ 8 have breast    │              │ 992 do not have  │
        │ cancer           │              │ breast cancer    │
        └──────────────────┘              └──────────────────┘
                    ◄ - - - (  all have  ) - - - ►
                            ( mammograms )

┌──────────────────┐ ┌──────────────────┐  ┌──────────────────┐ ┌──────────────────┐
│ 1 tests negative │ │ 7 test positive  │  │ 70 test positive │ │ 922 test negative│
│                  │ │                  │  │                  │ │                  │
│ 13% false        │ │ sensitivity 87%  │  │ 7% false         │ │ specificity 93%  │
│ negative         │ │                  │  │ positives        │ │                  │
└──────────────────┘ └──────────────────┘  └──────────────────┘ └──────────────────┘

                         ┌──────────────────────┐
                         │ 77 total test positive,│
                         │ 91% are false,         │
                         │ 9% are correct         │
                         └──────────────────────┘
```

Based on data from Gigerenzer, 2002, pp5-6, 40-49.

cancers found in younger women are of this type. A common benign type is called ductal carcinoma in situ (DCIS). If 1000 women participate in screening for 10 years, 500 will receive a positive diagnosis, of which 90% will be false. Just 1 woman in 1000 might be saved from dying of breast cancer, but as will be seen, will die of treatment. Women aged 50-69 who have annual mammograms may increase their life expectancy by 12 days! Gigerenzer confirms that women under 40 will get no benefit at all. He gives a benefit for women over 50, but even he failed to obtain and use all-cause mortality. And even he also followed the discredited linear no-threshold hypothesis, indicating an incorrect number of radiation-induced cancers from mammographic Xrays (see Myth 8), (Gigerenzer, 2002, p68-69).

In a survey, 145 American women 40-49 years old were asked how many women like them would not die as a result of breast cancer if screened by 10 years of annual mammography compared with those who were not screened. Their mean answer was 60 in 1000. (Gigerenzer, 2002, p73). The truth is NONE. While just one life in 1000 would *not* be lost to breast cancer in this young group of those *who were screened,* because of the low incidence, this would be balanced by the appearance of one death due to the trauma of diagnosis or the treatment.

Gigerenzer also found that the brochures women are given on mammography almost never give the lifetime risk of dying from breast cancer, the relative or absolute risk reduction of death from breast cancer, the NNT, the fraction of women who would need further examination, or the false positive or false negative rates (Gigerenzer, 2002, pp74-77). Even he failed to include the lack of reduction of *all-cause* mortality by mammographic screening. As noted in Myth 8, both a recent tome on cancer treatment and one on gynecology quoted lower relative risks of dying of breast cancer of 0.75 to 0.80 with no inkling for either the physician or the patient that there was no change in the *all-cause* mortality attributable to annual mammography.

More recently two scientists evaluated all published mammography trials to check on their quality. Separate findings for breast cancer death and all-cause death were carefully considered. As noted in Myth 8, it was reported that the all-cause mortality after 13 years of follow-up of 3 clinical trials of medium quality was *unchanged* (RR = 1.00). The two best-quality trials, both Swedish, failed even to find a significant effect on death from breast cancer (RR = 0.97), (Olsen & Gøtzsche, 2001). Lower quality trials usually cited to justify screening showed RR = 0.75 for breast cancer mortality, but showed RR = 1.06 for all-cause mortality, meaning that even these lower-quality trials did not support annual mammography for life extension. The common problem with these trials was poor randomization between the control and treatment groups. An additional bias surfaced: it was found that when researchers were uncertain about the cause of death, they were more likely to ascribe it to breast cancer if the woman had been in the control group than if she had been in the mammography group (Gøtzsche & Olsen, 2000).

The directors of some of the trials objected to this negative evaluation, so they re-evaluated the Swedish trials with the result that, after 16 years of follow-up, the all-cause mortality was *still* unchanged (RR = 0.98)! The breast cancer deaths were lower (RR = 0.79), but the only significant effect was in women ≥55 years old (Nystom et al., 2002).

An "independent" panel of medical experts in the USA reviewed the work of Gøtzsche & Olsen, 2000, and agreed with it, intending to rewrite the section on mammography for the National Cancer Institute (www.cancer.gov). Before this, the website as accessed on 21 Nov 2000 had the claims that regular mammograms in women aged 40-49 reduced the chances of dying from breast cancer by 16%, and for women 50-69 by 25-30% (Charatan, 2002). There was no sign of all-cause death rates, a sure sign of ignorance at best or fraud at worst. So did anything change by the time the website was accessed on 25 Mar 2004? It then read: "Several large studies conducted around the world show that breast cancer screening with mammograms reduces the number of deaths from breast cancer for women ages 40 to 69, especially those over age 50. Studies conducted to date have not shown a benefit for regular screening mammograms, or for a baseline screening mammogram, in women under age 40." (http://cis.nci.nih.gov/fact/5_28.htm) Note that the "16%" and "25-30%" lower relative risk of breast cancer death are now gone, perhaps a belated recognition that they never existed. Still no sign of all-cause mortality. Could it possibly still be ignorance?

As accessed on 30 Mar 04, the website of Imaginis Corp., a privately held corporation, while mainstream in outlook, appeared to be realistic about the limitations of all types of breast imaging techniques (http://imaginis.com/breasthealth/nuc_med.asp?mode=1). It cites a study on 75 women carried out at the Los Robles Regional Medical Center, CA, in whom there were signs of breast cancer with mammograms or physical examinations. There were 30 who were finally diagnosed with breast cancer, of which 27 (90%) were positively identified with scintimammography (see below), and only 19 (63%) of the 27 were identified with mammography.

Joann G. Elmore, MD, and co-workers carried out a retrospective observational study on matched groups of women aged 40-65 enrolled in 6 health plans in WA, OR, CA, MA and MN, and followed for 15 years. The control group had half as many mammograms and clinical breast examinations as the "active" group in the 3 years before the onset of breast cancer. There was no statistically significant difference in breast cancer deaths between the groups with more or less mammography. In a vivid example of ignoring "evidence-based medicine", Dr. Elmore encourages everyone to continue with the current screening recommendations (Elmore et al., 2005). In the editorial in the same issue of the journal, Russell Harris, MD, wrote that: "Regardless of the reasons for the lack of efficacy, the study should not change current practices of breast cancer screening." Is this insane? See below for the result of clinical breast examinations in this study.

Professor Malcolm Law, London School of Medicine, notes that screening has gut appeal, but unproved value. Encouraging people to decide for themselves is ducking the issue, which is that cancer screening in people with no symptoms is useless. This even included breast self-examination (Law, 2004).

David Plotkin, MD, an experienced specialist in breast cancer, wrote that abandoning widespread mammography in the USA would be a good idea, because it is useless for prolonging life, but that its restriction to just very high-risk women is unlikely to be accepted; the oversold juggernaut is unstoppable. He notes that Michael Baum of the British Institute of Cancer Research, who helped set up the mammography screening program in the UK, resigned because he was disturbed about the claims of no benefit of mammography (Plotkin, 1996).

In overall agreement, John R. Lee, MD, et al. wrote:

> "For a breast cancer tumor to become large enough to be detected by palpation, the cancer has usually been growing for about ten years. If found one year earlier by mammography, the cancer has been growing for about nine years, which is plenty of time to spawn metastases if the [particular] cancer is prone to do that. The one-year difference between palpation and mammography detection is ultimately of little importance... [This one year gap is the 'lead-time' bias of claims made for improved cancer cure rates. See Myth 10.]

> "Since there is no reliable evidence that mammography screening decreases breast cancer mortality [and none whatever that all-cause mortality is improved, see above], mammography screening for breast cancer is unjustified. This means that physicians should not order routine mammography screening." (Lee et al, 2002, p11).

## So Why Did Breast Cancer Mortality Rates Fall Between 1990 and 2000? (from Kauffman & McGee, 2004)

In 1935, 26.2 out of 100,000 women in the USA died of breast cancer. In 1992, after adjustment for age because women were living longer, 26.2 out of 100,000 women died of breast cancer (Plotkin, 1996). Non-cancer deaths caused by treatment were not determined.

The British medical statistician Richard Peto and coworkers noted that the breast cancer mortality rate between 1990 and 2000 in women 50-69 years old dropped by 30% in the UK and 25% in the USA, and attributed this to improvements in the many types of treatment interventions, each responsible on its own for only a moderate reduction. The early portion (from 1990-1993) of the rate decrease was described by Bailar and Gornik, who also noted the then recent "substantial increase in the use of mammography among women over 50". When something positive occurs in medicine attempts are usually made to explain the observation or claim the credit. The implication was that increased use of mammography was contributing to a reduction in the breast cancer mortality rate somehow, but without significant reductions in all-cause mortality, as shown above. What could give such a result?

*Surgery?* For at least the past quarter-century the treatment of breast cancer by surgery has been applied at about the same rate, certainly in the UK and USA. While a 1969 study showed that fewer radical mastectomies were performed in the UK than in the USA, a 25-year follow-up described in a randomized trial found no significant difference in disease-free survival time between radical (also called Halsted: lymph nodes also removed) and total mastectomy in women with either positive or negative lymph nodes (positive indicates metastases). Earlier evidence had shown that radical, total and segmental mastectomy (lumpectomy) gave the same all-cause mortality (Plotkin, 1996). Because of the steady rate of surgery as the primary treatment during the last 30 years in the UK and USA, it is unlikely to be responsible for the recent drop in breast cancer mortality regardless of how radical a procedure is performed. Despite the shift in recent years to less extensive surgical procedures (lumpectomy and skin-saving), this change has not altered the all-cause mortality, and could hardly have lowered breast cancer mortality by being less aggressive, thus surgery is not really a "variable" in the time period of concern. Therefore, the changes toward needle biopsy from surgical biopsy and lumpectomy instead of the more extreme excisions could not explain the drop.

Skin-saving operations accompanied by clever reconstruction do give a much better cosmetic and psychological outcome in recent years (Link, 2002, pp68-77), but are not likely to have altered breast cancer mortality much.

*High-dose radiation?* The cumulative doses of Xray or gamma radiation delivered to treat breast cancer are usually in the range of about 4,500-6,000 cGy (rads). This total amount of radiation is given in doses of about 200 rads per day. Treatments are given five days a week for five to six weeks. The addition of high-dose radiation to total mastectomy did not significantly change the cancer free survival times in the 25-year follow-up of the randomized trial cited above. This is the key evidence. In the Early Breast Cancer Trialists' Collaborative Group's comprehensive overview of all available adjuvant radiotherapy trials for breast cancer started between 1961 and 1990, the absolute survival gain was 1%, and the absolute reduction in breast cancer deaths was 4%. The recent Danish Breast Cancer Cooperative Group trial seemed to show a reduction in breast cancer deaths of 8%. These small reductions cannot explain the larger reductions in breast cancer mortality observed in the 1990s (25-30%).

Even John S. Link, MD, a mainstream oncologist who routinely uses mammography and high-dose radiation, admits that the protection it confers on breasts lasts only 5-7 years, claiming that the risk of another cancer by then returns to the level of the non-irradiated breast (Link, 2002, p116). He does not mention the increase in fatal heart disease caused by radiation (see above), or other damage, or unchanged all-cause mortality.

*Chemotherapy?* Because of the extreme side-effects of the typical cytotoxic drugs, no truly double-blind placebo-controlled trials have actually taken place for the adjuvant (that is, accompanying surgery) chemotherapy of breast cancer, and probably never will be again because of the ethical dilemma of providing placebos with similar side-effects to those of the drugs. This is in addition to lead-time bias, stage migration, publication bias and selection bias common to drug trials in cancer. In addition, there was a near cessation of placebo-controlled trials of chemotherapy in 1980 for so-called ethical reasons. The most influential trial, from the National Cancer Institute of Milan, Italy, reported impressive results from lymph node-positive women to cyclophosphamide + methotrexate + 5-fluorouracil (CMF) after 1 year; but after 9 years, as reported in 1984, there was only a 12% improvement in relapse-free survival, and this only in premenopausal women, not in the much greater number of postmenopausal ones. However, the Guy's-Manchester and West Midlands trials showed no significant benefit even in premenopausal women.

The Early Breast Cancer Trialists' Collaborative Group's meta-analysis of all the trials begun before 1985 showed cancer-free survival advantages of about 6% absolute after 10 years follow-up, a gain of only 0.6% per year with no overall survival advantage, that is, no improvement in all-cause mortality. Newer chemotherapeutic regimens have improved an end-point called "time to progression" by only a few weeks despite some impressive figures for "relative risk reduction". According to a review from the National Cancer Institute (US): "...among patients with newly diagnosed stage 1 breast cancer, for whom 5-year overall survival is greater than 90%, a 2- or 3-drug chemotherapy regimen lasting 4 to 6 months, with its adverse effects, offers an absolute survival benefit of just 1% to 2%".

Newer drugs that reduce the amount of vomiting and and maintain red blood cell production in bone marrow make chemotherapy easier to endure, but would not alter the long-term outcome of it.

*Chemoprevention?* In their report on the Royal Marsden Hospital trial, Powles et al. (1998) showed that there was no effect of tamoxifen on breast cancer incidence in healthy women followed for 6 years. This was confirmed by the study by Veronesi et al. of 4 years duration, but not by the Breast Cancer Prevention Trial (BCPT) of the US National Cancer Institute of 3 years on average of treatment. However, the absolute reduction of breast cancer incidence in the BCPT was from 1.2% to 0.6%, and it must be mentioned that side-effects nullified even this result so far as indicating any overall treatment value (Pritchard, 1998). A more favorable review of this trial seemed to suffer from underplaying inadequate randomization and arbitrary alteration of data for the control group (Gail et al., 1999).

Adding to this poor performance, long-term tamoxifen users had more endometrial cancer. Serious endometrial cancer occurred in 17% of users for 2 years or more vs. 5% for non-users (Bergman et al., 2000). A meta-analysis of trials on 37,000 women who used tamoxifen to treat breast cancer for 1-5 years found that the mortality from all causes other than breast or endometrial cancer after 10 years was 59% (EBCTCG, 1998).

*Low-dose radiation from diagnostic Xrays?* As was noted in Myth 8, low-doses of Xrays for tuberculosis diagnosis and control reduced breast cancer rates by the amount observed by Peto et al. for mammography. The substantial increase in the numbers of women aged 50 or more who underwent mammography in the 1980s-1990s provided the exposure. The hypothesis that radiation hormesis from low-dose Xrays was the main reason for lower breast cancer mortality in the 1990s was published in a peer-reviewed journal (Kauffman & McGee, 2004). *For now this appears to be the most plausible reason for the drop in breast cancer rates in the 1990s.*

The reduction in the Xray dose in mammography from about 2 rads for the total examination in the 1970s to about 0.4 rads by 1995 also reduces the hormetic effect postulated above (and see Myth 8). But the main reasons for the failure of mammography are the traumatic experiences brought about by the many false positives, and the general failure of treatment beyond lumpectomy. It is well-known that both radiation and chemotherapy cause more heart deaths (Moss, 2000, pp171-191; Cuzick, et al., 1994).

To prevent a small tumor that is removable by lumpectomy from growing to the size requiring more major surgery, early detection is still desirable, but annual mammograms are not the ideal approach.

## If Not Mammography, What Early Detection Method Could be Used Instead?

*Breast self-examination.* According to John Lee, MD, assuming you are an adult woman:

"If you stop having mammograms [which he advises], it becomes essential that that you examine your own breasts thoroughly at least once a month [contrary to Malcolm Law, MD]. If you're premenopausal, you should examine them shortly after your period, when hormone levels are low, so that premenopausal lumps aren't confused with a cancerous lump. You should also examine your breasts in the mirror and look for any unusual skin abnormalities or dimpling. After a few months you'll become very familiar with how your breasts feel, and you'll be able to detect very small abnormalities...

"Lumpy breasts are often diagnosed by doctors as 'fibrocystic breast disease', but this is not a disease. It can be a symptom of underlying metabolic imbalance in a woman's hormones. These breast lumps are tender but benign [harmless]. They're composed of dense, fibrous tissue and variably sized cysts that arise from fluid engorgement of either breast duct segments or lobes. If the cyst is large enough, an experienced physician can usually tell by squeezing a lump whether it's solid or fluid filled.

"Most cysts go away at the end of your [menstrual] cycle, within a few days of when bleeding begins. If a lump stays around for a few months, even if you're using progesterone cream, then you should see a doctor. If he or she says that the lump is fluid-filled, then it can be drained with a needle in the doctor's office. If the lump is solid, then you should have it biopsied [by the thin needle method]. Cancerous lumps generally feel solid and hard and are usually not painful." (Lee et al, 2002, p11-12, 79-80).

As noted above, you are unlikely to miss a hard lump more than a year before a mammogram might find it, especially with consistent practice, because you would be more sensitive to a change in your breasts than a medical professional who sees you once a year.

*Breast examination by medical professional.* This is called palpation to give it a professional sound. An experienced professional might, by being a little rougher than you, find a more deeply-seated lump, or confirm one you found. There is nothing wrong with having this done once per year, or more often if you found something suspicious yourself. The next moves are the same as given above by Lee — wait for the end of your menstrual cycle, and try progesterone cream.

In the Canadian National Breast Screening Study cited above, women aged 50-59 were randomly assigned to either annual physical examination alone or with mammography. After 7 years and 5 rounds of screening the numbers of deaths for both groups was nearly identical. "Current evidence suggests that screening by physical examination is as effective as screening mammography in reducing mortality from breast cancer." (Mittra, 1994). Note that even in this article, it is not clear whether reduction in mortality from breast cancer meant all-cause mortality after a diagnosis of breast cancer. Mittra did report that in the Breast Cancer Detection Demonstration Project in the USA on 280,000 women 34-74 years old, an "uncontrolled" study, which probably means that the subjects were not randomized, the 10-year survival with physical examination was 77%, while with mammography was 85%. Biases were supposed to have created the difference. Mittra also hinted that the Health Insurance Plan trial in which the intervention group had both mammography and physical examination (see above) might have owed its slight success to the latter.

In the study by Elmore et al. (2005) noted above for no benefit of mammograms, clinical breast examinations of women 50-65 years old cut their risk of death from breast cancer by 39% (RR = 0.61) if they were in a higher risk sub-group due to heredity, and this was just statistically significant. However, all-cause mortality was not given. Based on other data in given in Myth 8 and here it is very likely that there was less or no reduction in all-cause mortality. There was no benefit for women 40-49 years old.

*Ultrasound.* Also known as sonography or ultrasonography, this is frequently used to further evaluate breast abnormalities found by palpation or mammography. It is excellent at imaging cysts, which are round, fluid-filled pockets inside the breast, and always non-malignant. The next moves are the same as above. Some women actually prefer the pain of mammography, because it is impersonal and fast, to the prolonged personal attention, however painless, of ultrasound, which does utilize a gel that is often needlessly quite cold when applied to the breast before the movable sensor is used. A test costs about $150 and requires about 20-30 minutes.

The ultrasound images are even more blurry than mammograms, but have better contrast. Ultrasound may guide a physician on where to place the needle for a biopsy. The FDA has not approved ultrasound by general screening, but it is commonly used after palpation and/or mammography. An ultrasound interpretation is very judgmental. It is less reliable for deep-seated tumors; it cannot detect calcium deposits on tumors; and is subject to many false positives and negatives. (http://imaginis.com/breast health/ultrasound.asp)

*Thermography.* Appealing because it is so non-invasive, thermal imaging or infrared imaging of the breast was approved by the FDA in 1982. It may operate on the principle that tumors with faster metabolism than that of the surrounding tissue are slightly warmer. Nevertheless, according to the American College of Radiology, thermography is so inaccurate as to have no value as a screening, diagnostic, or adjunctive imaging tool. It has a false positive rate of 25%. (http://imaginis.com/breast health/thermal_imaging.asp?mode=1)

*T-scan breast imaging.* Also called electrical impedance scanning (EIS), this works by creating an image "map" of the breast using a sensor placed on the breast that detects small changes in electric current originating from 1 volt applied either with an arm patch or a hand-held cylinder. Since cancerous tissue conducts electricity differently than healthy tissue, tumors are made to show up as bright white spots on a monitor. This device can confirm the location of abnormal areas that were detected by a conventional mammogram. The scanner sends the image directly to a computer, allowing the radiologist to move the probe around the breast to get the best view of the area being examined. The device may reduce the number of biopsies needed to determine whether a mass is cancerous. It may also improve the identification of women who should have a biopsy.

This was approved by the FDA in 1999 as an adjunct to mammography. In 2000 it was available at only 35 facilities worldwide. Regardless of FDA approval, no rates of sensitivity (lack of false positives) or selectivity (lack of false negatives) were found for this technique (see Figure 9-1). (http://imaginis.com/breast health/t-scan/index.asp?mode=1)

*PET Scan.* The positron emission tomography (PET) scan creates computerized images of chemical changes that take place in tissue during the metabolism of glucose. The patient is given an injection of a substance that contains glucose molecules to which a radioactive fluorine-19 atom is attached. The radioactive glucose can help in locating a tumor, because cancer cells take up or absorb (metabolize) glucose faster than other tissues in the body. After receiving the radioactive injection, the patient lies still for about 45 minutes while the drug circulates throughout the body. If a tumor is present, the radioactive glucose will accumulate in the tumor(s). The patient then lies on a table, which gradually moves through the PET scanner 6 to 7 times during a 45-minute period. The PET scanner is used to detect the radiation. A computer translates this information into the images that are interpreted by a radiologist. Very bright areas in the image are easy to interpret.

212

PET scans may play a role in determining whether a breast mass is cancerous. However, PET scans are more accurate in detecting larger and more fast-growing tumors than they are in locating tumors that are smaller than 8 mm and/or less fast-growing. They may also detect cancer when other imaging techniques show normal results. Other forms of PET scans may be helpful in evaluating and assigning the stage of recurrent disease (cancer that has come back) as metastases.

An NCI-sponsored clinical trial is evaluating the usefulness of PET scan results in women who have breast cancer compared with the findings from other imaging and diagnostic techniques. This trial is also studying the effectiveness of PET scans in tracking the response of a tumor to treatment. The PET scan procedure is too expensive to be used routinely. (http://cis.nci.nih.gov/fact/5_14.htm)

*Scintimammography.* Also called nuclear medicine breast imaging and Miraluma™ as the DuPont Pharmaceutical trade name, this process is most appropriate for dense breast tissue that makes mammograms hard to endure and interpret. It was approved by the FDA as an adjunct to mammography and palpation.

To perform the examination, a radioactive tracer, technetium-99, a gamma ray emitter of very short half-life, is injected into the arm opposite to the breast being studied. The tracer travels around and is absorbed preferentially by cancer cells, much as in a PET scan. A gamma camera detects the emitted gamma rays by scintillation counting, conversion of some of the energy of the gamma rays into light pulses (the "scinti" of scintimammography). There is no breast compression.

Scintimammography is of most use in younger women or any with dense breast tissue, when multiple tumors are suspected, and to find a tumor after mastectomy when the ability of this method to distinguish a cancer from scar tissue of equal density is of value. Like some forms of PET scan, this procedure can detect metastases to underarm lymph nodes. It costs $200-400 per exam and takes 45-60 minutes. It is not good with small abnormalities. Its sensitivity, as noted above, was as high at 90% in one trial, and far better than mammography in this trial. There are no long-term studies of overall benefit available. (http://imaginis.com/breasthealth/nuc_med.asp?mode=1)

*Magnetic Resonance Breast Imaging.* Usually referred to as MRI or MR, this was approved by the FDA in 1991 as a supplemental tool after mammography. The procedure does not involve any breast compression, but there is an injection of a magnetic tracer called gadolinium DTPA, followed by a wait for it to spread. In the presence of a powerful magnetic field tiny radio waves emitted are detected. Images can be taken in any plane and from any orientation without needing the subject to move. MRI is effective in women with dense breast tissue or with implants. It can find metastases in lymph nodes, small tumors, and is more sensitive than mammography in that fewer false negatives are seen, but there are some false positives. The procedure takes 30-90 minutes and costs $1000, another reason for not using it for mass screening besides limited availability. A biopsy of an MRI-detected abnormality can be hard to place properly, especially when mammography and ultrasound cannot find the location at all. (http://imaginis.com/breasthealth/mri.asp?mode=1)

*Computer-Aided Detection (CAD) Technology for Mammography.* As evidence of the deficiencies of mammography, new computerized image processing devices are used to enhance the mammographic image, even marking suspicious areas on the digitized mammogram.

Approved by the FDA in 1998, CAD mammography, in 1 trial carried out in 12 centers, was able to detect 90% of the cancers that were overlooked in mammograms! This would make the sensitivity 96-99%, far better than conventional mammograms, but there are more false positives.

This process raises the cost by only $10-15 per exam.

(http://imaginis.com/breasthealth/cad.asp?mode=1) Still, one would think that CAD mammography would be preferable to the conventional form *after* a suspicious lump had been found by palpation or some other method, or *after* a positive test result was obtained by a non-imaging method.

*Ductal Lavage.* This is a minimally invasive procedure intended for very early detection of breast cancer. Most women will not have any discomfort with the procedure, which begins with the application of anesthetic cream to the nipple area, then drawing out some nipple fluid from each of the milk ducts. Samples are sent to the pathology lab to identify any abnormal cells. When the ducts most likely to have produced these cells are identified, normal saline solution is used to wash the duct by means of an inserted catheter (no pain, more anesthetic is used). The cells obtained are sent to the pathology lab to confirm the presence of cancerous cells.
(http://imaginis.com/breasthealth/ductal_lavage.asp)

This procedure is not yet widely available, but probably will become so. It is intended for very early detection in women with a family history of breast cancer or those who have the BRCA1 or -2 gene mutations associated with higher breast cancer rates. Pro-Duct Health, a company co-founded by Susan Love, MD, the inventor of the procedure, provides more information at http://www.producthealth.com/

However, the AMAS test described below seems preferable.

*AMAS Test.* At present, one of the best screening methods for breast cancer *or almost any other internal cancer,* one that has been available for 11 years, the Anti-Malignin Antibody in Serum (AMAS) test, is carried out on a few mL of drawn blood. The sample must be handled in a particular way and mailed to Oncolab, Inc., 36 The Fenway, Boston, MA 02115. (617-536-0850; www.amascancertest.com). A phone call will provide the location of the nearest physician or lab to you who can handle the test. The test costs $135, but the blood draw and shipping bring the total to about $200. A kit must be ordered with full instructions if the lab of your choice does not stock them.

The antibody is found in increased concentration when some form of cancer is present. It can also be used to check on whether a treatment is working, but, of course it cannot protect you from the side-effects of the treatment; however, it might indicate that treatment can stop earlier than the oncologist would otherwise think. The test is not reliable with advanced or terminal cancer; it is an excellent means of obtaining an early warning of cancer. The AMAS test is protected by US Patent 5,866,690 (February 2, 1999).

Biopsies of 43 women with suspicious mammograms revealed that 32 actually had cancer, showing a 23% false positive rate among these mammograms for the 11 women who had benign tumors. For those with breast cancer, 31 of 32 were positive in the AMAS test (sensitivity 97%, only 3% false negative), while 4 of the 11 who had benign tumors were AMAS positive (either a 36% false positive rate, or more likely, an early warning of cancer of some type not found by biopsy). No % value for the specificity of the AMAS test was given in the abstract of the report in *Cancer Letters* (Thornthwaite, 2000).

Blinded determinations were carried out by laboratories in 4 different locations during 20 years of responses to the AMAS test in 8,090 randomized cancer patients and controls. These included 1,175 with breast disorders. The AMAS levels were not increased in healthy controls, or in patients with inflammatory conditions, benign tumors, or in remission, but AMAS levels were increased 2-5 fold when an active malignancy was present. At the time of the primary diagnosis of active cancer the sensitivity was 98.2% (<2% false negatives) and the specificity was 91.4% (<9% false positives). At recurrence the sensitivity was 96.2% and the specificity was 100%. Accuracy was similar in malignancies other than breast (Bogoch & Bogoch, 1998). Oncolab Company literature claims that *duplicate* tests have specificity and sensitivity rates of over 99%.

"Many doctors are unaware of this test [even after 11 years] and may not be inclined to order it. It then becomes a challenge either to convince your doctor to order the test or to find a doctor or a walk-in health clinic that will." (Bognar, 1998).

Allan E. Sosin, MD, founder of The Institute for Progressive Medicine, Irvine, CA, had used the AMAS test for years, but stopped because there was too much trauma from putative "false positives" when imaging methods later could not find the tumor. Either patients must be warned of the number of false positives, or have the test repeated after a positive, or both.

Some severe criticism of the AMAS test has been made on theoretical grounds by Ed Friedlander, MD, who noted the absence of experiments on certain specific types of cell staining. He also noted the lack of a % value for specificity in Thornthwaite's paper, while ignoring the 4 of 11 positives presented that are not necessarily false in this group, and he mistakes the 97% sensitivity in a group of women with positive biopsies for breast cancer as "...telling almost everybody that he or she has cancer...", calling this finding, which he misrepresents, "...a classic quack fallacy...". He does not address the 20-year results noted above. His website was accessed on 12 Apr 04 (http://www.pathguy.com/malignin.htm).

This writer has no financial interest, direct or indirect, in Oncolab.

*****

As you can see, the *imaging* methods all have their problems, and the most fundamental information needed to make a decision on which, if any, to use, their sensitivity and specificity, are not readily available, even on the NCI website, or not available at all, except, of course, for mammography and the AMAS test. Being able to locate a new tumor amid implants or scar tissue by methods other than mammography is valuable. An imaging method is needed to locate tumors found by the use of the AMAS test. It cannot be repeated too often that accurate early detection is of limited use with an affliction that has no satisfactory treatments at present beyond lumpectomy. If new treatments are developed that will increase the 10-year survival time, preferably without serious side-effects, then really early detection would actually be a benefit.

If you have a suspicious lump or a positive AMAS test, you can bring this list of imaging methods to your oncologist or radiologist and ask why one imaging method was chosen over the others. You will learn a lot from the type of answer or lack of answer.

## Statistical Games with DCIS

Other than cysts, a form of cancer that may remain benign for years or forever is called ductal carcinoma *in situ* (DCIS). The *in situ* means that it has not spread. According to Dr. John Lee:

"The breast cancer industry has been playing a statistical shell game...by including DCIS as a breast cancer diagnosis when in fact it's rarely fatal, with or without treatment. Many oncologists like to say that DCIS is '99 percent curable.' (Since DCIS wasn't detectable—and thus not diagnosed or treated—until the advent of mammograms, we don't even really know the true nature or course of untreated DCIS, because it has always been treated if diagnosed [somehow].) ...some 30 percent of [so-called] breast cancers are DCIS.

"Given that DCIS is rarely fatal, let's make some gross generalizations to illustrate a point. If we simply eliminate DCIS from breast cancer statistics, and thus subtract 30 percent of those who have survived breast cancer from the statistics, we would then not have a recent drop of 20 percent (as claimed by some) [as noted above, Richard Peto and coworkers claimed a drop of 25-30%] but rather a rise of 10% in breast cancer mortality rates. This is a crude way of making the point, but it's important to consider when a doctor is using these types of statistics to justify a treatment. For example, let's say a doctor justifies putting you on tamoxifen to prevent breast cancer [not DCIS] based on the now much-quoted 'fact' that breast cancer deaths have dropped 20 percent thanks to tamoxifen...[see above for the real story]... If you know going into the doctor's office that this is a highly questionable statistic, you'll be more empowered to make the right decision for yourself. In fact, we suspect that if women with low-grade DCIS weren't subjected to tamoxifen, chemo, and radiation, their survival rate would stay the same—but the women would not be damaged for life by the treatments.

"But even experts debate whether DCIS is really a cancer... If DCIS becomes even the tiniest bit invasive, then it's automatically no longer considered [to be] DCIS... the women who receive mastectomies, radiation, and chemotherapy for a 'cancer' that is '99 percent curable' (as many DCIS experts like to say) may not find it amusing...

"...we really have little idea what the natural course of DCIS is if it's left alone...One study published in...1996 took all women diagnosed with DCIS between 1983 and 1991, regardless of treatment (or no treatment), and found that their survival rates were ranged from 100 to 104 percent. This meant that these women were less likely than the general population to die of breast cancer *or* other causes...

"Tragically, because DCIS calcifications tend to be scattered around in the breast tissue, in the 1980s women were often prescribed a mastectomy for treatment of this non-cancer, because it's so difficult to remove all of the breast tissue with microcalcifications. This is a brutal form of overtreatment that leaves women psychologically and physically scarred for life. It has become much less common, but it's still done with women who have a lot of calcifications." (Lee et al., 2002, pp13-14, 52-55).

In contrast to these reasoned observations, John S. Link, MD, cardiologist and author, who prides himself on not overtreating women for breast cancer wrote: "Women who desire a mastectomy in spite of a good response to systemic [chemo]therapy or who require mastectomy because of remaining...DCIS [!] often can have immediate [breast] reconstruction, without concern for the healing problems secondary to chemotherapy... Additionally, women who have cancers with an associated...DCIS component, involving a large area of the breast duct system, require large amounts of tissue to be removed." Dr. Link, incidentally, while acknowledging the false negatives of mammography, treated it as an inevitable test, and did not remark on the false positives or the lack of life-extension its use engenders (Link, 2002, pp24-25, 64, 69).

A report on the Breast Cancer Detection Demonstration Project in the USA on 280,000 women said that 42% of the tumors detected by mammography could not have been detected by physical examination. It turns out that 3/4s of these were DCIS. Other studies have shown that up to 66% of tumors detected were DCIS. It was considered doubtful that the lead time of about 2 doublings in the number of cells in the tumor before treatment provided by mammography would lead to a significantly greater reduction in mortality (Mittra, 1994).

## Summing Up

The pain of mammograms is not accompanied by the gain of any lifespan. Undergoing annual mammography does not improve all-cause mortality after a diagnosis of breast cancer. The most careful examination of mammography trials does not even support a lower breast cancer mortality. If there is a lower breast cancer mortality, some of it may be attributed to the hormetic effect of the Xrays used in mammography. Another reasonable explanation is that aggressive treatment of the many false positives from mammography, which are mostly DCIS, is replacing cancer deaths with deaths from treatment.

Many or most of the claims for benefits of mammography or other breast imaging techniques tout lower breast cancer mortality without even providing all-cause mortality. Major texts on gynecology and oncology do exactly this, and many or most gynecologists and oncologists are unaware of the omission and hard-sell the supposed lower breast cancer mortality.

Monthly breast self-examination makes one very aware of any change. An experienced health professional may find a deeper abnormality by being a little rougher. There is no significant benefit of mammography in detection beyond what palpation provides, since the DCIS mainly located by mammography is not malignant.

Several of the alternative imaging methods are of value after an abnormality has been detected by palpation, especially as a guide for placement of the needle used for a biopsy. Dense breasts, or the presence of implants, or of scar tissue favor the use of non-mammographic imaging methods, or at least a computer-enhanced mammogram. Because of the low incidence of breast cancer in women under 50 years old, no imaging method used annually will be of much benefit or be cost-effective in these women.

For women who cannot shake off their unfounded faith in the value of annual mammography, at least they should not begin until over 50 years old, unless family history or the presence of pro-breast cancer genes indicate the possible value of an earlier start. These women should remember that the chances of a false positive after 30 mammograms is about 88%. No trials indicating any benefit of pre-emptive mastectomy have been seen, which is still promoted for women with a bad family history or pro-cancer genes.

A major reason for the poor results after detection and diagnosis of breast cancer is that the standard treatments beyond lumpectomy do not work. More specifically, shrinkage of tumors or halting their growth and metastases is usually accomplished (see Myth 10), but the side-effects are so bad that all-cause mortality is not improved because of the toxicity of the routine treatments presently used.

Another reason is that cysts and DCIS are often claimed to be more than they are, and women who have them are overtreated.

The benefits of tamoxifen are minimal at best, and are accompanied by serious side-effects.

With early detection, even by palpation, the 5-year survival rate of breast cancer is over 50% even without treatment (some say 90%), so one now should demand the 10-year survival rate claimed for any detection, imaging, or treatment method. The major delayed toxicities of radiation and chemotherapy often strike between the 5th and 10th years.

For the earliest detection, including of other types of cancer, the AMAS test is the most effective, costs little more than a mammogram, and takes only the time to have some blood drawn. If this test is positive, some imaging method is then needed to locate the tumor(s), and it need not be ordinary mammography.

The expenditures on screening mammography are a serious waste of health insurance.

Some ideas on the prevention of breast cancer are addressed in Myth 10.

Redundant though it may be, again be warned that, at the present time, all claims of benefit of imaging, tests, or treatment beyond lumpectomy that are given as lower breast cancer mortality or higher survival rates from breast cancer are useless unless the 10-year *all-cause* mortality or *all-cause* survival rates are presented.

## Acknowledgements for Myth 9

William A. Reinsmith, DA, Fred Ottoboni, PhD, MPH, Alice Ottoboni, PhD, Alayne Yates, MD, and Frances E. H. Pane, MSLS, provided extremely valuable editorial advice and/or key references.

## References for Myth 9

Bailar JC III, MacMahon B (1997). Randomization in the Canadian National Breast Screening Study; a review for evidence of subversion. *Canadian Medical Association Journal* 156(2):193-199.

Bergman L, Beelen MLR, Gallee MPW, et al. (2000). Risk and prognosis of endometrial cancer after tamoxifen for breast cancer. *Lancet* 356:881-887.

Bognar D (1998). *Cancer. Increasing Your Odds for Survival.* Alameda, CA: Hunter House, Inc.

Bogoch S, Bogoch ES (1998). A quantitative immune response in human cancer: antimalignin antibody. *Cancer Detection and Prevention,* 22(suppl. 1). Seen at http://www.cancerprev.org/Journal/Issues/22/101/11/2702

Charatan F (2002). US panel finds insufficient evidence to support mammography. *British Medical Journal* 324:255.

Cuzick J, Stewart H, Rutqvist L, et al. (1994). Cause-Specific Mortality in Long-Term Survivors of Breast Cancer Who Participated in Trials of Radiotherapy. *Journal of Clinical Oncology* 12(3):447-453.

EBCTCG, Early Breast Cancer Trialists' Collaborative Group (1998). Tamoxifen for early breast cancer: an overview of the randomised trials. *Lancet* 351:1451-1457.

Elmore JG, Reisch LM, Barton MB, et al. (2005). Efficacy of breast cancer screening in the community according to risk level. *Journal of the National Cancer Institute* 97(14):1035-1043).

Gail MH, Costantino JP, Brynant J, et al. (1999). Weighing the Risks and Benefits of Tamoxifen Treatment for Preventing Breast Cancer. *Journal of the National Cancer Institute* 91:1829-46.

Gigerenzer G (2002). *Calculated Risks: How to Know When the Numbers Deceive You.* New York, N.Y: Simon & Schuster.

Gøtzsche PC, Olsen, O (2000). Is screening for breast cancer with mammography justifiable? *Lancet* 355:129-134.

Kashikar-Zuck S, Keefe FJ, Kornguth P, et al. (1997). Pain coping and the pain experience during mammography: a preliminary study. *Pain* 73(2):165-172.

Kauffman JM, McGee CT (2004). Are the biopositive effects of Xrays the only benefits of repetitive mammograms? *Medical Hypotheses* 62(5), 674-678.

Law M (2004). Screening without evidence of efficacy. Screening of unproved value should not be advocated. *British Medical Journal* 328:301-302.

Lee JR, Zava D, Hopkins V (2002). *What Your Doctor May* Not *Tell You About Breast Cancer. How Hormone Balance Can Help Save Your Life.* New York, NY: Warner Books.

Link JS (2002). *Take Charge of Your Breast Cancer,* New York, NY: Henry Holt.

Lomborg B (2001). *The Skeptical Environmentalist.* Cambridge, England, UK: Cambridge University Press.

Mittra I (1994). Breast screening: the case for physical examination without mammography. *Lancet* 343:342-344.

Moss RW (2000). *Questioning Chemotherapy,* Brooklyn, NY: Equinox Press.

Nystrom L, Andersson I, Bjurstam N, Frisell J, Nordenskjold B, Rutqvist ER (2002). Long-term effects of mammography screening: updated overview of the Swedish randomised trials. *Lancet* 359(9310):909-919.

Olsen O, Gøtzsche PC (2001). Cochrane review on screening for breast cancer with mammography. *Lancet* 358:1340-1342.

Phillips K-A, Glendon G, Knight JA (1999). Putting the risk of cancer in perspective. *New England Journal of Medicine* 340(2):141-144.

Plotkin D (1996). Good News and Bad News about Breast Cancer. *Atlantic Monthly* 277(6):53-82.

Porter-Steele N (1996). Breast pain causes noncompliance with mammography and self-examination. *Canadian Medical Association Journal* 155:632-633.

Powles T, Eeles R, Ashley S, et al. (1998). Interim analysis of the incidence of breast cancer in the Royal Marsden Hospital tamoxifen randomised chemoprevention trial. *Lancet* 352:98-101.

Pritchard KI (1998). Is tamoxifen effective in prevention of breast cancer? *Lancet* 352:80-81.

Robin ED (1984). *Matters of Life & Death: Risks and Benefits of Medical Care,* Stanford, CA: Stanford Alumni Assoc.

Skrabanek P, McCormick J (1989). *Follies and Fallacies in Medicine,* Glasgow, Scotland, UK: Tarragon Press.

Thornthwaite JT (2000). Anti-malignin antibody in serum and other tumor marker determinations in breast cancer. *Cancer Letters* 148:39-48.

# Myth 10: Cancer treatments are better than ever, and have cure rates of 60%.

*I knew that even after decades of intense research, there...had been no treatment advances beyond the highly toxic drugs developed before 1965. What I didn't know was how fiercely the cancer establishment would resist the efforts of an outsider... to come up with new ideas for treatment.*
*---Candace B. Pert, PhD, Biology (Pert, 1997)*

## Spacedoc Speaks Out

Cancer is not one disease; it is hundreds of diseases making generalizations difficult. We have made progress in a few cancers such as early Hodgkin's lymphoma and testicular tumor, but for the overwhelming majority such as lung, breast and bowel cancers our survival figures are not much different from those observed many years ago. Doctor Kauffman has done an incredible job of summarizing just where we are today. His major contribution in this chapter is helping the reader understand confusing and misleading terminology. The use of the term cure rarely applies to a cancer survivor. The correct term for judging effectiveness of cancer control is the five-year survival rate, that fraction of patients alive after five years from diagnosis. When a cancer expert says current treatment has a 60% success rate, he means 60% will still be alive after five years but in many, the cancerous cells still silently lurk.

Kauffman points to other pitfalls of false claims and misleading cancer survival information when alarmists talk of increasing cancer deaths from a specific type of cancer without age adjustment. As our population ages, so must the specific deaths, yet when corrected for age, these apparent epidemics become usual and customary trends. To one unfamiliar with the twists and turns of bio-statistics, it is easy to be confused. We desperately need reviewers such as Kauffman who are thoroughly trained in statistics and epidemiology to lead us by the hand as we try to absorb the immense amount of, at times conflicting, data on this subject.

Having been through my own PSA crisis, I agree that our sudden surge of prostate cancer is nothing more than the inevitable consequence of having initiated widespread PSA screening programs a result of which is earlier detection of cases that might have taken years to manifest otherwise. And, of course, in my age group [over 70], many would "pop off" with stroke and heart attack allowing our prostate cancers to remain hidden.

And no one will argue with the side effects of traditional radical surgery, radiation therapy and the "seeds". When I told my urologist I wanted the "seeds", he first asked me how long I expected to live. He then proceeded to remind me that the side effects of radiation burns to the bladder and bowel would start in roughly eight years. I said, "According to the literature the seeds don't do that". He laughed and reminded me that with the bladder and bowel only a millimeter or so from the prostate margins you cannot seed-irradiate the entire prostate without hitting those other vital structures. So there I was between a "rock and a hard place".

Then this doctor described for me the revolutionary new approach of radical laparoscopic prostatectomy. "We'll deliver the entire prostate through your navel and send you home within 24 hours with five band-aids on your abdomen and practically no discomfort. I went home in 14 hours assured that when I finally depart this place, it will likely be from heart attack or stroke but it will not be from prostate cancer. So for prostate cancer the scales of choice have shifted recently because of technological innovation, but, as Kauffman reminds us, for much of cancer the treatment effects on life quality are so frequently discouraging that treatment often is a "coin toss".

So, much of our apparent therapeutic progress in cancer is nothing more than earlier detection. Various groups in our society will be either alarmed or pleased depending on their interpretation of the cancer statistics, but nowhere will you find a better review.

------Duane Graveline MD MPH

## Overview

Cancer experts claim current treatment approaches achieve a 60% "success" rate, but this should not be confused with a true "cure" rate. What they are referring to is the 5-year survival rate. This is the fraction of patients alive after 5 years from diagnosis. This positive outcome is said to have improved from about 39% in 1962 to 50% by 1975 to 60% by 1995. Even this modest progress will be seen to be a result of earlier and earlier diagnosis with very little improvement due to the benefit of mainstream types of treatment. This seeming improvement is actually caused by what is called lead-time bias, a result of earlier detection. Other types of bias exist in clinical trials.

Advice on cancer prevention usually neglects the fact that most cancers are genetically based. Lung cancer, malignant melanoma of the skin, and possibly breast cancer may involve some genetic susceptibility along with the exposure to the external agent. There are some work-exposure-related cancers that are now very rare in developed countries. Advice not to eat animal fat has no basis in fact, and there are plenty of plant-derived carcinogens. Advice to avoid or seek sun exposure is often not accompanied by specifying the types of cancer that sunlight will affect one way or the other.

The common mainstream treatments may stop solid tumors from growing, or even shrink them, but the treatments themselves are delayed causes of cancer, causing new types in 5-15 years. Treatments to prevent recurrence, such as tamoxifen, do so for limited periods, but cause other types of toxicity. Poorly applied hormone replacement therapy caused some breast cancer, dementia and heart disease.

Oncologists usually mislead patients about the benefits of mainstream treatment, and minimize the delayed effects and the side-effects. They disparage all alternative treatments regardless of evidence, and conspire to prevent low-cost trials of alternative therapies from being carried out on patients not damaged by mainstream treatments. Most alternative cancer treatments are of no value, but many are non-toxic, so that a higher quality of life can be enjoyed while one is hoping for a remission. A few non-toxic alternative treatments are proven to be effective, and there is always the chance that some more really beneficial treatment from any source may appear.

Some accurate and unbiased sources of information on cancer treatment do exist. One must seek these out and act on them rather than being processed routinely by The Cancer Industry.

## Cure, Incidence, and Death Rates in Cancer

On Jan 18th, 2003, Barrie R. Cassileth, MD, spoke about cancer treatment at a meeting of a Philadelphia area skeptics group. She is the director of the Complementary Medicine Center at the Memorial Sloan-Kettering Cancer Center (MSKCC). She was an excellent speaker with an earnest and confident manner, and maintained absolutely perfect poise during a long questioning session. One of the questions was on the cure rate at MSKCC: what was the overall cure rate there for cancers in general? She answered that MSKCC had an overall cure rate of 60% for cancer. On being asked by me whether this was a 5-year survival rate, she affirmed that 60% was the cure rate. In fact, a recent press release from the USA Department of Health and Human services seemed to confirm her opinion by stating: "The 5-year survival rate for all cancers improved from 51 percent in the early 1980s to

| Table 10-1. Changes in 5-Year Survival Rates for 20 Types of Solid Tumors, Comparing 1950-54 with 1989-95. Data from Welch et al., 2000. | | |
|---|---|---|
| Primary Cancer Site | 5-Year Survival, % | |
| | 1950-54 | 1989-95 |
| Prostate | 43 | 93 |
| Melanoma | 49 | 88 |
| Testes | 57 | 96 |
| Bladder | 53 | 82 |
| Kidney | 34 | 61 |
| Breast | 60 | 86 |
| Colon | 41 | 62 |
| Rectum | 40 | 60 |
| Ovary | 30 | 50 |
| Thyroid | 80 | 95 |
| Larynx | 52 | 66 |
| Uterus | 72 | 86 |
| Cervix | 59 | 71 |
| Mouth | 46 | 56 |
| Esophagus | 4 | 13 |
| Brain | 21 | 30 |
| Lung | 6 | 14 |
| Stomach | 12 | 19 |

almost 60 percent in the early 1990s... ...since the 1971 National Cancer Act [the War on Cancer], much of the research into early cancer detection and treatment has paid off." (Table 10-1), (Welch et al, 2000).

Calling the 5-year survival rate, the % of those treated (or not) who are still alive after 5 years without recurrence of cancer the "cure rate" has been called statistical sophistry (Lerner, 2002, p29). H. Gilbert Welch, MD, calls 5-year survival rates "...the world's most misleading number" (Welch, 2004, pp129-149). Due to improved or more frequently used diagnostic methods, cancers might be detected a year or more earlier than had been the norm. This would automatically lead to claims of another year or more of survival since diagnosis, assuming the treatment method did not change. But there is no more time of survival, really, just earlier detection and diagnosis. Understanding this "lead-time bias" is very important, especially because many in the medical or reporting professions do not understand it.

What is a cure? This term was best applied to an infectious disease, such as pneumonia or syphilis. These were contracted by people only when the particular bacterium was introduced from an outside source. After treatment with a penicillin, the symptoms disappeared and the bacterium could no longer be found in the patient if looked for. If there were no contact with the particular bacterium at a later date, even many years later, the disease would not return. This is a cure. The 5 year "cure" rate for cancer is simply the percent of people who are alive 5 years following a diagnosis of cancer, and it has nothing to do with whether cancer is present at the 5 year mark.

At present only temporary healing can be expected from most treatments of cancer, whether mainstream or alternative. The same or other cancer can return at any time, and the treatment may be repeated, and so on. Cancer, of course, is any uncontrolled cell growth leading to solid tumors that interfere with some organ's function, or to production of too many white blood cells (leukemia). There are many rare forms, such as thymic cancer, many of which are so rare that no serious studies of the effects of the standard surgery, chemotherapy and radiation have been done. About 20 forms are considered common and listed in tables of incidence and treatment, usually by location, such as liver cancer (Table 10-1). Even breast cancer is not quite the same in any patient, and is said to have hundreds of forms, based on various tests on genes and receptors (Link, 2002, pp20-21).

Another term that is used by oncologists to encourage or confuse cancer victims is the response rate. When asked by a patient, "What are my chances with chemotherapy?", the answer is likely to be 60%. The patient thinks that means a cure rate, the odds of a cancer disappearance. Response rates to standard treatments for common cancers range from 60-90%, yet cancer-free survival is 0-20% (Moss, 2000, pp56-57). For cancer as much as for any other affliction, the all-cause death-rates or years of life remaining must be given with and without the planned treatment. Or how many years of *quality* lifespan will be gained with treatment. Patients who do not receive this type of information have been misled — or worse.

Ever the optimist, the oncologist John S. Link, MD, wrote that 80% of women today are cured of breast cancer, meaning to most patients that they will live the rest of their lives without a recurrence, rather than that the 5-year survival rate is 80% (Link, 2002, p59). Putting it this way is not the same as calling it a 5-year survival rate. However, Table 9-1 (Myth 9) shows that 40% of women diagnosed with breast cancer do die of it, not 20%. Others die of treatment, so the cause of death becomes something other than breast cancer in perhaps 10-30%, so a total of 50-70% of women diagnosed with breast cancer (not DCIS, see Myth 9) die early because of it, not 20% as Link implied by what he wrote.

*****

Professional scaremongers, especially pseudoenvironmentalists, have caused alarm by spreading fears that the total number of new cancer cases is at an all-time high in industrialized countries, and that most of the increase in cancer is caused by pesticides or other pollutants. A typical false alarm is to spread the idea that cancer deaths had doubled in the USA between 1950 and 1998, an increase of 100%. The doubling is true, as shown by the top (white) line in Figure 10-1, but what does it mean? Epidemiologists and others have known for at least a century that the meaningful way to to measure disease or death in any population group is to calculate the incidence rate of the disease or the death *rate.* The death (mortality) rate, for example, is the number of deaths in a given year divided by the size of the population in which those deaths occurred. It is usually expressed as the number deaths per 100,000 of population in a given year; this is the mortality rate. Since the population of the USA also doubled in the same time period, broadcasting only the change in the total number of deaths is a form of amateurism at best and deliberate dissemination of misinformation at worst.

When the crude cancer death *rate* is plotted (pale gray line in Figure 10-1) the increase is a lot less dramatic, being about 33%. But cancer is primarily a disease of old age. With so many more people in the USA reaching old age because of better food, better food additives, such as vitamin D and folic acid, taking supplements such as vitamin C and not dying of infectious diseases, more are living long enough to contract cancer and die of it, or of its treatment. This is allowed for by an age adjustment. When this was done, there was no difference in the cancer death rate over the half century period in Figure 10-1 (dark gray line). More impressive, when cancers due to smoking are removed, the age- and smoking-adjusted rate shows a 33% drop! No cancer epidemic after all! (lower black line in Figure 10-1). So all the frenzied explanations of drastically increased cancer deaths caused by pesticides, bad food, no exercise, etc., are mostly a waste of your time because there is no increase in most cancer death rates not caused by smoking or sunbathing. However, it must be repeated that cancer treatment causes non-cancer deaths, so if these are counted it is possible that the lowest line on Figure 10-1 would not show a decrease in what might be called "deaths due to cancer *or its treatment*", even when adjusted for age- and smoke-related cancers.

Figure 10-1. All-cancer mortality in USA from 1950-1998 per year. Top line: actual deaths. Second line: unadjusted all-cancer death rate. Third line: Age-adjusted all-cancer death rate. Fourth line: Age- and smoking-adjusted all-cancer death rate. From Lomborg, 2001, p217.

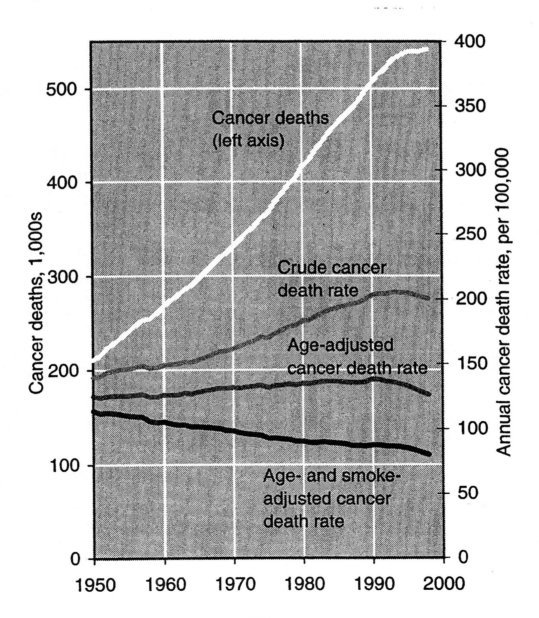

As a specific example of "progress" with one common cancer type, let us look at leukemia in the USA (Figure 10-2). The alarmists would broadcast that deaths from leukemia have more than doubled from 1950 to 1997 (white line, left scale), and this is true, but misleading, as for all cancers. The leukemia death *rate* rose 27% (gray line, left scale). When adjusted for the higher ages of people dying of leukemia in the later years, this rate is seen to have fallen about 14%; so there is no epidemic (lower black line, left scale). False alarms on the supposed increase in leukemia because of increased use of pesticides have thus been exposed, discrediting some famous environmentalists, including Rachel Carson (Lomborg, 2001, pp218-219). The number of people newly diagnosed with leukemia per 100,000 population in a given year, the incidence rate, is given by the thin black line near the top Figure 10-2, right scale). Note that the incidence line is roughly parallel to the death rate line. This indicates that there has been no improvement in treatment for this type of cancer, in this case between 1973 and 1997. It must be conceded that between 1960 and 1973, chemotherapy was developed which caused long-term remissions for a type of childhood leukemia (Moss, 2000, p27).

Even normally reliable publications fumble when cancer is involved. An article in *New Scientist* showed parallel lines on a graph of all cancer incidence and of cancer mortality in the USA from 1975 to 2000 without the slightest inkling that this meant that the treatments discussed in the article, on the whole, do not work (Cohen, 2004).

A glance at Figure 10-3 shows that, of the 6 most common types of cancer in men, only lung and bronchial cancer deaths increased greatly (up 1500%), while those from stomach cancer plunged by 88%, a little-known fact for which no good explanation exists. Figure 10-4 shows a similar story for lung and bronchial cancer deaths in women (up 1700%). Several other types of cancer death rates plunged before radiation treatment was at all common, and before any chemotherapy had begun. These welcome drops are still as puzzling as the ones in men.

Figure 10-5 shows the now unsurprising (except to tobacco companies) relation between smoking rates and age-adjusted lung cancer death rates. The peak deaths for males occurred 19 years after the peak for smoking rate. If females follow suit, the peak death rate for them will have occurred in 2004. If the expected trends continue, the demands on Medicare and national health services outside the USA may drop significantly. There is no effective treatment for lung cancer.

Now have a look at properly age-adjusted incidence rates (Figure 10-6). Here is the kind of "evidence" that can spark false alarms and panic spending by politicians. Starting at the top white line, it appears that there was an incredible prostate cancer epidemic in the early 1990s. This actually coincided with the sudden acceptance and wide application of the prostate specific antigen (PSA) test around 1988. This test was applied to many asymptomatic men for the first time during the first 10 years this test was used, and it detected a prevalence of prostate cancer or prostatitis that was unexpected, but mostly not lethal. No epidemic.

Next it appears that breast cancer incidence increased by 57% between 1977 and 1997 (black line). This coincides with the great increase in mammography (see Myth 9). About half of the so-called cancers detected are the benign DCIS, and many of the rest merely had been caught 1-2 years earlier than by palpation. Other imaging methods reviewed in Myth 9 also appeared during this period and detected DCIS or very small tumors earlier than had been the case before. Result: no real epidemic.

No such changes in detection appeared for most of the other types of cancer shown in Figure 10-6, so the incidence has remained about the same. For lung cancer, the vertical scale compression in Figure 10-6 and the shorter time period are responsible for the apparent difference compared with Figures 10-3 and 10-4. The case has been made that the increase in female genital cancer is due to the use of tamoxifen (Bergman et al., 2000). The case has been made that much breast cancer is due to poorly applied hormone replacement therapy, as practiced with estrogens mixed with patented unnatural progestins. Experts wrote that this would not have happened if non-patentable progesterone had been used instead (Lee et al., 2002).

So the only cancer epidemics in the USA seen in the last half of the twentieth century were caused by smoking, sunbathing and prescription drug side-effects (see below). The first is already receding because smoking is less prevalent; but the latter are still increasing.

Figure 10-2. Leukemia mortality in USA from 1950-1997 by year. Top white line: actual leukemia deaths. Middle gray line: unadjusted leukemia death rate. Third black line: Age-adjusted leukemia death rate. Top thin black line: Age-adjusted leukemia incidence. From Lomborg, 2001, p218.

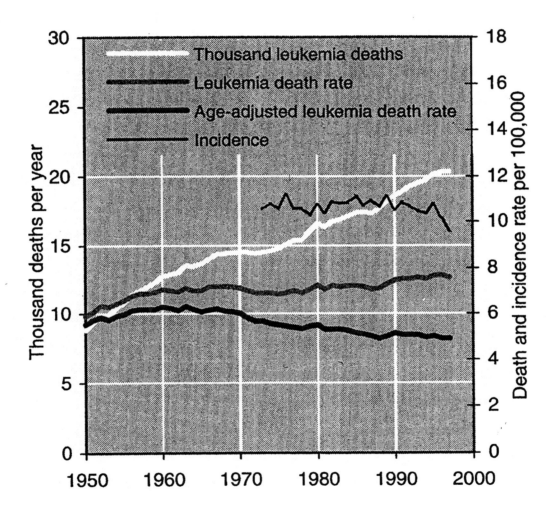

### Why Do 5-Year Survival Rates Seem to be Improving?

If 100 people initially diagnosed with cancer are treated in any manner, and 50 are still alive after 5 years from the diagnosis, this is called a 5-year survival rate of 50%. There is a finagle factor in 5-year survival rates that does not exist in incidence or mortality rates besides the effect of earlier detection. It was voiced by Dr. Hardin Jones, Professor of Medical Physics at the University of

California, Berkeley, at a meeting of The American Cancer Society in New Orleans in March, 1969, and on numerous other occasions since 1956:

"First, [he said], the notion that patients treated by conventional therapies live longer than the untreated victims is biased by the methods of defining the groups. Thus, [Jones claimed], if a person in the *untreated* category dies at any time while he or she is being studied, this is recorded as a death in the control [untreated] group, and is registered as a failure of the no-treatment approach. If, however, patients in the the treated category die during the course of treatment (before the course of treatment is completed), their cases are rejected from the data since 'these patients do not then meet the criteria established by the definition of the term 'treated.' A patient dying on day 89 of a prescribed 90-day course of chemotherapy would be dropped from the list of treated patients. The longer the treatment, the greater becomes the error.

Figure 10-3. Cancer mortality in men from the most common types in the USA from 1930-1998 by year. Age-adjusted. From Lomborg, 2001, p220.

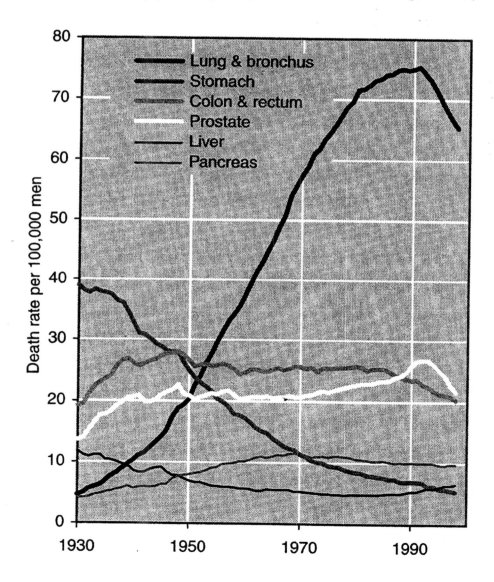

Figure 10-4. Cancer mortality in women from the most common types in the USA from 1930-1998 by year. Age-adjusted. From Lomborg, 2001, p220.

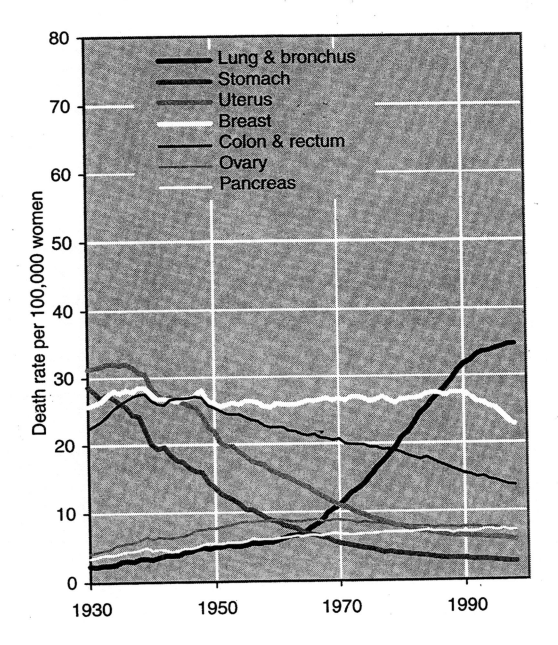

"With this effect stripped out,...the common malignancies show remarkably similar rates of demise, whether treated or untreated.

"Second,...beginning in 1940, various low-grade kinds of malignancies were redefined as cancer. From that date, the proportion of 'cancer' cases being cured increased rapidly, corresponding to the fraction of questionable diagnoses included.

"Third, Jones's research showed no relationship between the intensity of treatment and survival rates. Radical surgery, for instance, did not seem to be more successful than more limited operations that removed only the tumor and small amounts of normal tissue.

"Fourth, there is no proof that early detection affects survival. Serious attempts to relate prompt treatment with chance of cure have been unsuccessful.

"Jones concluded that evidence for benefit from cancer therapy had depended on systematic biometric errors...The possibility exists that treatment makes the average situation worse. To reporters Jones once stated that, in his opinion, radical surgery does more harm than good, and, as for radiation treatment, most of the time it makes not the slightest difference whether the machine is turned on or not." (Moss, 1999, pp32-33)

Figure 10-5. Cigaret consumption from 1900-1999 and death rates from lung and bronchial cancer from 1900-1998 in the USA by year for men (black lines) and women (white lines). Age-adjusted. From Lomborg, 2001, p220.

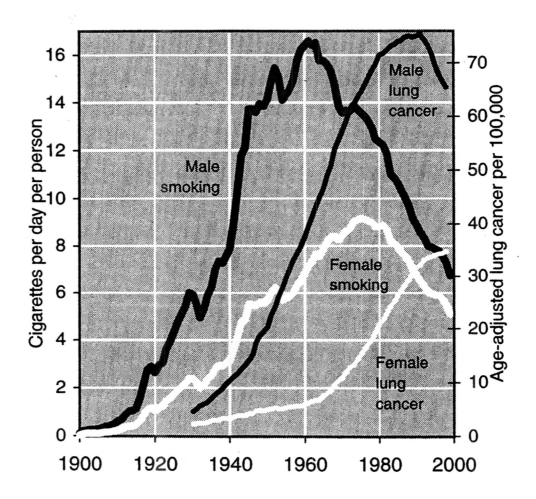

No studies have really invalidated Jones's positions, which apply to age-adjusted values.

This was solidly confirmed for both more radical surgery and for radiation treatment of breast cancer in a recent paper, compared with less radical surgery and no radiation (Fisher et al., 2002). Jones's comment on the different method of counting deaths in control and treated patients is based on the unfamiliar, hidden policy of not counting the deaths in treated patients if the treatment is incomplete. This is worse policy than ignoring dropout rates in trials of less lethal drugs in order to hide the number of adverse effects (see Myths 3 and 4).

Another aberration in the 5-year survival rates was another adjustment to rates not only adjusted for age, but for increased rates of non-cancer death, since a survivor of cancer treatment is more likely to be run over by a truck, or die of CHF or CVD, for example. This change helped to conceal some of the non-cancer deaths caused by treatment, and it was made because the 5-year survival rate in whites in 1973 was 38.5%, yet after 5 years of the War on Cancer, it had only reached 40.1% in 1978. This was too pathetic a result for the cancer warriors, so they made this change "for greater accuracy", and they began to report on white citizens only, who have lower cancer rates than Afro-Americans, so that the 5-year survival rate magically climbed to 50% by 1974-6 with this adjustment (Moss, 1999, pp35-39). These changes have obscured the lack of progress in cancer treatment, or prevention (except for lung cancer).

Figure 10-6. Cancer incidence of the most common types in the USA from 1973-1997 by year. Age-adjusted. From Lomborg, 2001, p223.

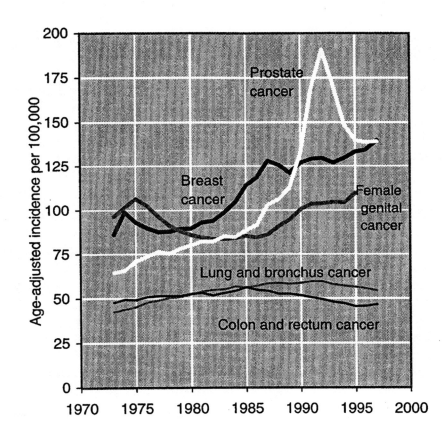

By the year 1995 the claim was made that the 5-year survival rate had climbed to 60% overall. A look at Table 10-1 seems to indicate that the War on Cancer, whose name was allowed to vanish in the 1980s, is being won and won big. But is it?

As indicated in Myth 9 the improved breast cancer 5-year survival rate was due to earlier detection by mammography, and the classification of the non-malignant DCIS as cancer. The "incidence" went up between 1950 and 1996 by 55%, while the mortality rate dropped by 8% (Welch et al., 2000). The increase in incidence is completely an artifact of the detection of DCIS by mammography, and 1-2 year earlier detection of actual cancers. The mortality rate counts only deaths caused directly by breast cancer. As noted before, treatment changes the cause of some deaths, as many as 30% of deaths, to some other cause (Table 9-1), such as heart failure or suicide.

For prostate cancer, the "incidence" rose by 190% from 1950 to 1996. Nearly all of this is based on early detection, first by the rectal physical examination, and most by the PSA (prostate specific antigen) test (Figure 10-6). Nearly all the positive tests contributing to the "incidence" are based on detection in asymptomatic men. Prostate cancer mortality actually increased by 10% during this period, indicating that treatments from radioactive implanted "seeds" to finisteride (Proscar™) are of little to no use. Men are subject to a 1 in 10 threat of being diagnosed with prostate cancer during a lifetime. Actual autopsies show that 1 in 2 men have the disease at death, while only 1 in 33 (3%) actually die of it (Bostwick et al., 1999, pp xxi,32-33). As with other cancers, the 3% figure does not allow for a change in the cause of death due to treatment. Prostate cancer usually proceeds so slowly, while the benefits from early mainstream treatment are so meager, that the US Preventive Services Task Force concluded that routine screening for prostate cancer be abandoned (Woloshin & Schwartz, 1999). Malcolm Law, Professor of Preventive Medicine, London School of Medicine, UK, wrote:

"The serum concentration of prostate specific antigen can predict mortality from prostate cancer. [But] there are no published randomised trials that the earlier detection improves prognosis, yet in the United States and Italy a third or more of healthy men aged over 50 have had prostate specific antigen measured in the past two years. In Britain, on the other hand, only 5% have, and the available evidence on prostate specific antigen testing in reducing mortality indicates that the British are right to reject it... [The test has]...a false positive rate as high as 18% in men over 70...

"At present the one certainty about prostate specific antigen testing is that it causes harm. Some men will receive treatment that is unnecessary..., and the treatment will cause incontinence, impotence, and other complications." (Law, 2004).

H. Gilbert Welch, MD, MPH, Co-Director of the Veterans Administration Outcomes Group and Professor at Dartmouth Medical School, NH, USA, wrote:

"Most of the million men whose prostate cancer is found because of superior screening [since 1988] have [sic] to undergo some sort of treatment, whether radical surgery or radiation. A few (less than 1 percent) die from surgery, but many experience significant complications: 17 percent need additional surgery because they have difficulty urinating after surgery; 28 percent must wear pads because they have the opposite problem—they cannot hold their urine; and more than half are bothered by a loss of sexual function (inability to have an erection). Among men undergoing radiation, 19 percent still suffer from radiation damage to the rectum two months afterward, and over a third report diarrhea or bowel urgency as much as two years later.

"...right now we need to be clear about the way it [the PSA test] has been used so far: it has been making men sick." (Welch, 2004, p63).

For lung cancer, the "incidence" rose 249% from 1950-1996 while lung cancer mortality rose 259%. This is a sure sign of the ineffectiveness of treatment. The more than doubling in the 5-year survival rate from 6% to 14% (Table 10-1) is of no value for judging the war on cancer, since this result is due entirely to earlier detection by more skillful or more frequent use of chest Xrays!

For malignant melanoma, the incidence rose 453% from 1950-1996 while the cancer mortality from it rose 161%. The incidence parallels the use of sunscreens as discussed below (Garland et al., 1993). Lower mortality shows that surgery is an effective treatment.

According to Welch et al., 2000, none of the improved 5-year survival rates indicate improved treatments, and all of them are the result of earlier detection. Welch et al. see the 5-year survival rate as a valid measure only in randomized trials, not for promoting actual treatments; but Jones's observations are not addressed. Since evidence I have been made aware of indicates that the delayed side-effects of radiation and chemotherapy become apparent largely between the 5th and 10th year after treatment, the 5-year survival rate was a clever choice, and might better become a 10-year survival rate. "The most basic measure of progress against cancer is age-adjusted mortality... The use of mortality as the chief measure of progress against cancer, rather than incidence or survival, focuses attention on the outcome that is most reliably reported and is of greatest concern to the public: death." (Bailar & Gornik, 1997).

As an illustration of the limitations of the 5-year survival rate in indicating mortality or quality of life, of the side-effects of treatment, and of the change of cause of death by treatment, here is an example of an actual patient experience from our "empathetic" mainstream oncologist, Dr. John S. Link:

"A few years ago I took care of a woman named Alice who had newly diagnosed breast cancer. Together we developed a comprehensive plan that gave her an excellent chance of survival [no time frame was given]. She received a wide local excision of her primary tumor with a sentinel lymph node sampling, six months of chemotherapy followed by radiation for approximately six weeks, and then took an oral medication, tamoxifen, for five years. She did relatively well during the active phases of the treatment: surgery, chemo, and radiation. But once she completed the active treatment, she went into a fearful, anxiety-dominated depression. Alice was forty-six years old, and though recovered from her treatment and in excellent physical health, she was sure her life was over, that she was dying of breast cancer. I treated her with several antidepressant drugs with little success, and I then referred her to a psychiatrist. Nothing seemed to help much. She became fixated on making the five-year anniversary without relapse. I suspected that was because her mother had had breast cancer, had relapsed after four years, and ultimately died of the disease.

"As Alice waited for the five-year mark, it seemed that she almost stopped living. She developed an almost superstitious quiet. It seemed as if she was afraid to do anything lest it somehow provoke a recurrence. She dropped out of all her social activities. She had divorced ten years before her diagnosis and had been involved with a very supportive man. After she was diagnosed, she ended the relationship. Her two grown children lived far away and were not aware of how the cancer had altered her life, which was now consumed by her health concerns and her fear of relapse. I encouraged her to get involved in support groups, but she refused. She became more withdrawn and reclusive, and her two children came to see me out of concern for their mother. I explained that she had an excellent chance of being cured and that I was worried about her inability to live life more fully. For many patients, the close encounter with the reality of death that the experience of breast cancer forces upon them also results in a profound commitment to live life to its fullest. These patients don't just survive, they thrive. They have fought so hard for the quantity of their lives that they insist the quality be the best. Not so for Alice. She was almost fifty years old and she was consumed by depression and anxiety. At some point I suggested that she get a dog... to encourage her in investing in a relationship. She did get a small dog, which seemed to ease her loneliness and bring her joy.

"On her fifth anniversary, she came to the office and we gave her a small party to celebrate the milestone. She told us that she was feeling more optimistic about the future and that she was ready to really start living again. The following week she had a massive cerebral hemorrhage [stroke]. She died three days later. Her children requested a postmortem examination. No evidence of breast cancer was found." (Link, 2002, pp60-62).

Dr. Link thought the lesson to be learned was that the patient must buck up regardless. Nowhere did he even hint that antidepressant drugs such as the SSRIs (Prozac™ type) can cause stroke, but it has been reported (Cohen, 2001, pp44-45). Nowhere did he concede that Alice was depressed because of the side-effects of treatment, either directly, or because Alice never had a single day of quality life once treatment had begun, or that she may have died of treatment. Obliquely, Dr. Link was blaming the victim.

Long ago a young radiologist, in the privacy of his home, told me what he was taught to say to any of his patients who complained about a common side-effect of cancer treatment: "There was a one in a million chance that could happen, just one in a million."

Even when the mortality rate is shown in any promotion of a cancer treatment, rather than the 5-year survival rate, what is usually shown is cancer mortality, not an all-cause death rate. The cancer warriors take full advantage of their ability to knock out cancer in selling their skills, while concealing the fact that their efforts cause non-cancer deaths.


Cancer Prevention

Many examples of positive and helpful findings on prevention are given here. But there is plenty of mythology in opinions of what will prevent cancer. Some typical examples are presented to show the level of false claims and confusion on this topic.

*Low-level ionizing radiation.* Myth 8 showed that low-level ionizing radiation below a certain level *prevents* cancer, just the opposite of the dogma that radiation at any level *causes* cancer. The risks of medical diagnostic radiation are often exaggerated, because they are usually in the beneficial range of exposure (Kauffman, 2003).

*Sunlight.* The longer-wavelengths of ultraviolet (UV) light from the sun are called, collectively, UVA. The next-shorter-wavelengths are called UVB, and these UVB rays are what are absorbed by the older versions of commercial suntan lotions, now called sunblock preparations. Many of the newest ones absorb most of the UVA rays as well and have the words "broad spectrum" on the container. Numerous research papers have shown that the UVB portion of sunlight interacts with a form of cholesterol in our skin to produce vitamin D. This vitamin prevents or limits the growth of malignant melanoma (the more deadly skin cancer), as well as cancers of the breast, colon and prostate. This is in addition to the well-known prevention of osteoporosis by vitamin D. The incidence of these cancers is lowest in the sun-drenched countries near the equator. Some researchers think that the heavily pigmented skin of Afro-Americans and dark Asians living far from the equator prevents vitamin D formation, and is indirectly responsible for the higher incidence and more rapid spread of cancers in Afro-Americans, whose skin is adapted to more intense sunlight. Caucasians who apply sunscreen lotions that block only UVB are preventing vitamin D formation. Also, the big exposure to UVA without sunburn made possible by older sunblocks is thought partly responsible for causing malignant melanoma. Men are more likely to get malignant melanoma on their backs, women on their legs. Most men go through life with their backs covered and protected from the sun's rays. Gradual and repeated exposure of caucasians to direct sunlight, always avoiding burning, without sunblock, is strongly recommended, rather than a big dose of sun on weekends in summer (Eades & Eades, 2000, pp241-256; Garland et al., 1993). Even old-style sunblocks with SPF 8 cut vitamin D production by

3/4 after exposure to artificial sunlight (Holick, 2004). Newer sunblocks with SPF 25 would be even worse. Outdoor workers have a decreased risk of melanoma compared with indoor workers, suggesting that chronic sunlight exposure can have a beneficial effect. Research shows that there is a genetic susceptibility to melanoma (Rivers, 2004). The easily treatable types of skin cancer, the ones called basal and squamous cell carcinomas, are the ones caused by exposure to UVB.

William B. Grant, an independent researcher based in Newport News, VA, has done an ecologic study that agrees with the findings of Garland et al. and of Eades & Eades. Breast cancer mortality rates among 16 developed Western countries are lowest in the most southerly ones: Greece, Spain and Portugal, while being highest in the most northerly of the bunch: Denmark, Netherlands, Belgium and the UK (Grant, 2002). People in countries closest to the equator receive the most sunlight, including the beneficial UVB. The incidence of some 16 different types of cancer has been linked with vitamin D insufficiency. Light-skinned people living more than 40° from the equator probably do not receive enough sunlight for adequate vitamin D production in winter. Those living more than 50° from the equator may not get enough sun all year round. Dark-skinned people living more than 30° from the equator may find that they need vitamin D in diet or supplements all year round, since D deficiency may cause several of the problems of the dark-skinned living in areas with limited sun (Gillie, 2004).

"A. Bernard Ackerman, MD, is an exceptionally distinguished dermatologist and one of the world's foremost authorities on the subject of skin cancer. In 1999, after a long career in academic medicine, he founded and became director of the Ackerman Academy of Dermatopathology in New York. Dr. Ackerman advises people to stay out of the sun in order to avoid premature aging of their skin. He also says that if you are very fair, you can prevent squamous cell carcinoma, a less dangerous cancer, by avoiding sunlight... (Squamous cell carcinomas, although they can be disfiguring, are rarely life-threatening and easily treated.) But don't make the mistake of thinking that by avoiding sunlight *or using sunscreen* you will be protected against deadly melanoma. This, he says, is a myth" (Moss, 2004).

Were you convinced of the value of gradual exposure to unfiltered sunlight? And the lack of value of sunblocks? Two meta-analyses trials on the use of sunblock vs. incidence of melanoma found no association! One, from the College of Public Health and the College of Medicine, University of Iowa at Iowa City, Iowa, USA, searched for trials, and found 18 of a quality level to be worth citing. Fully 11 of the trials showed a positive association of sunblock use with melanoma. Only in people who were very sun-sensitive was use of sunblock associated with less melanoma. Yet their conclusions were: "No association was seen between melanoma and sunscreen use." An astute comment was made that most of the studies were conducted with old sunblock formulations that had no UVA protection, while newer formulations have some (Dennis et al., 2003). The second meta-analysis, this one from Harvard Medical School and Beth Israel Deaconess Medical Center, Boston, MA, USA, found some flaws in the first meta-analysis, but came to similar conclusions: sunscreen use protected only the most sun-sensitive people from melanoma. "We should continue to advocate that our patients avoid sun exposure to prevent skin cancer, including melanoma. Measures should include avoiding midday sun, wearing protective clothing, and the proper use of sunscreens." (Bigby, 2004). Both meta-analyses ignored the benefits of natural production of vitamin D in the skin and the consequent protection from many kinds of cancers! Since the newer formulations with UVA protection have not been tested in proper trials, you cannot be certain that they will prevent melanoma. You *can* be certain that desirable vitamin D production will be inhibited.

Get out in the sun, but not so much as to be burned. Use sunblock of SPF 15 or higher whose label says that it will absorb both UVA and UVB for longer exposures to sun. Follow the advice on how much time in the sun for your skin type in the book *The UV Advantage* by Michael Holick, PhD, MD.

*Work-Related.* In the past, exposure of chemical workers to vinyl chloride and 2-naphthylamine, among other things, did cause specific types of cancers. Mining of coal and other minerals with certain kinds of dust, including radioactive particles, caused mostly lung cancer. Precautions taken in many countries have minimized exposure to carcinogens in the workplace to the point where this type of exposure is usually not a concern at present.

While the uncommon amosite, crocidolite and amphibole forms of asbestos used in the past caused a form of lung cancer, mostly in smokers, the common chrysotile form is not dangerous, and, in fact, less so than the rock wool or fiberglass replacements for it (Ray, 1990, pp83-86). The lawsuits seemingly proving otherwise, at great expense to all of us, are often used as examples of "junk science in the courtroom".

*Exercise.* Aerobic exercise is unhesitatingly recommended for prevention of breast cancer. Studies are said to support this assertion, and it is said to be advocated by the American Cancer Society; but no citations to trials are given (Kushi, 2002, p141; Block, 2002, p223). John R. Lee, MD, et al. strongly advise *moderate* exercise for prevention of breast cancer, citing a RR = 0.8 from a Nurses Health Study, but with no absolute risks given (Lee, 2002, pp15,37,63). John S. Link, MD, wrote that there is *no* evidence that exercise *prevents* breast cancer (Link, 2002, pp115-116). Martin Milner, ND, cited 4 papers with epidemiological evidence that several types of cancer had lower rates in athletes who engaged in *extreme* exercise (Diamond, et al., 1997, p296).

A study that received plenty of attention because of its publication in the *New England Journal of Medicine* was carried out on 25,624 women who were followed for a median of 14 years by which time 351 serious breast cancer cases had been diagnosed. The results showed that *moderate* exercise was of no significant benefit, only that *extreme* exercise was, especially for thin, premenopausal women, to give RR = 0.67 for all women, ranging from 0.23 for the thinnest to 1.38 for the fattest. This last finding was missing from the Abstract of the paper (Thune et al., 1997). An Editorial in *NEJM* on this paper was very cautious in interpretation, noting that a number of variables that might have been used in the adjustments of the raw data were not; yet this Editor gave a resounding "yes" to the hypothetical question of what a woman asking her physician whether to exercise to prevent breast cancer should be told (McTiernan, 1997). Among several sharp readers who saw flaws in the study, at least one noted a lack of adjustment for smoking frequency (Jackson, 1997); the authors responded by making the adjustment, which showed no big effect. Another saw possible differences in frequency of mammography between groups that might indicate poor randomization (Woloshin & Schwartz, 1997). Most important and germane to a main theme of this book was the observation that *extreme* exercise gave an absolute reduction in breast cancer of only 0.5% overall, that is, 98.5% of the non or moderate exercisers did *not* get breast cancer after 14 years of observation, while 99% of the *extreme* exercisers did not (Goldenberg, 1997).

So the lack of absolute risk in the seemingly most promising trial and the failure to caution obese older women about the dangers of exercise in the *NEJM* paper were misleading, but the true trial result was extracted from the data in this paper — there is no worthwhile correlation between exercise and prevention of breast cancer. Very possibly the slight benefit in extreme exercisers was increased exposure to sunlight, or less bra use among the thin, premenopausal women.

*Brassiere Wearing.* In their 1995 book: *Dressed to Kill,* Sidney Singer and Soma Grismaijer reported on a study they had carried out in the USA in the early 1990s. The Singers queried 4,500 (sometimes reported as 4,700) women in 5 cities across the USA about their habits in purchasing and wearing bras. Half had breast cancer and half did not. Though their study did not take into account other lifestyle factors, such as the level of obesity or amount of sunbathing, the results are too striking to be denied: (http://www.007b.com/bras_breast_cancer.php)

- 3 out of 4 women who wore their bras 24 hours per day developed breast cancer.
- 1 out of 7 women who wore bras more than 12 hour per day but not while sleeping developed breast cancer.
- 1 out of 152 women who wore their bras less than 12 hours per day got breast cancer.
- 1 out of 168 women who rarely or never wore bras acquired breast cancer.

Singer wrote, on 27 Feb 98 in a review of his own book on www.Amazon.com, that lymphatic vessels are easily constricted by by external pressure, such as from a bra. This compression prevents proper draining of the breast tissue, causing tenderness, pain, cysts, and finally, cancer. These breast problems are only found in bra-wearing cultures. Women who do not wear bras have the same breast cancer incidence as men. Singer noticed that the Maoris of New Zealand integrated into white culture have the same rate of breast cancer, while the marginalized aboriginals of Australia have practically no breast cancer. The same was true for "Westernized" Japanese, Fijians and other bra-converted cultures. Alas, none of this made it into a peer-reviewed journal. Is there any confirmation?

Two researchers from the Department of Epidemiology, Harvard School of Public Health, found, by studying 3,918 women with breast cancer and 11,712 controls, that premenopausal women who do not wear bras had less than half the risk of breast cancer compared with bra wearers (RR = 0.44, $p$ = 0.09). Among postmenopausal women, most of whom used bras, larger cup size was associated with increased risk of breast cancer ($p$ = 0.026). Obesity accounted for only part of the difference (Hsieh & Trichopoulos, 1991). There are a number of supportive (pun intended) studies with indirect evidence (http://www.breathing.com/articles/brassieres.htm).

So here is a breast cancer preventive that will actually save you money. Do not wait for The Cancer Industry to confirm that you can minimize breast cancer by wearing a bra less than 12 hours per day.

*Diet.* A popular book on alternative cancer treatments cites a 1982 study of a Committee of the National Research Council claiming that 60% of all cancers in women and 40% in men "may be due to...high-fat diet[s]" (Diamond et al., 1997, pp605). This is the type of oversimplification that is expensive and deadly. An extensive review showed that fats or oils containing omega-6 fatty acids (soybean, safflower, corn, grapeseed) are carcinogenic and increase metastases, while fats containing omega-3 fatty acids (in flaxseed and perilla oils, or EPA and DHA from fish) were protective, and saturated and monounsaturated (olive oil) fatty acids were neutral. Since 1950 the intake of omega-6 fatty acids in Japan is up 3.5 times, and the incidence of western-type cancers has tripled (breast, colon, prostate, pancreatic, non-smoking-related lung), (Okuyama et al., 1997). A study of post-menopausal women in Spain showed that those who had the lowest omega-6 to omega-3 ratios in their tissues had the lowest rates of breast cancer (Ottoboni & Ottoboni, 2002, p37).

In the American Cancer Society's book *Prostate Cancer* a section exists called Dietary Common Sense. The best part said that there is no scientific evidence that dietary strategies affect the onset of prostate cancer let alone controlling or reversing it. Unfortunately a statement followed advocating a diet made of fresh fruit, whole grain foods, fiber, and "good" proteins, but very low in fat. Myth 2 showed that this is an obesity- and diabetes-promoting diet in the many people who are genetically so disposed; no consideration was given to this, or to grain allergies. The culprit in fat was said to be alpha-linolenic acid, an omega-3 fatty acid found beneficial in preventing heart deaths. This fatty acid was said to be present in red meat, whole milk products, butter and processed soybean oil (Bostwick et al., 1999, p189). The fact is that none of these foods are significant sources of linolenic acid! Of this food group, only unprocessed, unhydrogenated soybean oil contains it (Enig, 2000, p136).

After admitting that the evidence for its effectiveness in prevention is lacking, John S. Link, MD, said he was not opposed to "...a well-balanced, low-fat diet..." for victims of breast cancer, but he presented no evidence from trials (Link, 2002, pp115-116). Obviously, a well-balanced diet could not be low in fat.

John R. Lee, MD, was far more realistic, noting that the early studies linking fat consumption with breast cancer have been disproven at least since 1996. He advocates avoiding refined carbohydrates, soy protein and *trans* fats, and emphasizes unprocessed food and whole grains, ignoring their effect on obesity, diabetes and celiac disease. Later an almost macrobiotic high-carbohydrate diet is recommended along with plenty of fiber. Here, too, very little evidence from trials was presented (Lee at al., 2002, pp25-26,34-36,241-290).

There was no association of total dietary fat with the *incidence* of breast cancer in any of 7 trials examined in a meta-analysis. The simpleminded approach of early researchers in using available fat (based on sales) rather than on fat actually eaten, and lumping all fats together was partially responsible for the spurious advice that cancer could be prevented by eating less fat. Eight of 11 clinical trials were said to have found that a high-fat diet increased mortality *after* a diagnosis of breast cancer; but this opinion did not distinguish between types of fat, and comes from a reviewer committed to vegetarian diets, including omega-6 vegetable fats (Kushi, 2002, pp116-125).

One of the most influential epidemiological studies was conducted by scientists at Harvard Medical School and other major medical institutions. A prospective analysis of the relation between dietary fat intake and breast cancer risk among 90,655 pre-menopausal women in the Nurses' Health Study II, followed for eight years, showed, according to the results in the abstract of the paper in the *Journal of the National Cancer Institute:* "...Relative to women in the lowest quintile of fat intake, women in the highest quintile of intake had a slight increased risk of breast cancer (RR = 1.25, 95% CI = 0.98 to 1.59; *p* trend = 0.06). [This meant that there was 1 chance in 20 that the actual RR did not fall between 0.98 and 1.59, and that the trend was not quite statistically significant.] The increase was associated with intake of animal fat but not vegetable fat; the [multi-variables adjusted] RRs for the increasing quintiles of animal fat intake were 1.00 (the benchmark from the lowest fat intake), 1.28, 1.37, 1.54, and 1.33 (95% CI = 1.02 to 1.73; *p* trend = 0.002)..." The conclusions in the abstract are: "Intake of animal fat, mainly from red meat and high-fat dairy foods during pre-menopausal years, is associated with an increased risk of breast cancer." (Cho et al., 2003). The absence of absolute risk levels is misleading. Their Tables 1 and 2 allow us to calculate what the chances are *not* to get breast cancer based on the unadjusted data. Following are the median energy percentage intake as animal fat/percentage who did *not* get breast cancer for each quintile of animal fat intake: 12% energy as animal fat/99.3% with no breast cancer, 15/99.2, 17/99.2, 20/99.1, 23/99.3. Clearly there is no difference of any significance here, and there was *no* trend, since the highest animal fat intake gave the same result as the lowest animal fat intake (Kauffman, 2004).

In 1965, Ernst Wynder, MD, of the American Health Foundation gave a talk at a meeting in which a slide was shown to indicate that animal fat and colon cancer were correlated when many countries were compared. The data looked odd to Mary G. Enig, PhD, who found that the fat was mostly partially hydrogenated *(trans)* vegetable fats, including 89% of the fat listed for the USA. Later, other researchers from both Hawaii and the NIH explored diet and colon cancer prevalence among Hawaiians of Japanese descent, actually finding that the highest risk was from macaroni, green peas, green beans and soy, yet the conclusions drawn were that beef consumption was related to the prevalence of colon cancer. Kenneth Carroll, PhD, a Canadian biochemist, found that more cancer was observed in test animals the more unsaturated the dietary fat was, while the least cancer-promoting oil was the mostly saturated coconut oil (Enig, 2000, pp81-83).

In Dr. Wolfgang Lutz's practice (see Myth 2), of 36 women just operated on for breast cancer and placed on a low-carbohydrate diet (or who were already using such) 35 had no recurrence or metastasis of their cancer after an unspecified time. The 1 exception was found to have had lymph node involvement right after surgery. In a study cited by Allan & Lutz, no association between meat consumption, regardless of cooking method, and breast cancer was found. They also cited the older Nurses Health Study in which there was no difference in colon cancer risk on high or low fiber diets. An Australian study was cited in which fecal markers of colon cancer were more prevalent with a high-carbohydrate diet than with a high fat diet (Allan & Lutz, 2000, pp173-177).

Milk fat contains several ingredients shown to prevent cancer in test animals (Parodi, 2004). One of them is the 4-carbon butyric acid-containing fat also present in butter.

An observational study carried out at the National Cancer Center in Tokyo, Japan, showed that the incidence of liver cancer was lower by 1/2 to 3/4 in coffee drinkers . Compared with non coffee drinkers, those who drank 1-2 cups per day had a RR = 0.52, 3-4 cups per day had RR = 0.48, and those who drank 5 or more cups per day had RR = 0.24. Wow! The absolute risk of liver cancer in this population was 547 per 100,000 over 10 years for non coffee drinkers, and only 215 per 100,000 for daily coffee drinkers as a whole (Inoue et al., 2005).

Drinking fluoridated city water increases cancer rates by about 10%. Common orange tea contains 3 times as much fluoride as fluoridated water, while coffee does not (see Myth 11).

Most natural carcinogens are found in plants. For example, tannins occur widely in plant foods and we ingest them daily in tea, coffee, and cocoa. Tannic acid has caused liver tumors in experimental animals, and may be linked to esophageal cancer in humans. Cycad plants, such as the sago palm and burrawang, are important food sources in tropical regions. Cycads contain cycasin and related azoxyglycosides that were found to cause liver and kidney tumors when fed to rats. Safrole, which is a liver carcinogen in rats, is found in sassafras tea, cinnamon, cocoa (trace), nutmeg, and other herbs and spices. Black pepper was found to be carcinogenic to experimental mice. Piperidine and alpha-methylpyrroline are secondary amines derived from black pepper which can be nitrosated *in vivo* to N-nitrosopiperidine, a strong carcinogen. Nitrosation is the addition of a nitroso group (—N=O) to an amine, and is a common reaction in our bodies. Aflatoxins and ochratoxin A are natural toxins made by fungal food contaminants that also cause cancer in animals and humans. Although not of plant origin, heterocyclic amines in overcooked (burned) meats *have* been associated with stomach and other cancers (http://extoxnet.orst.edu/faqs/natural/natcarc.htm).

The tendency among authorities to blame meat and fat for almost any ailment is as ubiquitous in cancer as for CVD. In fact, there is little evidence for such blame; on the contrary, many researchers point out that the favorite nutrient of cancer cells is glucose, most of which originates from the carbohydrates in plants. Carbohydrate consumption in general is positively related to cancer incidence (Ely, 1996). A macrobiotic diet is merely an ultra-high carbohydrate diet with few processed foods. There is no evidence presented that it will prevent or cure cancer by those who recommend it (Kushi, 2002, pp131-136). There is some evidence that *trans* fats of plant origin can cause cancer and that omega-3 fats prevent cancer (Kushi, 2002, p129; Ottoboni & Ottoboni, 2002, pp31-35). There is also a plausible claim based on clinical experience that gluten, wheat, or cow's milk allergies that can lead to celiac disease, irritable bowel syndrome (see Myth 2), or autoimmune diseases, can also lead to cancer (Reading, 1999, pp138-139,147,251-253).

Okinawans' calorie intake is 20% less than the national average for Japan. Protein and fat intakes are about the same, while carbohydrate intake is lower in Okinawans. The cancer mortality rate for Okinawans 60-64 years old is 69% of that of Japanese as a whole (Weindruch, 1988, p302). Was this due to lower energy intake, as the authors claimed, or lower carbohydrate intake?

A recent study on diet and breast cancer in Mexican women with 475 cases and 1491 controls showed that those women eating the most carbohydrate, the highest quartile, were more than twice as likely to contract breast cancer as those in the lowest quartile after a number of plausible adjustments; this result was highly statistically significant. The abstract of the article indicated that consumption of sucrose and fructose were the types of carbohydrates most associated with breast cancer; however, a Table in the body of the article indicated that starch was also highly associated. So much for the health value of "complex carbohydrates" (see Myth 2). Fiber consumption was much less associated with breast cancer, and fat not at all (Romieu et al., 2004).

So the high-carb, high omega-6 oil diet recommended so strongly by the USDA and others is just as deadly in causing cancer as it is in causing cardiovascular problems.

*Supplements.* At one extreme, John S. Link, MD, wrote that no supplements prevented cancer (Link, 2002, pp115-116). In the American Cancer Society's book *Prostate Cancer,* only an inconclusive study on vitamin E was cited (Bostwick et al., 1999, p41). At the other extreme, Keith I. Block, MD, wrote an entire chapter on the supposed benefits of many supplements (actually on micronutrients) in cancer without citing a single controlled study that included all-cause death rates. He relied on surrogate endpoints and projected survival rates (Block, 2002, pp214-244). John R. Lee, MD, recommended 25 supplements for prevention of breast cancer without citing a single controlled study (Lee et al., 2002, pp283-290).

Vitamin A has been investigated for decades with inconclusive results, possibly because precursors and derivatives of it were used in some studies (Moss, 199, pp227-233).

Vitamin C intake from food of >50 mg/day in 11,348 free living US adults aged 25-74 years and followed for a median of 10 years was correlated with lower cancer rates than vitamin C intake of <50 mg/day, and rates were lower still with vitamin C supplements in addition, but in none of the cancer sites were the overall RRs (0.75-0.85) statistically significant (Enstrom et al., 1992). A meta-analysis of 12 case-control studies on dietary factors and breast cancer, directed from the University of Toronto, Canada, found that vitamin C intake had the most significant and inverse relation with breast cancer. Those with the highest intake (mean 305 mg/day) had a RR = 0.69 ($p = < 0.0001$) compared with those with the lowest intake (mean 59 mg/day), (Howe et al., 1990). Note that the highest intake is still only 1/8 of the lowest intake recommended by Linus Pauling for adult humans (Pauling, 1986, p78).

Robert C. Atkins, MD, investigated supplements as well as diet. He cited a study showing that a 1-year supplementation with 750 µg of vitamin B12 and 10-20 mg of folic acid, presumably daily, reversed the precancerous changes noted in smokers' lung cells (displasias). Atkins also reported that vitamin D lowers the rates of breast and ovarian cancer, and that calcium lowers rates of endometrial, pancreatic and colon cancer (Atkins, 1998, pp72,108-109,124). Atkins also noted that good RCTs showed that saw palmetto supplements help 90% of the men with prostatitis, improving urine flow and minimizing the number of trips to the toilet. Several other supplements are usually used in addition (Atkins, 1998, pp348-349, 400-401).

Vitamin D from sunlight or supplements had been shown to prevent cancers of the breast, ovary, prostate and brain, as well as leukemia (Atkins, 1998, pp 108-109). The prevailing anti-supplement dogma suggests that 400 IU per day, the amount usually added to a quart of milk in the USA, is the maximum safe dose. Actually, there is no support for this in studies. A dose of summer sun that produces a tan and not sunburn may give a serum level of vitamin D equal to that of oral doses of 10,000-20,000 IU. Patients in trials have been given 50,000 IU daily for 8 weeks with no ill effects. Elderly and dark-skinned people living more than 30° from the equator may make only 1/4 as much vitamin D from sunlight as a pale 20-year-old (Holick, 2004). So the most reasonable dose of supplemental vitamin D may range from nil for pale young people near the equator to as much as 2000 IU per day when none of these conditions apply (Atkins, 1998, pp 110). Cod liver oil, a good source of vitamin D, is now available in a more agreeable form than in the past. The older limits on supplemental vitamin intake of 400 IU per day and sun exposure have no scientific basis. Besides reducing cancer incidence, 700-800 IU per day of vitamin D supplements halved the number of hip fractures in elderly men and women in two placebo-controlled trials (Holick, 2003).

If you cannot get enough vitamin D from sunlight, supplements. or tanning beds, eating salmon or sardines and some other foods will provide decent amounts (Holick, 2003, p150 ).

Vitamin E, the commercial alpha-tocopherol of unspecified purity, which is not at all the natural mixture of 8 related compounds, cut prostate cancer incidence by 1/3 in a trial on 29,133 male smokers in Finland. How disappointing then that there was no significant drop in prostate cancer among those smoking for <36 years (Heinonen et al., 1998).

One of the best trials of a supplement for cancer prevention, selenium, produced results that were unrelated to the original reason for doing the trial. A total of 1312 patients at 7 dermatology clinics in the eastern USA, mean age 63, 3/4 male, who had a history of basal cell or squamous cell carcinoma, the easily treated skin cancers caused by UVB, were randomized, and half were given 200 µg of selenium orally as 0.5 g of brewer's yeast and the rest were given identical-appearing placebo. After a mean treatment period of 4.5 years and followup of 6.4 years, it was discovered that the original object of the trial had failed — there was no difference in incidence of basal cell or squamous cell carcinoma. These researchers kept their eyes open and reported that 108 people died in the selenium group against 129 in the control group (all-cause death RR = 0.84). There were 29 cancer deaths in the selenium group against 57 in the controls (cancer RR = 0.51 with selenium). Some of the details on specific cancers are important: the incidence of lung, prostate, colorectal and esophageal cancers were much reduced in the selenium group, while breast cancer tripled, and melanomas and other types of cancer did not change much (Clark et al., 1996). So selenium may be a men-only choice, not that any vendor makes the distinction. It is important to remember that this study used high-selenium yeast, which is still widely available. Yeast may contain other anti-cancer substances besides selenium. In addition, approximately 40% of the selenium compounds found in high-selenium yeast have not been chemically identified. It is therefore possible that the more common supplements such as sodium selenite or selenomethionine (also called selenomethylcysteine) would not be as effective as the preparation used in this study (Gaby, 2001).

*Hormone Replacement Therapy (HRT).* An entire book exists that blames most breast cancer on improperly applied hormone replacement therapy, in which estrogens are used with the patentable unnatural progestins, rather than with a balanced amount of progesterone. The authors even indicate that lumpy breasts will often respond to topical progesterone cream after a few months at most (Lee et al., 2002). Mainstream oncologist John S. Link admits that postmenopausal women on HRT are taken off it when diagnosed with breast cancer, and has no idea that there might be a difference between progestins and progesterone (Link, 2002, pp66,86).

Actually, when 5 high-quality studies on HRT were analyzed, including on estrogens (such as Premarin™), the risk after 15 years of use was 1.6 for breast cancer, and the risk after 25 years was 2.0, meaning 20% of women would be diagnosed with breast cancer rather than 10% not using HRT. This may mean that a third to a half of breast cancer is caused by HRT, but not "most" of it. HRT also raises the incidence of endometrial (uterine) cancer 6-8 times (Wolfe S, Sasich, 1999, pp714-717), but only if estrogen is given without progesterone.

Alayne Yates, MD, by e-mail on 23 May 04, noted that estriol, a weak estrogen that pregnant women produce in copious amounts, has recently been made available in a mixture with two other naturally occurring estrogens called Tri-est™. "The theory behind tri-estrogen is a simple one: By taking it, you get the benefits from three different estrogens, and they are in a ratio similar to that which your body produces. The bulk of tri-est is estriol, which is the weakest form of estrogen produced on our bodies -- and, as mentioned before, not only is it the least likely to cause breast cancer, some studies have shown that it actually helps prevent it. So by taking all three estrogens --

very small doses of the stronger ones and a higher one of the weakest one, you can eliminate menopausal symptoms, fight osteoporosis and heart disease and help prevent the increased risk of breast cancer. It's a great theory, and one that bears watching. The only problem: As with other newer forms of estrogen, there haven't been any long-term studies done on this." (http://www.earlymenopause.com/hrt_triest.htm)

## Mainstream Cancer Treatments

*Oncologist Optimism.* With few exceptions oncologists will exaggerate the benefits of mainstream treatments including tumor removal and beyond, and minimize the side-effects. A great example was given in the Introduction involving Michael Gearin-Tosh, who was diagnosed with multiple myeloma when he was 54 years old, and told to begin chemotherapy within a week. He asked how much longer he would live if he accepted chemotherapy. "Nobody knows, but longer...2-3 years at most... Refuse our treatment and you will be dead in less than a year" he was told. Eight years later, with alternative therapies, he was still alive and employed. When patients ask how effective a cancer treatment will be, the usual answer is a "cure" rate related to the 1989-95 column in Table 10-1. These are not cure rates, they are 5-year survival rates. When patients ask "how many" similar patients respond to treatment, meaning what fraction respond, the answer is likely to be the same fallacious "cure" rate.

Contrarily, if a patient refuses to follow the oncologist's advice, or suggests an alternative treatment, the first response is often a death threat from the oncologist. If the patient is persistent, the oncologist may refuse to serve the patient any longer. This horror was addressed directly by Stephen M. Fulder, MA, PhD, in his book *How to Survive Medical Treatment:*

"The need for full and balanced information is obviously even more important and helpful in the case of cancer than where less serious decisions have to be made. It is unfortunate, therefore, that doctors are particularly likely to pull the wool over your eyes in relation to cancer. This is partly because they themselves find it difficult to cope with with the emotional intensity of clear statements. It is partly because they need to believe in unrealistic expectations in order to keep the entire cancer-treatment machine rumbling along. Sometimes they simply don't know or they may feel that the patient doesn't want to know. Therefore they will typically downplay the disease, or lie about it to both patients and family, or worse, to the patient only while telling the truth to everyone else. According to a recent poll in New York, if you were dying only one in four doctors would tell you. Be aware of the temptation that everyone feels to avoid the truth. Even in the very worst case, where the doctors would give the patient only a very short time to live, knowing the truth allows the patient to question toxic, hopeless treatments and explore gentler ways to treat himself...

"Oncologists are always in dispute about treatments among themselves, and always trying out new treatment combinations which have not necessarily been fully evaluated. Some believe in the psychological aspect and will work with counselors and psychologists. Others think that cancer is entirely due to random factors and [that] patient weaknesses are humbug. Some oncologists will be prepared automatically to give highly toxic drugs believing that the ends always justify the means. Others will not do so. For example removal of the entire breast of women with diagnosed breast cancer used to be the norm until it was discovered that removal of the lump only ('lumpectomy') gave the same 5-year survival figure...

"Second opinions are essential. If this results in a conflict between two authoritative views, it is usually better to choose the opinion that advises the less drastic treatment, given the current confusions." (Fulder, 1994, pp129-130).

The so-called success of mainstream treatments is based on anecdotes about patients who have had remissions. Take another look at Table 10-1. Even 50 years ago, many types of cancers had 5-year survival rates over 40%, in fact, 12 of the 20 types did, even when there was no treatment beyond surgery. This natural survival of a significant number of cancer patients provided many examples that were supposed to indicate success, and does so to this day regardless of the effects of radiation and chemotherapy.

Oncologist optimism, while it lasts, does have a positive psychological effect, which should not be minimized. However, burnout among oncologists is now admitted freely. Some of them liken their efforts to those of the orchestra on the Titanic, playing while the ship sank.

*Surgery.* The good news is that surgery is better than ever. Malignant melanoma is said to be "curable" if caught early (Moss, 2000, p130). Other skin cancers respond well to surgery. Skin-saving operations are done more often. Reconstructions are better than ever. Colon re-sections can have a patient back in action in a week or two...sometimes. However, Myth 9 showed that breast cancer operations beyond lumpectomy are not more effective, and usually will not prevent metastases. Newer prostate operations can be less devastating, for example, the laparoscopic procedure of John Heaney, Chief of Urology, Dartmouth Hitchcock Medical Center, Lebanon, NH. The key is to find how fast a particular tumor is growing, which might entail a several-month wait, and then decide whether either slow tumor growth or a patient's advanced age might make any operation "just a pain" (Plotkin, 1996).

The bad news is that cancer surgeons rush to operate: "...getting this thing out before it spreads". They solemnly tell family members in the waiting room: "Well, we got it all." Actually, the surgeons have no idea how many metastases have already begun, and at least a third of these operations are an expensive waste when done on slow-growing tumors or in very old patients (Plotkin, 1996).

*Radiation, high-dose.* The dismal result of 6000+ rads applied to a human body in a few weeks has been documented (Moss, 1999, pp59-72). Heart deaths often result, but are not attributed to cancer treatment, as noted in Myth 9. Halting tumor growth is commonly observed, but this does not mean lengthening life, or having any quality of life after irradiation. Exceptions are in Hodgkin's disease and lymphosarcoma where radiation may allow years of additional life, and even in advanced prostate cancer with *temporary* implantation of radioactive seeds, and maybe in cancer of the vocal cords. It is impossible to give high-dose radiation, usually from gamma rays from cobalt-60, without damaging normal cells, causing inflammation, nausea, bone marrow destruction, and compromising the immune system (McTaggart, 2001, pp85-93). If the latter leads to a fatal infection, the cause of death will be listed as due to the infection, not irradiation or cancer. Radiation does not distinguish between cancer or healthy cells, nor does careful aiming eliminate all exposure of healthy cells. One specific study found that adjuvant radiotherapy for breast cancer was associated with the development of lung cancer in 19 of 31 patients a median of 17 years later. Of the 19 patients, 15 developed lung cancer in the lung nearest the irradiated breast, while the other 4 did so in the other lung ($p = < 0.001$), (Wiernik et al., 1994).

*Chemotherapy.* The key reference here is Ralph W. Moss's book *Questioning Chemotherapy* (Moss, 2000). For 50 years, success in cancer treatment, usually called "cures", has been claimed for cell-killing (cytotoxic) drugs. You may recognize the names of a few old ones: methotrexate, 5-

fluorouracil (5FU), cyclophosphamide, and the newer cisplatin. This latter has been claimed to have been a great success with testicular, ovarian, lung, neck, and bladder cancers. One chemotherapist at the National Cancer Institute called the platinum-containing agents "the most important group now in use for cancer treatment". In fact, cisplatin is one of the 5 worst drugs in causing nausea and vomiting, deafness, damaged kidneys, and destroying bone marrow, leading to life-threatening infections. If a cancer patient on cisplatin dies of any of these things, one of *them* will be listed as the cause of death, not the drug or the original cancer. Of 79 Canadian lung cancer specialists asked whether they would participate in a drug trial involving cisplatin, 64 said they would not because of its toxicity. And 58 found all cancer drug trials unacceptable because of ineffectiveness and toxicity. While kidney damage is usually the reason that the use of cisplatin must be reduced in dose or stopped, the less frequent side-effects are cardiac arrhythmias, brain damage, glucose intolerance leading to diabetes, inflammation of the pancreas, and in patients surviving all that, leukemia (Moss, 2000, pp40,109,184).

Newer drugs that have received publicity appropriate to landing a human on Mars, such as paclitaxel (Taxol™), docetaxel, Herceptin™ and oxaliplatin have no to marginal advantages over older agents (Moss, 2000, pp i-xvii).

"Chemo Brain" is now a recognized side-effect of chemotherapy in general. This condition is a combination of forgetfulness, inability to concentrate, and depressive feelings. After years of being dismissed as a figment of patients' imaginations or as a result of anxiety or depression, "chemo brain" is beginning to be taken seriously by cancer doctors and researchers. Indeed, it appears to be fairly common, affecting as many as 16 to 40 percent of women undergoing chemotherapy for breast cancer, says Dr. Ian Tannock, the Daniel E. Bergsagel Professor of Medical Oncology at Princess Margaret Hospital and Professor of Medicine and Medical Biophysics at the University of Toronto. So far, most studies of "chemo brain" have been in women with breast cancer, but "chemo brain" can affect both men and women. (http://www.myhealthsense.com/F030701_Chemo.html) Personality changes toward irritability are also noticed.

True, some oncologists are aware of the problems, and give lower doses of drugs; some patients are not so seriously affected, but what is gained? Only weeks to months of life at best, and all of it of poor quality, according to Ralph W. Moss: "The medical profession and the media applaud the introduction of each new anticancer drug. Each one in turn is hailed as a breakthrough, and then all but forgotten as another 'miracle drug' appears on the scene. This process has gone on since at least the start of the 'War on Cancer' in 1971. We are told of increasing response rates with some of these agents. But whether improvements in 'responses', 'activity', 'disease-free' or 'progression-free' survival convey any real survival value is still a matter of debate. If there is a survival advantage [even ignoring quality-of-life], it is generally so small that it is undetectable through the normal route of clinical trials [RCTs]" (Moss, 2000, pp xvii, 29-30).

The latest "huge breakthrough" in lung cancer occurred around the middle of 2005:

"In the world of cancer chemotherapy, progress is made in small increments rather than giant leaps. The use of what is called 'adjuvant' chemotherapy – that is, chemotherapy given after the surgical removal of the tumor to assist in 'cleaning up' any possible remaining tumor cells – often results in at best a disappointing 7-10 percent improvement in overall survival.

"Sometimes no benefit at all can be demonstrated. Until very recently, such was the situation with the commonest form of lung cancer, non-small cell lung cancer (NSCLC). Over the past decade, randomized, controlled trials of adjuvant chemotherapy in NSCLC have repeatedly failed to show any significant survival advantage at all for this treatment. But last month saw the publication in the New England Journal of Medicine of the results of a study that showed an unequivocal survival advantage – a full 15 percentage points - for patients with successfully resected early lung cancer who were given adjuvant chemotherapy.

"That this represents good news is not in doubt. However, it is important to keep a sense of proportion when it comes to interpreting these results. The number of lung cancer patients who stand to benefit from this kind of treatment is very small – less than 10 percent of the total number of patients with this disease. And while any increase in survival time is to be welcomed, adjuvant chemotherapy of this cannot help the majority of patients with NSCLC.

"Yet to read some of the headlines and listen to some of the medical commentary on this research, one could have been forgiven for thinking that lung cancer would soon be a thing of the past. In an accompanying editorial in the New England Journal of Medicine, Dr. Katherine Pisters, a specialist in lung cancer at the M. D. Anderson Cancer Center in Houston, TX, wrote that the study's results were 'astonishing" and "remarkable.'

"The remarkable thing, as far as I am concerned, is not the result of the study but this kind of immoderate reaction. Is such unbridled enthusiasm really warranted? And, more important, is it in the best interests of patients and their families? When hope gives way to hype, no one is well served." (Ralph W. Moss, Ph.D. Weekly www.CancerDecisions.com Newsletter #192 07/10/05)

The 10-year survival rates for patients after beginning chemotherapy for metastatic cancer beginning in the breast, prostate, lung, or gastrointestinal system have been reported for 3 time periods: 1978-86, 1987-93 and 1994-2002 (see Table 10-2). The score for breast cancer is truly dismal: 11% alive after 10 years in the earliest period, then 8%, then 7% in the most recent period. For the other 3 organs there is not much change: all low single digits. The 5-year figures are equally dismal (Blech, 2004).

**Table 10-2. Ten-Year Survival Rates (% alive) for Patients on Chemotherapy for Common Metastatic Cancers (adapted from Blech, 2004).**

| Time Period of Treatment | Original Cancer Location | | | |
|---|---|---|---|---|
| | Breast | Prostate | Lung | Gastrointestinal |
| 1978-1986 | 11% | — | 3% | 4% |
| 1987-1993 | 8 | 2 | 1 | 5 |
| 1994-2002 | 7 | 3 | 2 | 5 |

However, there has been some success with chemotherapy in acute lymphocytic leukemia in children, and less success in adults, but good improvements in survival in those with chronic myelogenous leukemia have been possible with Gleevec™. Even less success is seen with Hodgkin's disease and a dozen very rare types (Moss, 2000, p27-28), but perhaps enough to warrant using chemotherapy.

\*\*\*\*\*

If you decide on a mainstream treatment, check the literature as well as you can, especially the books by Ralph W. Moss and his website www.cancerdecisions.com. There are many books dealing with treatments for each type of cancer (see Appendix A). Get second opinions, even for the severity of surgery. Consider joining a support group before you choose treatment to see what others have felt about each treatment. Make sure that the support groups is not funded by the purveyors of the treatment. You cannot be forced to undergo mainstream treatment for cancer. There have been cases when parents were forced to put their child through such treatment. If you are faced with such a thing, maybe you can find some relatives in another country.

Pain of cancer or its treatment is poorly handled by oncologists. At least half of patients with cancer experience moderate to severe pain, and one quarter die in severe pain even though medication is available to treat them. "When a doctor starts talking to a patient about making them [sic] comfortable, patients think they are going to die." (Cohen, 2004)

Many cancer patients are aware of all these problems, and it is said that half of all American and UK cancer patients are using alternative methods concurrently with mainstream ones, or instead. And many will not tell the oncologist about the alternatives for fear of being dumped.

The Cancer Industry now admits that other approaches, such as enhancing the body's immune system or cutting the supply of blood or glucose to tumors are valid approaches.

## Alternative Cancer Treatments

There are several problems with alternative or complementary cancer treatments.

First, most of them do not work, but most are not toxic, so little damage is done, and the placebo effect remains. But oncologists berate patients who take this route, saying that the delay in getting mainstream treatment allows the cancer to grow or spread; thus the patient is blamed if the mainstream treatment does not do all the oncologist says it will do because it was begun "too late."

Second, non-patentable treatments are expected to be subjected to randomized clinical trials (RCTs), while cytotoxic treatments have not been subjected to RCTs in the USA since about 1980. This is an effort by The Cancer Industry to make the cost of developing and confirming a non-mainstream treatment as high as possible (Moss, 2000, pp xvii-xix). This is not just a reaction to financial competition; mainstream practitioners really resent the reminders that their treatments are so destructive, even when the cancer is halted (Lee et al., 2002, pp14-15).

Third, most cancer patients who are "allowed" to try alternative treatments by their mainstream oncologists are only "permitted" to do so after they have been pronounced terminal or incurable or untreatable. These patients are often the only ones an alternative researcher can get — ones already damaged by mainstream treatment.

Two examples are given below of alternative treatments of terminal cancer patients and vehement opposition to them: (1) megadoses of vitamin C, and (2) antineoplastons. In the first example, Linus Pauling ran afoul of mainstream medicine with vitamin C and was opposed by Charles Moertel of the Mayo Clinic, destructively in public media, but politely in medical journals. In the second example, Stanislaw Burzynski, MD, was vilified and harassed by both the FDA and the self-appointed debunker, Saul Green, PhD, of www.Quackwatch.com.

*****

*Vitamin C in terminal cancer patients.* Scotland was the world capital of cancer, with 9 times the incidence of some other countries, such as Mexico, providing plenty of cancer patients in the Vale of Leven District General Hospital in Loch Lomondside. There, in 1971 Ewan Cameron, MD, working with Linus Pauling, PhD, two-time Nobel Prize winner, began to give high doses of vitamin C to terminal cancer patients, based on a theory of Cameron's.

Their early trials on 50 terminal cancer patients were reported in 1973 in the journal *Oncology* and in 1974 in the journal *Chemical-Biological Interactions*. Early observations of life-extension were reported. Objections to the methods used made Cameron and Pauling tighten up their protocol. In their 1976 paper in *Proceedings of the National Academy of Sciences*, they made the mistake of writing that all the patients in the study, 100 treated with vitamin C and 1000 controls, had first been treated in a conventional way with surgery, radiation and drugs, both cytotoxic and hormonal. As an example, they wrote that all 11 breast-cancer patients in the treated group had already had mastectomy, radiation and hormones; but all had relapsed by the time they were declared terminal and began vitamin C. Actually, use of toxic therapies was far lower in Scotland, just a few %, unlike in the USA. They were careful enough to note that the vitamin C group received it intravenously at 10g/day for 10 days and orally at that level until death. The sodium salt of vitamin C (ascorbic acid) was actually used intravenously — sodium ascorbate. The control group was selected by examination of hospital records by Frances Meuli, MD, of New Zealand, who found patients of matching cancer type, including leukemia, as well as age, sex, and the date of the declaration of "untreatable" or of hospital admission for terminal care. The mean survival time of the controls was 50 days and all died within a year, while 90% of the treated group survived for a mean of 210 days and 10% were still alive for 200-841 days, and had better quality of life as well. It was readily admitted that no formal process of randomization was carried out, and there was obviously no blinding (Cameron & Pauling, 1976).

Experienced investigators expressed doubts that patient selection had been unbiased, so Cameron & Pauling replaced 10 of the 100 treated patients with 10 new ones who had less rare forms of cancer and for whom better-matched controls could be found. A fresh selection of matched controls was made by a new person in order to make the groups match better. The result was that the vitamin C treated group fared even better in this later version of the study: 22% survived more than 1 year from the beginning of treatment vs. 0.4% of the controls; 8 were still alive 3.5 years after being pronounced "untreatable". There was no mention of the route of administration in this paper (Cameron & Pauling, 1978).

Printed on the very next page of the journal, *Proceedings of the National Academy of Sciences,* was an editorial calling for a random assignment and double-blinding in any future trial of vitamin C, which had not been done, and using both a control and a treated group, which had been done. The implication was that Cameron & Pauling did not know how to run a trial (Comroe, 1978). In fact, they were doing as well as circumstances allowed.

Creagan & Moertel of the Mayo Clinic, Rochester, MN, USA, attempted to carry out a prospective study with good randomization on patients who had been irradiated and subjected to chemotherapy, the result of which was reported in the *New England Journal of Medicine* in 1979 as Failure of High-Dose Vitamin C (Ascorbic Acid) Therapy to Benefit Patients with Advanced Cancer: A Controlled Trial. Pauling wrote to the *New England Journal of Medicine* in 1980 to point out that he had communicated with Creagan & Moertel as early as 1977 indicating that none of the patients in the Scottish trial had received chemotherapy, which he noted wrecked the immune system; the Mayo Workers answered that they had been told otherwise, and that the 1976 paper of Cameron & Pauling indicated otherwise (Pauling, 1980).

Acting like good scientists, Creagan & Moertel et al. carried out a new prospective study on 100 advanced colorectal cancer patients with minimal symptoms. These were well-randomized and given capsules of vitamin C (not the salt) or of placebo (lactose) to provide 10 g per day orally, and assays were made on urine samples to make sure of compliance. "We felt ethically justified in studying this group of patients without first offering cytotoxic drugs because in our opinion there is no known form of chemotherapy for colorectal cancer that has been demonstrated to produce palliative benefit or extension of survival." Treatment was discontinued when cancer progression was noted or the patient could no longer take the capsules. "Somewhat more than half the patients who have discontinued participation in this study (58 of 98) have received subsequent chemotherapy." There was no change in the degree of relief of symptoms, and the vitamin C treated group had slightly shorter lifespan (Moertel et al., 1985).

Moertel appeared on the main TV networks to denounce vitamin C as "absolutely worthless" in cancer treatment. Between this PR campaign and the *NEJM* paper, most physicians of all types thought the controversy was at an end, and most still think so. Soon, at a meeting of the American Cancer Society, Pauling struck back by pointing out 3 flaws in the claims of Moertel et al. to have duplicated the conditions of the Cameron & Pauling studies. First, Moertel et al. gave vitamin C for a mean time of only 10 weeks, not for the life of the patient. None of the Mayo Clinic patients died while taking vitamin C. Second, none of the vitamin C was given intravenously, which does give a higher serum concentration, and there is a linear correspondence between that concentration and survival time (Cameron & Campbell, 1991). Third, there was a well-known rebound effect from sudden withdrawal of vitamin C, called rebound scurvy, and patients in this state, as well as an equal fraction of controls (58±1%) were given chemotherapy despite the clear opinion of Creagan & Moertel et al. that there was no hope of benefit from such.

Stung by Moertel et al., Cameron & now Campbell tried to improve the quality of their study by increasing the number of patients who received vitamin C to 294 and the number of controls to 1532 who did not. They used data from 3 hospitals in West Scotland, not just 1, and followed the patients for a 4.5-year period. A lot of patients were excluded for reasons not previously applied to bring the baseline characteristics of the two groups closer together, which was certainly achieved. The treatment group lived twice as long as the untreated, 343 days vs. 180 days. A manuscript was submitted to the journal *Cancer Research* first, then it was rejected after several months, a clear case of stonewalling in the name of peer review. Then it was rejected by *The Lancet* quickly, by *NEJM* after 5 revisions and a delay of 2.5 years (!), by *Cancer Research* again after months, by *The American Journal of Epidemiology*, and by the *British Medical Journal* quickly on the grounds that a "remarkable claim was being made". Finally, *Medical Hypotheses* accepted it readily after a total delay of about 8 years! (Cameron & Campbell, 1991).

N. Hugh Riordan et al., Bio-Communications Research Institute, Wichita, KS, USA, found that high enough concentrations of vitamin C were toxic to isolated tumor cells (Riordan et al., 1995). His later work, which was published under the auspices of the NIH, verified that intravenous vitamin C gave 6.6 times the plasma concentration of oral administration, and called for trials with intravenous administration (Padayatty et al., 2004). A Commentary in the *Journal of The American College of Nutrition* from 2 staff members of the NIH recognized the problems with the Mayo Clinic studies, and confirmed that intravenous ascorbate produces a plasma concentration that is toxic to some tumor cells, while oral administration does not. At long last in 2005, an *in vitro* study of sodium ascorbate, in concentrations that could be reached by intravenous administration and not orally, showed that several types of cancer cell lines were killed. Several non-cancerous cell lines were undamaged. Interestingly, this study was not primarily from the National Cancer Institute (NCI), but was spearheaded by Mark Levine and other researchers at the Molecular and Clinical Nutrition Section of the National Institute of Diabetes and Digestive and Kidney Diseases of the NIH, with support from the Radiation Biology Branch of the NCI and others (Chen et al., 2005).

Two smaller studies in humans confirmed the benefit of vitamin C (Padayatty & Levine, 2000). An article in *The Townsend Letter for Doctors and Patients* was even more negative about the Mayo Clinic trials, but did note that vitamin C was not beneficial in the treatment of leukemia (Gaby, 2001). So it seems that the value of vitamin C in providing life-extension of terminal cancer patients has been accepted by those who understand all the evidence. One such wrote that vitamin C should be among the *initial* treatments given to cancer patients, beginning with low doses if there are widespread metastases, and increasing the *oral* dose to just below the level that causes diarrhea, even if this is more than 10 g per day (Cathcart, 1981).

*****

*Antineoplastons.* The discoverer of antineoplastons, Stanislaw R. Burzynski, earned his PhD and MD degrees together in 1968 from the Medical Academy of Lublin, Poland, at age 24. His research for his doctorate in Biochemistry was on peptides, short chains of amino acids which are the building blocks of proteins. He noted that people with chronic kidney failure rarely develop cancer, and that these people have a superabundance of certain peptides in their blood. These peptides did turn out to have anti-tumor effects; Burzynski christened them antineoplastons.

Blood was an inconvenient source of antineoplastons, so Burzynski succeeded in finding them in the urine of healthy humans, and gradually identified about a dozen. These simple molecules, many related to phenylacetic acid, were found to stimulate the activity of "human suppressor genes", that is, ones that turn off the activity of oncogenes. Thus the antineoplastons seem to act as a normal control mechanism for cell division, so they are not cytotoxic and indiscriminate as are the usual antineoplastic (anticancer) drugs used in cancer chemotherapy. This early work was published in peer-reviewed journals; many of the early papers were in Polish. Mixtures of these antineoplastons isolated from human urine produced up to 97% inhibition of DNA synthesis and cell division (mitosis) in neoplastic cells in tissue culture (Burzynski, 1976).

Burzynski came to the USA around 1970 and worked at Baylor College of Medicine, Houston, TX. With others, he obtained, in 1974, a Research Grant from the National Cancer Institute (NCI) of 3-year duration. Individual antineoplastons were identified and, by 1980, synthesized. By 1977 he had published a study of the action of antineoplaston A on 21 patients considered end-stage and untreatable by conventional methods. It was reported that complete remission occurred in 4 cases, more than 50% remission in another 4 cases, and some improvement in another 4 cases. In 2 of the 5 patients who died, there was significant regression of the "neoplastic process", and the deaths were not due to cancer or to any toxicity of the treatment (Burzynski, 1977). Inexplicably by normal scientific standards, the grant was not renewed.

About this time Burzynski set up the Burzynski Research Institute in which cancer patients declared hopeless by mainstream practitioners were expected to pay for what was honestly called experimental treatment with antineoplastons. Success was considerable, especially for brain tumors in children (Burzynski, 1999). From the late 1970s to the present, every available government, state, and medical agency aligned with The Cancer Industry has done its best to shut down Dr. Burzynski's clinic. What made him a threat to the cancer industry from the beginning was the prospect that antineoplaston therapy represented a successful alternative to toxic and dangerous chemotherapy drugs, upon which a major part of The Cancer Industry's profits depend (Diamond, 1997). Like nutritional supplements, antineoplastons are natural products, and not patentable.

Attacks on Burzynski, both *ad hominem* and technical, have been launched from many directions. Burzinski attempted to complete New Drug Applications for the US Food & Drug Administration (FDA), and to have trials carried out by the NCI, as well as doing his own with whatever approval from the FDA he could manage to obtain. On one pretext or another the FDA brought Burzynski to trial several times for "administering unapproved drugs", and the FDA lost every case. The NCI is said to have faked clinical trials of antineoplastons in order to produce negative results (Haley, 2000, pp345-392; Diamond, 1997, 674-685,859-860). After 20 years of such struggle, along with publication of many more papers in peer-reviewed journals, Burzynski was asked by a reporter why he did not leave the USA; he replied that the science would prevail in the end.

The following short web page from www.Quackwatch.com was accessed in 2002. It's a supposedly sound skeptical attack on Burzynski, and is reproduced whole for accuracy and tone from: <http://www.Quackwatch.com/01QuackeryRelatedTopics/Cancer/burzynski1.html>
The bold letters in brackets [X] refer to specific inaccuracies found on this web page. Each is explained in a Comments section that follows.

247

"Stanislaw Burzynski and 'Antineoplastons'
By Saul Green, Ph.D."

"Unlike most "alternative medicine" practitioners, Stanislaw R. Burzynski has published profusely. The sheer volume of his publications impresses patients, but unless they understand what they are reading, they cannot judge its validity. To a scientist, Burzynski's literature contains clear evidence that his data do not support his claims. [A]

"Burzynski's Background and Credentials
Burzynski attended the Medical Academy in Lubin [sic],[B], Poland, where he received an M.D. degree in 1967 and an D.Msc. degree in 1968. He did not undergo specialty training in cancer or complete any other residency program. His bibliography does not mention clinical cancer research, urine, or antineoplastons during this period. [C]

"In 1970, Burzynski came to the United States and worked in the department of anesthesiology at Baylor University, Houston, for three years, isolating peptides from rat brains. (Peptides are low-molecular-weight compounds composed of amino acids bonded in a certain way.) He got a license to practice medicine in 1973 and, with others, received a three-year grant to study the effect of urinary peptides on the growth of cancer cells in tissue culture. The grant was not renewed. [D]

"In 1976, with no preclinical or clinical cancer research experience [E], Burzynski announced a theory for the cure of cancer based on his assumption that spontaneous regression occurs because natural anticancer peptides, which he named antineoplastons, "normalize" cancer cells. Since urine contains lots of peptides, he concluded that there he would find antineoplastons [F]. Less than one year later and based only on these assumptions, Burzynski used an extract from human urine ('antineoplaston A') to treat 21 cancer patients at a clinic he opened [G]. His shingle read, 'Stanislaw R. Burzynski, M.D., Ph.D.'

"Burzynski's claim to a Ph.D. is questionable. When I investigated, I found:
    •An official from the Ministry of Health in Warsaw informed me that when Burzynski was in school, medical schools did not give a Ph.D. [1]. [H]
    •Faculty members from at the Medical Academy at Lubin [sic], [B] informed me that Burzynski received his D.Msc. in 1968 after completing a one-year laboratory project and passing an exam [2] and that he had done no independent research while in medical school [3]. [I]
    •In 1973, when Burzinski applied for a federal grant to study "antineoplaston peptides from urine," he identified himself as "Stanislaw Burzynski, M.D, D.Msc." [4]

"Analysis of Antineoplaston Biochemistry

"Tracing the biochemistry involved in Burzynski's synthesis of antineoplastons shows that the substances are without value for cancer treatment. [J]

"By 1985, Burzynski said he was using eight antineoplastons to treat cancer patients. The first five, which were fractions from human urine, he called A-1 through A-5. From A-2 he made A-10, which was insoluble 3-N-phenylacetylamino piperidine 2,6-

dione. He said A-10 was the anticancer peptide common to all his urine fractions. He then treated A-10 with alkali, which yielded a soluble product he named AS-2.5. Further treatment of AS-2.5 with alkali yielded a product he called AS-2.1. Burzynski is currently treating patients with what he calls 'AS-2.1' and 'A-10.'

"In reality, AS-2.1 is phenylacetic acid (PA), a potentially toxic substance [K] produced during normal metabolism. PA is detoxified in the liver to phenylacetyl glutamine [sic] (PAG), which is excreted in the urine. When urine is heated after adding acid, the PAG loses water and becomes 3-N-phenylacetylamino piperidine 2,6-dione [sic] (PAPD), which is insoluble. Normally there is no PAPD in human urine.

"What Burzynski calls 'A-10' is really PAPD treated with alkali to make it soluble. But doing this does not create a soluble form of A-10. It simply reinserts water into the molecule and regenerates the PAG (Burzynski's AS-2.5). Further treatment of this with alkali breaks it down into a mixture of PA and PAG. Thus Burzynski's 'AS-2.1' is nothing but a mixture of the naturally occurring substances PA and PAG.

"Burzynski claims that A-10 acts by fitting into indentations in DNA. But PAG is too big a molecule to do this [L], and Burzynski himself has reported that PAG is ineffective against cancer [5,6].

"PA may not be safe. In 1919, it was shown that PA can be toxic when ingested by normal individuals. It can also reach toxic levels in patients with phenylketonuria (PKU); and in a pregnant woman, it can cause the child in utero to suffer brain damage. [K]

"Burzynski has never demonstrated that A-2.1 (PA) or 'soluble A-10' (PA and PAG) are effective against cancer [M] or that tumor cells from patients treated with these antineoplastons have been 'normalized.' Tests of antineoplastons at the National Cancer Institute have never been positive. [N] The drug company Sigma-Tau Pharmaceuticals could not duplicate Burzynski's claims for AS-2.1 and A-10. The Japanese National Cancer Institute has reported that antineoplastons did not work in their studies. No Burzynski coauthors have endorsed his use of antineoplastons in cancer patients. [O]

"These facts indicate to me that Burzynski's claims that his "antineoplastons" are effective against cancer are not credible. [P]

"About the Author
Dr. Green is a biochemist who did cancer research at Memorial Sloan-Kettering Cancer Center for 23 years. He consults on scientific methodology and has a special interest in unproven methods. He can be reached at (212) 957-8029. This article is adapted from his presentation at the American Association for Clinical Chemistry Symposium in Atlanta in July, 1997.

"References
1. Nizanskowski R. Personal communication to Saul Green, Ph.D., Jan 15, 1992.
2. Kleinrock Z. Personal communication to Saul Green, Ph.D., Nov 22 1993.

3.Bielinski S. Personal communication to Saul Green, Ph.D., Nov 22, 1987.

4.Burzynski S. HEW grant application 1973, item 20 (credentials).

5.Burzynski SR. Purified antineoplaston fractions and methods of treating neoplastic diseases. U.S. Patent No. 4,558,057, 1985.

6.Burzynski SR. Preclinical studies on antineoplastons AS-2.1 and AS-2.5. Drugs Exptl Clin Res Suppl 1, XII, 11-16, 1986.

This article was posted on June 25, 2001."

## Comments (Adapted from from Kauffman, 2002.)

[A] Green does not give any specific example to support this assertion. Julian Whitaker, M. D., for one, cites and accepts the evidence in at least one of Burzynski's papers (Whitaker, 1999).

[B] Green means Lublin.

[C] These two sentences are merely attempts at invalidation, since lack of experience in a sub-specialty does not disqualify a person from *beginning* the sub-specialty.

[D] Since Green did not give a reason for the non-renewal of the grant, this fact must be regarded as another smear.

[E] According to Daniel Haley, who devoted a 48-page book chapter to antineoplastons, Burzynski had suspected, before he left Poland, that his peptides had anti-cancer activity after noticing that one of them was almost absent from the blood of a prostate cancer patient. In 1974 he co-authored an article which reported that the peptides caused up to 97% inhibition of DNA synthesis and cell division in cancer cells in tissue cultures (Haley, 2000, p346). Thus Green's innuendo that antineoplastons (the anti-cancer peptides) sprang whole from nothing is probably false. Furthermore, Green's implication that clinical or pre-clinical experience is needed is false; anyone can come up with a treatment worth investigating.

[F] This innuendo is false. Burzynski had first isolated antineoplastons from blood, and looked for them in urine in order to have a more convenient source of them (Haley, 2000, p347), and by 1980, could synthesize them (Haley, 2000, p350).

[G] It is significant that Green did not reveal what happened to these 21 patients. It was reported that complete remission occurred in 4 cases, more than 50% remission in another 4 cases, and some improvement in another 4 cases. In 2 of the 5 patients who died, there was significant regression of the "neoplastic process", and the deaths were not due to cancer or to any toxicity of the treatment (Burzynski, 1977).

[H] According to Daniel Haley, Burzynski earned both his MD and PhD at age 24. Reacting to a paper in *JAMA* by this same Saul Green, Burzynski sent the *JAMA* a sworn statement from the President of the Medical Academy of Lublin confirming Burzynski's PhD in Biochemistry and MD with honors (Haley, 2000, pp345,362). Robert G. Houston, a medical writer, wrote in a letter to *JAMA* that "...Contrary to Green, I found Burzynski's doctoral dissertation in biochemistry listed in the bibliography that Green claims omits it." (Houston, 1993).

[I] An online search turned up 11 publications on research by Burzynski from 1964-1970, many in Polish.

[J] This statement smacks of one described above for EDTA chelation therapy in Myth 7, an intimation that understanding of Burzynski's synthesis of antineoplastons would somehow prove that they could not be effective treatments for cancer. Surely one can see that effectiveness of substances for cancer treatment is not related to a complete understanding of their biochemistry. Furthermore, the syntheses were by standard *in vitro* reactions, not biochemical (Burzynski et al., 1986).

[K] This innuendo fails to give any actual toxicity. According to the Merck Index, phenylacetic acid is used as an analgesic, antirheumatic and urinary antiseptic. Its sodium salt has been approved for human use by the FDA for treatment of hyperammonemia (Burzynski, 1993). Its $LD_{50}$ i. p. in mice is 2,710 mg/kg (Burzynski et al., 1986). (The $LD_{50}$ is the amount per weight of an organism to kill 50% of them.) By comparison, from the Merck Index, 9th ed., the common antineoplastic drug vincristine has an $LD_{50}$ i. v. in mice of 2mg/kg; this would extrapolate to just 100mg as the fatal dose for a human, making this FDA-approved drug several times as toxic as sodium or potassium cyanide.

[L] The structures of Antineoplaston A-10 and the DNA-intercalating agent Doxorubicin, "the most important anticancer drug available" (Foye et al., 1995, p839) are shown in Fig. 10-7 drawn to the same scale and style. It should be obvious that A-10 (also called PAG) is not too big to fit into (intercalate) with DNA, even if you do not fully comprehend these shorthand structures.

[M] Quite the contrary, Burzynski has reported promising clinical results with AS2-1 in refractory cancer of the prostate (Burzynski et al., 1990) and with synthetic A10 (Liau et al., 1987), and with both in primary brain tumors (Burzynski et al., 1999).

[N] According to Robert G. Houston, the NCI saw the results of antineoplaston treatments in 7 cases and concluded that antitumor responses occurred (Houston, 1993). In a press-release the NCI claimed that these were the only patients of about 3,000 who had benefited (a lie), that Burzynski had sent the NCI incomplete patient information (also untrue), and when NCI-sponsored trials were done, the patients selected by the NCI were much more advanced and sicker than ones Burzynski had agreed to have treated. The NCI used lower doses than Burzynski advised, and withdrew the 2 improving patients to damage the evidence! (Diamond et al., 1997, 674-685)

[O] Since coauthorship implies endorsement, the presence of coauthors with Burzynski in at least 11 papers in peer-reviewed journals on the use of antineoplastons in cancer patients contradicts Green's assertion. These authors include Burzynski B, Conde AB, Daugherty JP, Ellithorpe R, Kaltenberg OP, Kubove E, Liau MC, Mohabbat MP, Nacht CH, Peters A, Saling B, Stolzman Z, Szopa B, and Szopa M.

[P] Ample evidence has been given to show that much of what Green wrote on this webpage is questionable. To make an informed decision on the effectiveness of antineoplastons, Julian Whitaker, MD, over a 5-year period, visited the Burzynski Clinic 5 times, spoke with scores of patients, and evaluated their medical charts. He gave 4 examples of patients, 3 of them children, who were offered no hope of long-term survival by conventional cancer practitioners, then successfully treated with antineoplastons, and calls this treatment "the most significant breakthrough in cancer research ever" (Whitaker, 1999). "Antineoplastons do not work all the time — nothing does. But there is enough data and case histories to demonstrate conclusively that these medicines do represent a breakthrough" (Haley, 2000, p386). "For Dr. Burzynski's 3,000 patients, antineoplaston is a lifesaver; among ...alternative physicians, the treatment is gaining respect and credibility" (Diamond et al., 1997, pp684-685).

Fig. 10-7. Structural Formulas of Antineoplaston A-
and Doxorubicin

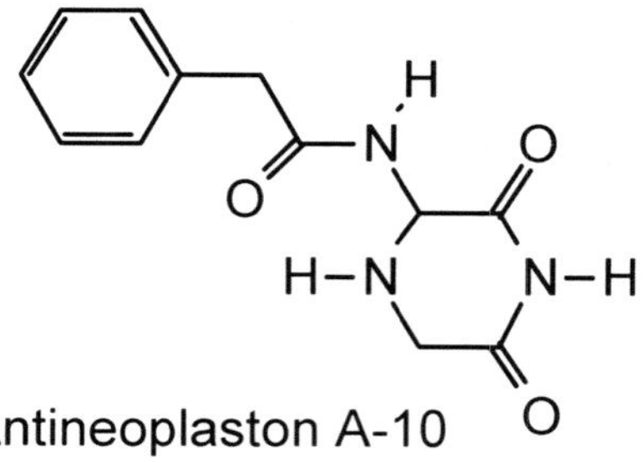

Antineoplaston A-10

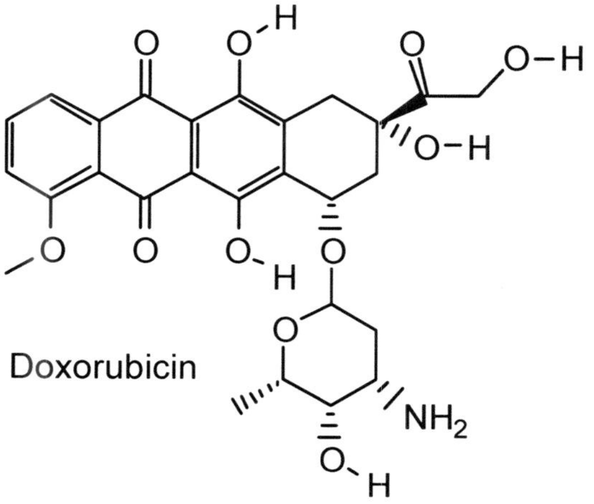

Doxorubicin

Ample evidence has been given here to show that much of what Green wrote on this webpage of www.Quackwatch.com is questionable at best. Despite vicious attacks and distractions, such as raids by FDA operatives on Burzinski's clinic, and confiscation of many of his records, his research and treatment continues on what is probably an affective approach to the treatment of many types of cancers. The most complete description of Burzinski, antineoplastons, and the actual results of treatment of cancer with them in individual patients may be found in a book by Thomas D. Elias, *The Burzinski Breakthrough*, Rev. Ed., Nevada City, CA: Lexikos, 2001.

*****

While it is valuable to have hurdles for a medical treatment, perhaps most so for cancer, these two examples show that any number of effective treatments that would not have been profitable enough for The Cancer Industry may have been lost because of mainstream opposition to them. According to Daniel Haley:

"In 1989, FDA Commissioner Frank Young proclaimed that FDA would approve a new drug if it proved effective in as few as 10 patients. Antineoplastons passed that milestone years ago, yet FDA still drags its feet. In 1996, former Commissioner David Kessler and Vice President Al Gore made a joint appearance stating that henceforth the FDA would move rapidly ahead to approve promising new cancer drugs. Did they mean anything except antineoplastons? Or is there basically just

252

the policy of former FDA official Dr. Crout, who said that he would approve nothing unless it was proposed by a large pharmaceutical company with unlimited resources?" (Haley, 2000, pp386-387)

Two excellent books (Haley, 2000; Moss, 1999) have covered this topic of attacking alternatives; but this recommendation does not mean that all the treatments described favorably in these books are certain to be effective .

## Promising Cancer Treatments

Obviously there are new claims of promising cancer treatments almost daily from both mainstream and alternative sources — too many to allow making an exhaustive list here. Many are too new to make available the key information: the 10-year survival rate, or the altered time to 50% deaths from all causes, or the duration of life gained. If the side-effects are bad enough, even good gains in lifespan might not justify submitting to the treatment. Just two promising treatments are discussed.

One of the most tantalizing variations on chemotherapy is insulin potentiation therapy (IPT), in use for decades, widely available, and even covered by health insurance, according to Robert J. Rowan, MD, who now writes the newsletter *Second Opinion*. While healthy cells burn both glucose and fat, cancer cells use glucose almost alone and in great quantities. When insulin is injected, it supposedly makes cancer cells more permeable, not only to glucose, but to the conventional chemotherapy drugs such as methotrexate, allowing as little as 1/4 to 1/10 of the normal dose to be used, almost eliminating side-effects, assuming the amount of insulin does not depress serum glucose levels too far. This is dealt with by injection of glucose. As is so common with promising cancer treatments, even ones that have been in use as long as IPT, 50 years, there are no controlled trials. At least one validation test was passed: there are several papers in good, peer-reviewed journals with case studies, including a recent review (Ayre et al., 2000). This procedure is widely available, with 115 practitioners now, and is not at all the purview of some lone practitioner in an island nation; for practitioners see: http://www.iptq.com/default.htm.

Some success has been claimed for the use of antiinflammatory drugs (aspirin and other NSAIDS) or supplements (such as omega-3 fatty acids, bromelain, and others) along with chemotherapy (Wallace, 2002). Here is another reason to avoid excess omega-6 fatty acids, which are metabolized to inflammatory eicosanoids (see Myth 2).

One of those island nation establishments for cancer treatment, Immuno-Technologies Laboratory (ITL) in the Bahamas, is actually using at least two types of immune system enhancement, a valid approach. A type of vaccine called dendritic cell vaccine made from a patient's own tumor is claimed to have value (http://www.immunemedicine.com/dendritic-cell-therapy.asp).

Investigate any treatments, mainstream or alternative, to the best of your ability.

## The Cancer Survival Personality

All of the observers in this field agree that an aggressive determination to "beat the cancer" does aid survival and remission odds.

"Researchers have looked for personality characteristics shared by all cancer patients. Although no personality profile fits all people with cancer, some psychological traits and stressful events are common among many people who contract cancer. These include:
  • having experienced a significant loss

• being overly critical toward oneself
• having a disturbed or emotionally sterile relationship with parents
• suppressing anger or strong emotions
• a loss of hope, depression, and being a self-sacrificing kind of person..."
"Self-doubt and criticism create stress that can negatively affect the immune system. Conversely, learning self-acceptance and self-love may help immunity and, at the very least, provide a more enjoyable life experience." (Bognar, 1998, pp169-171)

"It has been clearly demonstrated that those people who have a fighting, positive, active attitude to their disease are more likely to survive it whereas those who give up hope do not survive as long. 'Those who survived the longest were real troublemakers,' said Dr. Bernard Fox, Professor of Psychiatry at Boston University Medical school. 'They fought with their doctors, sought alternative opinions and methods of treatment. They refused to relinquish hope and struggled to survive.' It is now beginning to be accepted that there is no such thing as a 'spontaneous regression' [remission] which is a medical admission of ignorance about cancers which disappear by themselves. The cancers tend to disappear in people who have faith, independence, emotionally transforming experiences and active involvement in their disease. In a word, people who are really determined to live have a fighting chance to get over the disease." (Fulder, 1994, pp130-131).

The fight for accurate information is an important part of the struggle against cancer. Besides the citations in this and the last chapter, the books in Appendix A may be of use. At present, the best source of information on treatment is the pair of books by Ralph W. Moss: *The Cancer Industry,* 1999, and *Questioning Chemotherapy,* 2000. Moss's website is valuable: www.cancerdecisions.com. Using it, one may pay a fee for an individualized report on truly effective treatments of one's particular type of cancer from both mainstream and alternative sources.

### Summing Up

You can be sure that cancer cure rates are not 60% and that there has not been much change in 40 years. The 5-year survival rate is 60%, and has appeared to improve only because of earlier detection and some adjustments. A patient in a clinical trial dying just before a treatment program of even 6-12 months duration has been completed is *not* counted as a failure on the grounds that the patient had not completed the treatment program! A control patient dying of any cause is counted as a failure of non-treatment.

There is no epidemic of cancer at present except lung and malignant melanoma (skin cancer). The former is due to smoking and the latter, possibly, to too much UVA from sunlight, often caused by overexposure despite UVB "protection" from sunblock, which makes things worse by preventing vitamin D formation in the skin.

Since there is no epidemic of cancers of the gastrointestinal tract or other places where certain foods, pesticides or pollutants would be expected to manifest themselves, these factors can hardly be major causes of these types of cancers.

Low-carbohydrate diets may prevent some cancers, while low-fat diets will not. Polyunsaturated fats may be carcinogenic, while saturated fats are not. Vitamin C clearly can slow down some types of cancer if taken in sufficient quantity intravenously. Selenium is a worthwhile supplement in men.

Early detection is not prevention. When treatments are so poor, as the mainstream ones beyond surgery are at this time, there is almost no point in screening for the cancer. Certainly, it is beyond dispute that mammography in women and the PSA test for prostate cancer in men with no symptoms have no overall benefit. Since treatments for lung, liver and pancreatic cancer are so poor, there is not much use finding out early that you have one of them. Still, if one wants early detection with one simple test, the AMAS test is one of the best even if imaging techniques fail to find a tumor, or even if there are really too many false positives. On the other hand, in the opinion of Charles T. McGee, MD, pap smears have reduced the death rate from cervical cancer. Colonoscopy can find small cancers in polyps, and when these are removed, it is effective because the cancer has not yet spread. Also, surgical removal of melanomas is quite effective as a treatment.

Claimed reductions of mortality from cancer are of no use if the all-cause mortality rate remains the same or worsens, yet the first is usually the only sort of claim made for most treatments. The 5-year survival rate was cleverly chosen to mask the delayed destructive effects of radiation and chemotherapy. A 10-year survival rate would be better, but the added years of life gained of good quality would be most easily understood by patients. Mainstream treatments often provide only a few weeks to months more of poor quality life. Most slow-growing cancers should not be treated. Alternative treatments usually do not work, but at least are non-toxic. Some alternatives work well enough to cause complete remissions (antineoplastons and possibly coenzyme Q10). Others may provide 2-3 times as much lifespan after the patient is declared untreatable, such vitamin C, especially when taken intravenously as sodium ascorbate. Not all alternative practitioners are quacks, and good treatments not available in the USA may indeed be found outside the USA.

The highly toxic chemotherapeutic drugs developed in the 1950s and up to the present time kill all rapidly dividing cells in the body, which means not only cancer cells, but also many kinds of healthy cells. Unfortunately, the immune system, the body's natural defense system against cancer, is itself composed of rapidly dividing cells. So both the disease *and* the protection against the disease get zapped (Pert, 1997).

New treatments may appear at any time; find out whether your cancer is a candidate for one of them, but watch out for claims of merely stopping the cancer with no indication of toxicity or all-cause mortality rates. Watch out for 5-year survival rates given with no indication of how untreated patients fare. Determination to survive, willingness to travel for a treatment, and supportive family or friends will make a great difference to the outcome.

Acknowledgements for Myth 10

This chapter was critically reviewed by Frances E. H. Pane, MSLS, Alice Ottoboni, PhD, Fred Ottoboni, PhD, MPH, William A. Reinsmith, DA, Alayne Yates, MD, and Charles T. McGee, MD.

References for Myth 10

Atkins RC (1998). *Dr. Atkins' Vita-Nutrient Solution,* London, England: Pocket Books, Simon & Schuster.
Ayre SG, Garcia y Bellon DP, Garcia DP Jr (2000). Insulin, chemotherapy, and the mechanisms of malignancy: the design and the demise of cancer. *Medical Hypotheses* 55(4):330-334.
Bailar JC III, Gornik HL (1997). Cancer Undefeated. *Lancet* 336:1569-1574.
Bergman L, et al. (2000). Risk and prognosis of endometrial cancer after tamoxifen for breast cancer. *Lancet* 356:881-887.
Bigby ME (2004). The End of the Sunscreen and Melanoma Controversy? *Archives of Dermatology* 140:745-746.
Blech J (2004). Giftkur ohne Nutzen (Poison Cure without Utility). *Der Spiegel,* 4 Oct 04, Nr. 41, pp160-162.
Block KI (2002). Micronutrients: Vitamin and Mineral Supplementation in *Breast Cancer Beyond Convention,* Tagliafferi et al., Eds, New York, NY: Simon & Schuster.
Bognar D (1998). *Cancer: Increasing Your Odds for Survival,* Alameda, CA: Hunter House.
Bostwick DG, MacLennan GT, Larson, TR (1999). *Prostate Cancer,* New York, NY: Villard Books.
Burzynski SR (1976). Antineoplastons: biochemical defense against cancer. *Physiological Chemistry & Physics* 8(3):275-279.

Burzynski SR, Stolzman Z, Szopa B, Stolzman E, Kaltenberg OP (1977). Antineoplaston A in cancer therapy. (I). *Physiological Chemistry & Physics* 9(6):485-500.

Burzynski SR, Mohabbat MO, Lee SS (1986). Preclinical studies on antineoplaston AS2-1 and antineoplaston AS2-5. *Drugs Under Experimental & Clinical Research* 12 Suppl 1, 11-16.

Burzynski SR, Kubove E, Burzynski B (1990). Treatment of hormonally refractory cancer of the prostate with antineoplaston AS2-1. *Drugs Under Experimental & Clinical Research* 16 (7), 361-369.

Burzynski S (1993). Letter. *Journal of the American Medical Association* 269(4):475.

Burzynski SR, Conde AB, Peters A, Saling B, Ellithorpe R, Daugherty JP, Nacht CH (1999). A Retrospective Study of Antineoplastons A10 and AS2-1 in Primary Brain Tumours. *Clinical Drug Investigations* 18(1):1-10.

Cameron E, Pauling L (1976). Supplemental ascorbate in the supportive treatment of cancer: Prolongation of survival times in terminal human cancer. *Proceedings of the National Academy of Sciences* 73(10):3685-3689.

Cameron E, Pauling L (1978). Supplemental ascorbate in the supportive treatment of cancer: Reevaluation of prolongation of survival times in terminal human cancer. *Proceedings of the National Academy of Sciences* 75(9):4538-4542.

Cameron E, Campbell A (1991). Innovation vs. Quality Control: an 'Unpublishable' Clinical Trial of Supplemental Ascorbate in Incurable Cancer. *Medical Hypotheses* 36:185-189.

Cathcart RF (1981). Vitamin C, Titrating to Bowel Tolerance, Anascorbemia, and Acute Induced scurvy. *Medical Hypotheses* 7:1359-1376.

Chen Q, Espey MG, Krishna MC, et al. (2005). Pharmacologic ascorbic acid concentrations selectively kill cancer cells: Action as a pro-drug to deliver hydrogen peroxide to tissues. *Proceedings of the National Academy of Sciences* 102(38):13604-13609.

Cho E, Spiegelman D, Hunter DJ, et al. (2003). Premenopausal fat intake and risk of breast cancer. *J Natl Cancer Inst* 95:1079-1085.

Clark LC, Combs, Jr, GF, Turnbull BW, et al. (1996). Effects of Selenium Supplementation for Cancer Prevention in Patients with Carcinoma of the Skin. *Journal of the American Medical Association* 276:1957-1963.

Cohen JS (2001). *Over Dose. The Case Against the drug Companies.* New York, NY: Tarcher/Putnam.

Comroe Jr., JH (1978). Experimental studies designed to evaluate the management of patients with incurable cancer. *Proceedings of the National Academy of Sciences* 75(9):4543.

Dennis LK, Freeman LEB, VanBeek MJ (2003). Sunscreen Use and the Risk for Melanoma: A Quantitative Review. *Annals of Internal Medicine* 139:966-978.

Diamond WJ, Cowden WL, Goldberg B (1997). *An Alternative Medicine Definitive Guide to Cancer.* Tiburon, CA: Future Medicine Publishing.

Eades MR, Eades MD (2000). *The Protein Power LifePlan.* New York, NY: Warner Books.

Ely JTA (1996). Glycemic Modulation of Tumor Tolerance. *Journal of Orthomolecular Medicine* 11(1):23-34.

Enig, M. G. (2000). *Know Your Fats,* Silver Spring, MD: Bethesda Press.

Enstrom JE, Kanim LE, Klein MA (1992). Vitamin C intake and mortality among a sample of the United States population. *Epidemiology* 3:189-91.

Fisher B, Jeong J-H, Anderson S, Bryant J, Fisher ER, Wolmark N ( 2002). Twenty-Five-Year Follow-Up of a Randomized Trial Comparing Radical Mastectomy, Total Mastectomy, and Total Mastectomy Followed by Irradiation. *New England Journal of Medicine* 347(8):567-575.

Foye WO, Lemke TL, Williams DA, Eds. (1995). *Principles of Medicinal Chemistry,* 4th ed., Baltimore, MD, Williams & Wilkins.

Fulder SM (1994). *How to Survive Medical Treatment,* New York, NY: Barnes & Noble.

Gaby AR (2001). High-selenium yeast for cancer prevention. *Townsend Letter for Doctors and Patients,* August, pp4-6.

Garland CF, Garland FC, Gorham ED (1993). Rising trends in melanoma. An hypothesis concerning sunscreen effectiveness. *Annals of Epidemiology* 3(1):103-110.

Gilley O (2004). Sunlight Robbery: Health benefits of sunlight are denied by current health policy in the UK. Health Research Forum, 68, Whitehall Park, London N19 3TN, UK. Available at: www.healthresearchforum.org.uk. Accessed October, 2004.

Grant WB (2002). An Ecologic Study of Dietary and Solar Ultraviolet-B Links to Breast Cancer Carcinoma Mortality Rates. *Cancer* 94:272-281.

Haley D (2000). *Politics in Healing: The Suppression and Manipulation of American Medicine.* Washington, DC: Potomac Valley Press.

Heinonen OP, Albanes D, Virtamo J, et al. (1998). Prostate Cancer and Supplementation With alpha-Tocopherol and beta-Carotene: Incidence and Mortality in a Controlled Trial. *Journal of the National Cancer Institute* 90:440-446.

Holick MF (2004). Sunlight and vitamin D for bone health and prevention of autoimmune diseases, cancers, and cardiovascular disease. *American Journal of Clinical Nutrition* 80(suppl):1687S-1688S.

Houston RG (1993). Letter. *Journal of the American Medical Association* 269 (4):475-476.

Howe GR, Hirohata T, Hislop TG, et al. (1990). Dietary Factors and the Risk of Breast Cancer: Combined Analysis of 12 Case-Control Studies. *Journal of the National Cancer Institute* 82:561-569).

Hsieh CC, Trichopoulos D (1991). Breast size, handedness and breast cancer risk. *European Journal of Cancer* 27(2):131-135.

Inoue M, Yoshimi I, Sobue T, Tsugane S (2005). Influence of Coffee Drinking on Subsequent Risk of Hepatocellular Carcinoma: A Prospective Study in Japan. *Journal of the National Cancer Institute* 97(4):293-300.

Kauffman JM (2002). Alternative Medicine: Watching the Watchdogs at Quackwatch. Website Review, *Journal of Scientific Exploration* 16(2):312-337.

Kauffman JM (2003). Diagnostic Radiation: Are the Risks Exaggerated? *Journal American Physicians & Surgeons* 8(2):54-5.

Kauffman JM (2004). Bias in Recent Papers on Diets and Drugs in Peer-Reviewed Medical Journals, *Journal American Physicians & Surgeons* 9(1):11-14.

Kushi L (2002). Diet and Breast Cancer in *Breast Cancer Beyond Convention,* Tagliafferi et al., Eds, New York, NY: Simon & Schuster.

Law M (2004). Screening without evidence of efficacy. Screening of unproved value should not be advocated. *British Medical Journal* 328:301-302.

Lee JR, Zava D, Hopkins V (2002). *What Your Doctor May* Not *Tell You About Breast Cancer. How Hormone Balance Can Help Save Your Life.* New York, NY: Warner Books.

Lerner M (2002). Choices in Healing in *Breast Cancer Beyond Convention,* Tagliafferi M, Coehn I, Tripathy D, Eds., New York, NY: Atrai Books.

Liau MC, Szopa M, Burzynski B, Burzynski SR (1987). Chemo-surveillance: a novel concept of the natural defence mechanism against cancer. *Drugs Under Experimental & Clinical Research* 13 Suppl. 1:71-76.

Link JS (2002). *Take Charge of Your Breast Cancer,* New York, NY: Henry Holt.

Lomborg B (2001). *The Skeptical Environmentalist.* Cambridge, England, UK: Cambridge University Press.

McTaggart L, Ed. (2001). *The Cancer Handbook. What's Really Working.* 2nd ed., Bloomington, IL: Vital Health Publishing.

Moss RW (1999). *The Cancer Industry,* Brooklyn, NY: Equinox Press.

Moss RW (2000). *Questioning Chemotherapy,* Brooklyn, NY: Equinox Press.

Moss RW (2004). Weekly CancerDecisions.com Newsletter #146, 08/22/04.

Okuyama H, Kobayashi T, Watanabe S (1997). Dietary Fatty Acids — The N-6/N-3 Balance and Chronic Elderly Diseases. Excess Linoleic Acid and Relative N-3 Deficiency Syndrome Seen In Japan. *Progress in Lipid Research* 35(4):409-457.

Ottoboni F, Ottoboni A (2002). *The Modern Nutritional Diseases.* Sparks, NV: Vicente Books.

Padayatty SJ, Levine M (2000). Reevaluation of Ascorbate in cancer Treatment: Emerging Evidence, Open Minds and Serendipity. *Journal of The American College of Nutrition* 19(4):423-425.

Padayatty SJ, Sun H, Wang Y, Riordan HD, Katz A, et al. (2004). Vitamin C pharmacokinetics: implications for oral and intravenous use. *Annals of Internal Medicine,* 140(7):161.

Parodi PW (2004). Milk fat in human nutrition. *Australian Journal of Dairy Technology* 59:3-59.

Pauling L (1980). Vitamin C Therapy of Advanced Cancer. *New England Journal of Medicine* 302(12):694-695.

Pauling L (1986). *How to Live longer and Feel Better.* New York, NY: Freeman.

Pert, Candace B., *Molecules of Emotion,* New York, NY: Scribner, 1997.

Plotkin D (1996). Good News and Bad News about Breast Cancer. *Atlantic Monthly,* 277(6):53-82.

Ray DL, Guzzo L (1990). *Trashing the Planet,* Washington, DC: Regnery Gateway.

Reading C (1999). *Trace Your Genes to Health.* Ridgefield, CT: Vital Health Publishing.

Riordan NH, Riordan HD, Meng X, Li Y, Jackson JA (1995). Intravenous ascorbate as a tumor cytotoxic agent. *Medical Hypotheses* 44(3):207-13.

Rivers JK (2004). Is there more than one road to melanoma? *Lancet* 363(9410):728-730.

Romieu I, Lazcano-Ponce E, Sanchez-Zamorano LM, Willett W, Hernandez-Avila M (2004). Carbohydrates and the Risk of Breast Cancer among Mexican Women. *Cancer Epidemiology, Biomarkers and Prevention* 13(8):1283-9.

Wallace JM (2002). Nutritional and botanical modulation of the inflammatory cascade — eicosanoids, cyclooxygenases, and lipoxygenases — as an adjunct in cancer therapy. *Integrated Cancer Therapies* 1(1):7-37, discussion 37.

Weindruch R, Walford RL (1988). The Retardation of Aging and Disease by Dietary Restriction, Springfield, IL: Charles C. Thomas.

Welch HG, Schwartz LM, Woloshin S (2000). Are Increasing 5-year Survival Rates Evidence of Success Against Cancer? *Journal of the American Medical Association* 283:2975-2978.

257

Welch, H. Gilbert (2004). *Should I Be Tested for Cancer? Maybe Not and Here's Why,* Berkeley, CA, USA, University of California Press.

Whitaker J (1999). An Effective Cancer Therapy that Challenges Convention. *Health & Healing* 9(10):1-4.

Wiernik PH, Sklarin NT, Dutcher JP, Sparano JA, Greenwald ES (1994). Adjuvant radiotherapy for breast cancer as a risk factor for the development of lung cancer. *Medical Oncology* 11(3):121-125.

Wolfe S, Sasich LD (1999). *Worst Pills Best Pills*. New York, N.Y.: Pocket Books.

Woloshin S, Schwartz LM (1999). The U. S. Postal Service and Cancer Screening - Stamps of Approval? *New England Journal of Medicine* 340(11):884-887.

# Myth 11: Water Fluoridation Prevents Tooth Decay in Children and is Perfectly Safe.*

*Michael Easley, M.P.H., national spokesman on fluoridation for the ADA, posted the following on the internet for dentists in 1996: "...anti-fluoride cultists will not be dissuaded by the truth.... Let them spew their garbage, ignore them, and go on with your discussions as if they weren't there.... [T]heir twisted minds have accepted the notion that it is OK to lie, slander, libel, exaggerate, misquote.... [S]ee what kooks they really are." (Groves, 2001)*

*Aquafresh Fluoride Toothpaste, from GlaxoSmithKline Consumer Healthcare, © 2001, on label: "WARNING; Keep out of the reach of children under 6 years of age. If you accidentally swallow more than used for brushing, seek professional assistance or contact a poison control center immediately."*

### Brief Overview of Water Fluoridation

Steeped in the secrecy of wartime and cold war, born of aluminum production and uranium-235 enrichment for the Manhattan Project to make the first atom bombs, hazardous waste products containing fluoride were converted to purified sodium fluoride. This compound, still sold today as rat poison, was added to drinking water, beginning in 1945, "to prevent tooth decay in children". What a glorious goal of pollutant control combined with public benefit this would have been — if true.

Fluoridation of drinking water began 60 years ago in the United States, and it continues in 60% of public water supplies in the country today. Much of Australia, Canada, Ireland, and New Zealand have fluoridated water, but most developed non-English speaking countries have rejected this practice as nonbeneficial and probably harmful.

Current fluoridating agents, sodium hexafluorosilicate and hexafluorosilicic acid, which replaced sodium fluoride by 1980, differ from the calcium fluoride in naturally fluoridated water, which was the basis for claims of tooth decay prevention in early epidemiologic studies. Studies reported in the past 15 years support only possible slight benefits from water fluoridation for the deciduous teeth of 5-year-old children, although topical fluoride treatments may be effective. Older children and adults get no decay reduction according to the results of studies by researchers who are not supported by organizations who benefit financially from fluoridation.

Harmful effects include mainly bone and tooth fractures as well as increased cancer rates. Over 100 other problems have been linked to fluoride exposure. Perhaps the most serious is low thyroid gland function. (Shames & Shames, 2001, pp4,12-13,169-175)

Many clever schemes, legal and propaganda, are used to promote fluoridation, usually without ever having a local referendum.

Complex legal maneuvers have been used in an effort to prevent or stop fluoridation. Opponents have steadfastly prevented *all* of the drinking water in the developed world from being fluoridated.

The case against fluoridation has been weakened by opponents' condemnation of all organofluorine compounds, some of which are toxic, but many of which are beneficial, such as teflon.

Individuals can use several methods to remove fluoride from fluoridated water.

---

*Adapted from Kauffman, 2005.

## Some Terminology You Need to Know to Understand Fluoridation

Fluorine ($F_2$ or F—F) is element 9 in the Periodic Table. This means that each atom of fluorine, pretending that you could isolate the reactive stuff as atoms of plain F, has 9 protons in the nucleus. In the free element there are also 9 electrons, so a free fluorine atom has a charge of zero. Same goes for the normal molecule of the element $F_2$.

An ion is a form of element or group of elements with a charge. This charge is a result of the presence of more or fewer electrons, each with a charge of 1-, compared with the number of protons, each with a charge of 1+. The fluoride ion (F-) has one negative charge because 10 electrons are present, and they number one more than the 9 protons present.

A negatively charged ion must be accompanied by a cation such as sodium (Na+) as in sodium fluoride (Na+F- or NaF) to balance the charges. Unbalanced charges are energy-rich and unstable. One of the best examples of neutralizing unbalanced charges is a lightning bolt.

Other inorganics, such as liquid hydrofluoric acid (HF, often called hydrogen fluoride as a gas), hexafluorosilicic acid ($H_2SiF_6$), and compounds with a P—F bond, such as the sodium monofluorophosphate ($Na_2PO_3F$) used in toothpaste, form fluoride ion in water. Some organic compounds, which are by definition compounds of carbon, such as methansulfonyl fluoride ($CH_3SO_2F$) with an S—F bond and acetyl fluoride ($CH_3COF$) with a C—F bond, also form fluoride ion in water or alkali.

On the other hand, many organic compounds with carbon-fluorine (C—F) bonds are very stable to water, acid, base, enzymes and heat. The trifluoromethyl group ($CF_3$—) or the fluorophenyl group ($FC_6H_4$—) are often incorporated into drug molecules to make them more resistant to being metabolized. This is good because less drug can be used, so side-effects can be lower, and concentrations in the body will not vary as much. Organic polymers such as teflon, ($-CF_2-)_n$ and refrigerants (freons) with —$CF_2$— groups are usually extremely stable both chemically and thermally. These are properly called "fluoro compounds", not "fluorides", because they do not contain fluoride.

## Old Epidemiological Findings Favorable? to Fluoridation

By the early 1900s it was noticed that inhabitants of some areas of the United States, especially parts of Colorado and Texas, had mottled teeth (dental fluorosis), and that children with fluorosis tended to have fewer cavities. (Groves, 2001) Fluorosis was so common in these areas that it was called Colorado Brown Stain or Texas Teeth. (Bryson, 2004) In those days no one thought to follow children with dental fluorosis for long periods to see whether there were any long-term effects of any kind.

Usually the natural mineral fluorite, calcium fluoride ($CaF_2$) is the source of fluoride ion. Way back in 1935 C. H. Kick and colleagues reported on a study in which they fed rats each of three fluoride compounds, measuring how much of each was eaten, and calculated how much fluoride was retained. Calcium fluoride was fed for 11 days; no fluoride was retained. Sodium fluoride was fed for 18 days; one third was retained. Sodium hexafluorosilicate ($Na_2SiF_6$) was fed for 22 days; one third was retained. (Groves, 2001) The different results may be explained partially by the differences in solubility. Calcium fluoride is soluble in water only to 16 parts per million (ppm), or 16 mg per liter; sodium hexafluorosilicate to 650 ppm; and sodium fluoride to 42,000 ppm. So even by 1935 the existence of great differences in retention of fluoride ion or its precursor in the case of hexafluorosilicate were known.

So why not use calcium fluoride to fluoridate water? When it is present at a concentration to give 2-4 ppm fluoride ion in water in certain villages in China, calcium fluoride causes a crippling form of skeletal fluorosis, with extreme spinal curvature. (Foulkes, 2004) In those areas with severe fluorosis with 4 ppm or more fluoride in the water, children had IQs 5-19 points lower than in areas with 1 ppm fluoride or less. A cynic would say that calcium fluoride is not used to fluoridate water because it is not an industrial waste product and, therefore, costs too much. (Groves, 2001)

### Finaglers Facilitate Fluoridation Far and Wide

Industries that produced large quantities of fluoride byproducts were especially interested in the dental health effect and have been accused by antifluoridation activists of promoting water fluoridation as a method of toxic waste disposal. (Bryson, 2004; Foulkes, 2004) The purported value of fluoridation for dental health has, however, served to mitigate concerns about the toxicity of fluoride wastes, which will be discussed later.

Aluminum production, which increased greatly before and during World War II, utilized cryolite ($Na_3AlF_6$) as the solvent for the common ore of aluminum — bauxite, an oxide. The process of obtaining metallic aluminum by electrolysis of its oxide is one of the great inventions of all time, but there are emissions and leftovers. The big producers at the time were Alcoa, Reynolds and Kaiser. Zinc and fluorocarbon refrigerant production also soared with emissions of fluoride ion or its precursors.

An Alcoa-sponsored biochemist, Gerald J. Cox, fluoridated some laboratory rats in a study and concluded that fluoride reduced the number of cavities in their teeth, writing that: "The case should be regarded as proved." (Cox, 1939) On Sept 29, 1939, at a meeting of the American Water Works Association in Johnstown, Pa., "...Cox proposed that America should now consider adding fluoride to the public water supply." (Bryson, 2004) Did Cox report mortality or anything else for his rats? No! Was there a long-term pilot study on human prisoners, as was normal at the time? No! Thus, in a historic moment in 1939, the first public proposal that the U.S. should fluoridate its water supplies was made not by a doctor, or dentist, but by Cox, an industry scientist working for a company threatened by fluoride damage claims. Cox began touring the country, stumping for fluoridation. (Griffiths, 1992)

The Manhattan Project made use of uranium hexafluoride gas ($UF_6$), fluoroorganic lubricants for metal bearings exposed to $UF_6$, and other fluorine-containing materials. In the 1940s, certain major figures in the Manhattan Project and in fluoride-waste-producing industries succeeded in using some of those old epidemiological studies on calcium fluoride (Judd,1996) to allow public water supplies to have sodium fluoride added in order to prove that 1 ppm of fluoride ion would "prevent tooth decay in children." None of these or later studies followed other dental or medical outcomes of fluoride consumption over long periods, a flaw that remains in many medical trials to this day. (Kauffman, 2004)

Dr. Henry Trendley Dean, a U.S. Public Health Service researcher, at first opposed the addition of fluorides to city water supplies because he was aware of their toxicity. He later changed his mind, perhaps believing that mottled teeth were a small price to pay for less decay, or perhaps for other reasons. He later became the first Director of the National Institute of Dental Research (NIDR), and then, in 1953, a top official of the American Dental Association (ADA), two organizations unshakably committed to fluoridation to this day. (Bryson, 2004) They claim the credit for the drop in tooth decay in the United States during the past 50 years. It is now apparent that the NIDR was proposed and begun with the initial purpose of promoting water fluoridation. Since that time, Dean has confessed in court, twice, that early fluoridation studies of his did not support water fluoridation because of flawed statistics.

Once opposition by professionals was overcome, largely through the ADA and NIDR, the selling of fluoridation to the public was aided by hiring Edward L. Bernays, often called "the father of public relations," who had been hired earlier by the tobacco industry to persuade women to take up smoking. (Foulkes, 2004)

Fluoridation with fairly pure sodium fluoride (NaF) was begun in the United States in 1945. Beginning around 1950 hexafluorosilicic acid began to be used in place of NaF. Today, fluoridation uses hexafluorosilicic acid ($H_2SiF_6$) and its sodium salt ($Na_2SiF_6$) almost exclusively. These are not pure, but the acid is recovered in crude form by scrubbing the gaseous emissions from the treatment of phosphate ores with sulfuric acid. These phosphate ores, mainly from Florida, are the most important source of phosphate fertilizers. The crude ores contain a fixed amount of fluoride ion and variable amounts of lead, arsenic, beryllium, vanadium, cadmium, and mercury. (Groves, 2001) So where does the silicon (Si) come from? The emissions contain mostly hydrogen fluoride and were absorbed during the scrubbing into water mixed with sand ($SiO_2$), and thus hexafluorosilicic acid is formed, which became the main source of fluoride ion for drinking water fluoridation. Had the fluoride ion been left in the rock, the fertilizer would have been too toxic for any use.

Because of this change in fluoridation agents, old studies based on the use of natural calcium fluoride or on fairly pure sodium fluoride are irrelevant, even had they been done correctly. Calcium is a strong antagonist of fluoride, reduces its concentration in plasma, and inhibits its absorption from the intestine. (Teotia & Teotia, 1994).

According to Myron J. Coplan, Professional Engineer, hexafluorosilicic acid is supposed to dissociate into fluoride ion and silicic acid at 1 ppm in water. At higher concentrations it does not fully dissociate into fluoride, and it has its own separate toxicities. It is in equilibrium with hydrogen fluoride (hydrofluoric acid in water) and silicon tetrafluoride. These are both very toxic as well.

Fluoridation at 1 ppm fluoride reached its current extent in the USA by 1965. The proportion of fluoridated public water supplies is about 60% in the United States, 66% in Ireland, 55% in Canada, and 10% in England. Australia and New Zealand also use fluoridation extensively. At present almost none of the public water supplies in Austria, Germany, Luxembourg, Denmark, Finland, Norway, Sweden, the Netherlands, Switzerland, France, Italy, Belgium, Switzerland, Spain, Hungary, Portugal, Greece, Japan, and China are fluoridated. About half of these countries tried fluoridation, saw no benefit, and stopped it. (Groves, 2001)

U.S. studies on the toxicity of fluorine compounds, not necessarily the ones used to fluoridate water, have reportedly been suppressed, classified, censored, and removed from the National Archives. (Bryson, 2004) Some of this activity has been traced to Harold Carpenter Hodge, PhD, a biochemist and toxicologist at the University of Rochester, where he supervised experiments for the Manhattan Project. Some involved the injection of unsuspecting hospital patients with uranium and plutonium compounds. He later became Chairman of the National Research Council's Committee on Toxicology and the leading promoter of fluoridation in the United States during the Cold War. In 1953, Hodge, using data from a European study, estimated that the amount of daily fluoride intake for 10-20 years that would *not* cause crippling skeletal fluorosis was below 20-80 mg/day. It was later found that he had confused mg/kg with mg/lb. An American antifluoride campaigner, Darlene Sherrell, used the same European study from 1937 to estimate that skeletal fluorosis might be avoided with intakes of no more than 10-25 mg/day. Hodge later corrected his estimate. (Groves, 2001)

In 1975, the U.S. Food and Drug Administration (FDA) explicitly designated fluoride as *"not generally recognized as safe"* and permitted no fluoride whatsoever to be added to food or to over-the-counter dietary supplements. Nevertheless, the Department of Health, Education and Welfare (now Health and Human Services) exempted fluoridated water from this ban, including fluoridated water used to process food. (Groves, 2001)

In 1985, the U.S. Environmental Protection Agency (EPA) set 4 ppm (up from 2 ppm) as the safe level for fluoride in drinking water and prevailed in a lawsuit challenge. (Groves, 2001)

While the American Dental Association (ADA), the Centers for Disease Control and Prevention (CDC), and the NIDR of the National Institutes for Health (NIH) still support fluoridation, some 17 U.S. organizations have withdrawn their support since 1990, including the American Academy of Allergy and Immunology, the American Academy of Diabetes, the American Diabetes Association, the American Nurses Association, the American Psychiatric Association, the National Kidney Foundation, and the Society of Toxicology. (Groves, 2001)

Discussion of the scientific studies on fluoridation, as presented in the following sections, has been neglected by most of the media in the United States. The unique journal *Fluoride* is not covered by PubMed even though *Fluoride* is peer-reviewed and scholarly in tone.

## Does Water Fluoridation Prevent Tooth Decay?

Dr. H. Trendly Dean ran the first trial of fluoridation in Grand Rapids, Michigan, in 1945, declaring it a success in comparison with unfluoridated Muskegon, Michigan. Since that time, he twice confessed in court that statistics from the early studies were invalid. (Groves, 2001) Of some interest: Grand Rapids was still fluoridated in 2005. And now so is Muskegon.

Newburgh, New York, next to be fluoridated in 1945, was compared with Kingston, New York, as a control. Early reports were favorable. Naturally. But by 1989 workers at the New York State Department of Health found a difference of less than 1 fewer teeth decayed in 7-14-year-old children in Newburgh, slightly favoring fluoridation, but with no long-term report on side-effects. And by 1995 children's teeth in Kingston had slightly less tooth decay and half as much damage from fluoride. (Groves, 2001) This negative result could have been caused by a change in the fluoridation agent, or possibly by more accurate reporting.

North Shields, England, has no natural fluoride in its water, while South Shields has 1.4 ppm, presumably as calcium fluoride. While children of the same age had fewer decayed teeth in fluoridated South Shields, it was noticed that the onset of decay was merely delayed 3 years. (Groves, 2001) This finding by itself may invalidate the early Michigan and New York trial results and confirm the findings (Yiamouyiannis, 1990) that fluoride slightly lowers decay of deciduous teeth only.

A favorable report on fluoridation from New Zealand was found to be biased by the deliberate choice of the nonfluoridated communities with the highest tooth decay rates in comparison with the two fluoridated communities with the lowest decay rates. When all decay rates for all children in that area of New Zealand were compared, there was no difference with respect to fluoridation. Also, in New Zealand the number of decayed teeth per 5-year-old child has decreased steadily from 12 teeth in 1930 to 3 teeth in 1990. Neither the introduction of fluoridated water nor fluoridated toothpaste changed the downward slope of a graph of decay (see Figure 1). Had there been any effect of fluoridated water or fluoridated toothpaste on decay, the slope of the line would have become more pronounced in and after the year of introduction of either intervention. Because of this, John Colquhoun, initially appointed to *promote* fluoridation in New Zealand, now *opposes* it. (Colquhoun, 1997)

According to World Health Organization (WHO) figures, the most fluoridated country in the world, Ireland at 66%, does not have the least tooth decay. The five countries with less tooth decay (Finland, Denmark, UK, Sweden, and the Netherlands) had little or no water fluoridation (the rate was 10% in the UK). (Groves, 2001)

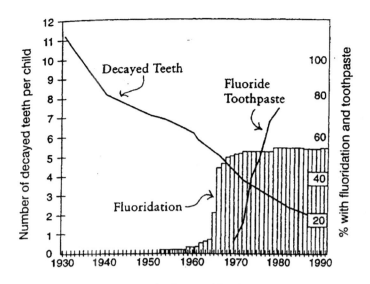

Figure 1. Tooth decay rates in 5-year-old children (left scale) vs. water fluoridation percentage (right scale) and fluoride toothpaste percentage (right scale). From Colquhoun,* cited in Groves,' reprinted with permission.

Chile began fluoridating water in 1985, but stopped it when the average of 6.0 decayed teeth per 12-year-old child, which dropped to 5.3 by 1991, increased to 6.7 in 1995.(Groves, 2001)

A study of 29,000 elementary school children in Tucson, Ariz., showed much more tooth decay when the fluoride level in the drinking water was higher (see Figure 2). (Judd, 1996) The extremes ranged from 6% of children with some decay in areas with water containing 0.0 ppm fluoride to 40% of children with some decay in areas with water containing 1.0 ppm fluoride.

Fluoridation was forced on parts of Japan during its occupation by the United States. A study reported in 1972 on 22,000 school children (median age 13, range 5-17) showed 90% with some tooth decay at 0.0 ppm fluoride. This high number was attributed to the absence of calcium in the water. A minimum in decay (38% of children) occurred with 0.3 ppm fluoride and more calcium content. This decay prevalence increased to 44% at 1.0 ppm fluoride and further to 55% with decay at 3.0 ppm fluoride and still more calcium (see Figure 3). Japan subsequently reduced the maximum allowed fluoride level to 0.05 ppm. (Judd, 1996)

The largest study on fluoridation and tooth decay involved 400,000 students (median age 13, range 5-17) in India (see Figure 4). The percentage of children with decay was 23% at 0.0 ppm fluoride; 35% at 0.7 ppm; and 75% at 2.75 ppm. (Judd, 1996; Teotia & Teotia, 1994) Other studies over a 30-year period prompted Teotia and Teotia to write: "...dental caries were caused by high fluoride and low dietary calcium intakes, separately and through their interactions.... The only practical and effective public measure for the prevention and control of dental caries is the limitation of the fluoride content of drinking water to <0.5 ppm, and adequate calcium...(> 1 g/day)."

Over a 20-year period from 1965-1985, the average number of decayed, missing, or filled teeth (DMFT) in 12-year-old children dropped by 50% in the United States. Proponents of fluoridation, and vendors of fluoridated dental rinses and toothpastes, took credit for this, very stridently. However, the following non-fluoridated countries had even greater reductions in DMFT during similar 20-year periods: the Netherlands, 72%; Sweden, 82%; Finland, 98%. (Judd, 1996; Kalsbeek & Verrips, 1990) No adjustments were made for some of the obvious confounders, such as consumption of refined carbohydrates and the other mineral contents of water supply. (Judd, 1996; Teotia & Teotia, 1994) Native Americans on reservations in this country have by far the most decay of any ethnic group in the United States, despite forcible fluoridation of their water and free dentistry for more than 50 years. (Judd, 1996)

264

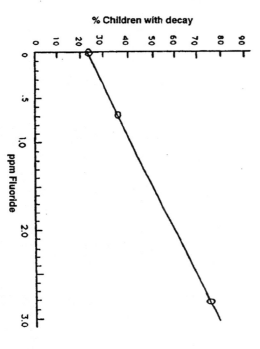

**Figure 2.** Study of tooth decay in 29,000 elementary schoolchildren in Tucson, Ariz., vs. fluoride content of their drinking water. Reprinted from Judd,[5] with permission.

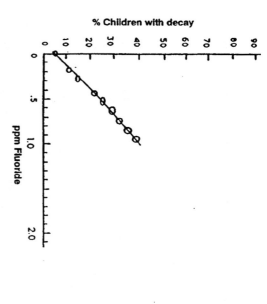

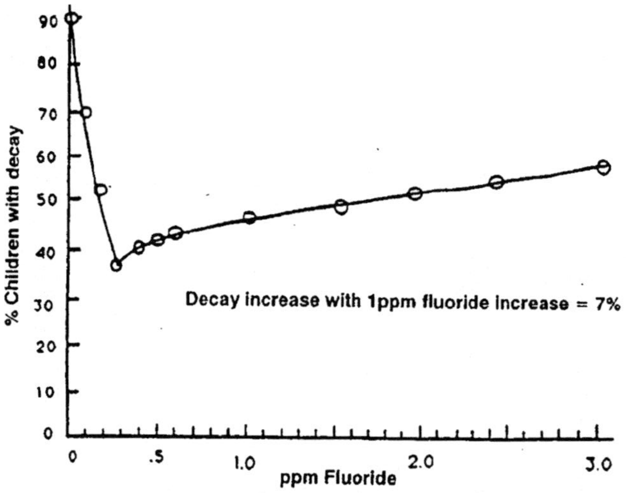

**Figure 3.** Study of tooth decay in 22,000 Japanese schoolchildren vs. fluoride content of their drinking water. Reprinted from Judd,[5] with permission.

**Figure 4.** Study of tooth decay in 400,000 Indian schoolchildren vs. fluoride content of their drinking water. Reprinted from Judd,[5] with permission.

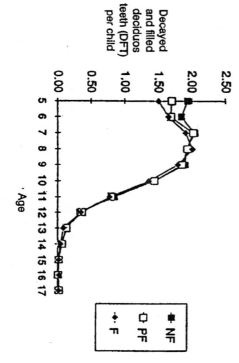

**Figure 5.** Decay of deciduous teeth in 39,207 white children in 84 areas in the United States. **F**, fluoridated; **PF**, partially fluoridated; **NF**, nonfluoridated areas. Reprinted from Yiamouyiannis,[6] with permission.

There was an overall increase in children 5-17 years old (median age 13) with tooth decay after initiation of water fluoridation. The tooth decay rate of children living in non-fluoridated American cities with average decay rates was 65% with natural fluoride levels of 0.4 ppm fluoride, but increased to 67% with fluoridation to 1 ppm. In high-decay cities, the decay rate of 71% with 0.4 ppm fluoride increased to 75% with fluoridation to 1 ppm, according to a 1990 study of 39,207 children, aged 5-17, in 84 areas in the United States. (Judd, 1996; Yiamouyiannis, 1990).

Reinterpretation of data from a 1986-1987 study by dentists trained by the NIDR showed that the decay rate of *deciduous* teeth in 5-year-olds was significantly lower in fluoridated areas (at 1.5 teeth per child) than in nonfluoridated areas (at 2.0 teeth per child), as shown in Figure 5. (Yiamouyiannis, 1990) Yes, this was an improvement of only 1/2 tooth per child! However, the decrease was no longer significant in 6-year-olds, and did not exist in children age 7 or older. Moreover, decay rates in *permanent* teeth in children aged 5-17 did not differ significantly at any age in areas with no, partial, or total fluoridation of water supplies (see Figure 6). (Yiamouyiannis, 1990) Earlier, widely accepted claims of caries reduction of 60% by fluoridation, published in the *Journal of the American Medical Association* and the *Journal of Dental Research* using data from the same source and widely quoted and accepted to this day, were not substantiated by Yiamouyiannis, who had to use the Freedom of Information Act to extract the raw data from the NIDR.

On the basis of observational studies, Hardy Limeback, BSc, PhD, DDS, head of the Department of Preventive Dentistry for the University of Toronto and President of the Canadian Association for Dental Research, announced a reversal of his earlier pro-fluoridation views. In an April 1999 interview, Dr. Hardy, once the primary promoter of fluoridation in Canada, stated: "Children under three should never use fluoridated toothpaste or drink fluoridated water. And baby formula must never be made up using Toronto tap water. Never." He remarked that "Vancouver, [British Columbia,] never fluoridated, has a lower cavity rate than Toronto, which has been fluoridated for 36 years [through 1999]." (Forbes, 1999; Limeback, 1999) In fact, the Canadian Province of British Columbia has the lowest rates of tooth decay in Canada. About 11% of B. C. is fluoridated, and the very lowest cavity rates were in the non-fluoridated areas. (Groves, 2001) In a recent article in the *Journal of the American Dental Association*, J. D. B. Featherstone wrote that:"Fluoride incorporated during tooth development is insufficient to play a significant role in caries protection." (Featherstone, 2000) In fact, fluoridation of municipal water supplies *increases* tooth decay overall in some studies and has not been demonstrated to be effective in prevention of decay in the most convincing studies, such as those of Colquhoun, Kalsbeek, and Yiamouyiannis, he concluded.

The effects of fluoridation were praised in a 2004 book, *Fluorides in the environment: effects on plants and animals,* by L.H. Weinstein and A. Davison, but expert reviewers considered the book to be blatantly biased. (Krook et al., 2004)

<u>Fluoride Supplements and Topical Application</u>

No adequate evidence for the effectiveness of fluoride supplements as pills or drops, or topical application of fluoride by means of toothpaste or dental rinses, has ever been presented. (Groves, 2001) Colquhoun's study concluded there was also no benefit from fluoridated toothpaste. (Colquhoun, 1997) Since the toxicity of fluoride ion and its precursors is beyond dispute, parents should not give children fluoride supplements that are to be swallowed to protect their teeth. The common brand, Luride™ Drops and Luride Lozi-Tabs from Colgate Oral Pharmaceuticals, have cautions not to use either of them in areas with fluoridated water, and to contact Pittsburgh Poison Control in case of trouble. The "benefits" are the ones not confirmed by Yiamouyiannis, and the listing of side-effects is woefully incomplete in the package insert or in the 1996 PDR.

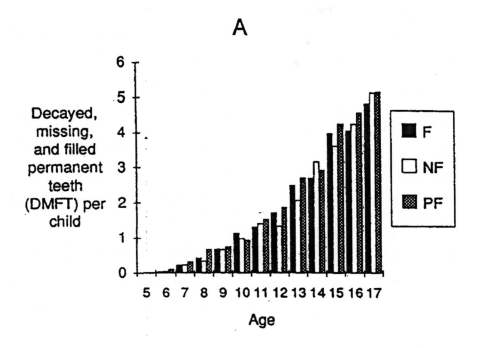

A

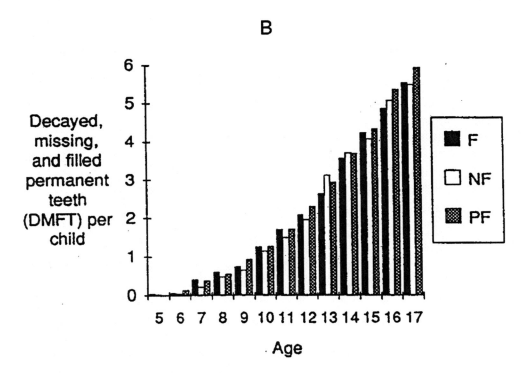

B

Figure 6. Tooth decay in fluoridated (F), partially fluoridated (PF) and non-fluoridated areas (NF). Permanent teeth in 39,207 white children in 84 areas of the USA. A: males; B: females. From Yiamouyiannis[12] with permission of journal *Fluoride.*

"Until recently, the rationale for most caries preventive programs using fluoride was to incorporate fluoride into the dental enamel. The relative role of enamel fluoride in caries prevention is now increasingly questioned, and based on rat experiments and reevaluation of human clinical data, it appears to be of minor importance...". (CDC, 2000) In fact, "...the prevalence of dental caries in a population is not inversely related to the concentration of fluoride in enamel, and a higher concentration of enamel fluoride is not necessarily more efficacious in preventing dental caries." (Fejerskov et al., 1981) Limeback found on reexamining the literature that topical effects of fluoride on newly erupted teeth were more likely to explain any benefit of fluoride than swallowing it in water or pill form. (Featherstone, 2000)

*In vitro* experiments showed that topical fluoride might protect tooth enamel by inhibition of bacterial metabolism, limiting acid generation by these bacteria. (Groves, 2001; Vanloveren et al., 1993) According to Gerard F. Judd, acid can react with the calcium hydroxyphosphate of tooth enamel to form calcium hydrogen phosphate ($CaHPO_4$), which is slightly water soluble. So it is likely that topical fluoride may achieve its anti-caries effect by its toxicity — to acid-producing bacteria. (Judd, 1996)

### Is Fluoridation Safe for the General Population?

In a report authored by Perry D. Cohn, Ph.D., M.P.H., for the New Jersey Department of Environmental Protection and the New Jersey Department of Health, the rates of bone cancer in fluoridated and nonfluoridated areas were compared. Both by counties or by municipalities, males under the age of 50 had 3 to 7 times as many bone cancers in the fluoridated areas. Males 10-19 years old fared the worst. (Cohn, 1992) An external review panel found no serious flaws with the study.

Dr. Chester Douglass, Chairman of the Department of Oral Health Policy and Epidemiology at the Harvard School of Dental Medicine, has received several years of large federal grants to study the possible relationship between bone cancer in boys and drinking fluoridated water. Reporting on the findings of his study supported by this funding, he told federal officials at the National Institutes of Health (NIH) unequivocally that there was no relationship. Douglass has made the same assertion to the National Academy of Sciences (NAS) panel now reviewing the safety of fluoridated drinking water. He is also the publisher of a Colgate-funded fluoride journal, a clear conflict of interest. The Environmental Working Group (EWG), a non-profit organization, has obtained documents suggesting that his reports to both the NIH and the NAS were falsified. The EWG discovered that the grant-funded publication Douglass cited found exactly the opposite of what Douglass said it found. In fact, the research was done by a former doctoral student of Douglass's and was the most rigorous study of its kind to date. EWG has filed an ethics complaint against Douglass with the National Institute of Environmental Health Sciences. (EWG, 2005)

Those bone cancers, called osteosarcomas, account for about 3% of all childhood cancers. The 5-year mortality rate is around 50%. Nearly all survivors have limbs amputated, usually legs. Remember Newburgh, NY? It had an incidence of 13.5% of bone structure defects, twice that of Kingston, NY, which was not fluoridated. Flaws were found in 5 studies in which no relation of fluoride to bone cancer was found. Available at: http://health-report.co.uk/fluoride_bone_cancer.htm as cited in EWG, 2005. So this is not a trivial matter.

Cancer rates in the ten largest fluoridated cities in the United States and in the ten largest unfluoridated cities were found to be the same before fluoridation began. After 20 years, the ten fluoridated cities had 10% higher cancer death rates than the unfluoridated cities. The cancers were found in the tongue, mouth, pharynx, esophagus, stomach, colon, rectum, pancreas, larynx, bronchi and lungs. When parts of Japan were fluoridated under U.S. occupation from 1945 to 1972, more uterine cancer deaths were observed. (Groves, 2001)

Hip fractures in two cities in Utah were compared: fluoridated Brigham City and unfluoridated Cedar City. In the fluoridated (1 ppm) city, the hip fracture rate in women around age 75 was twice as high as in the unfluoridated city. Men aged 80-85 also had twice the hip fracture rate in fluoridated Brigham City. (Danielson et al., 1992) The insidious nature of fluoride toxicity is that it does not cause bone density loss as found in osteoporosis by bone scans, but causes an increase in bone density with no clinical benefit. Fluoride makes both bones and teeth more brittle. (Groves, 2001; Lee, 1990). Early reports of supposed benefits of fluoridation to bone were quoted without citing later corrections, refutations or retractions. (Lee, 1990). Fluoridated adult teeth may fail by cracking, rather than from cavity damage.

Dr. A. K. Susheela of the India Institute of Medical Sciences in New Delhi found that fluoride severely disrupts formation of bone matrix, inhibiting the hardening of bones. She found that about 20 countries in the world have serious health problems due to excess natural fluoride levels in drinking water. Her work showed that high levels of fluoride in drinking water were associated with birth defects, stillbirths, and early infant mortality. (Groves, 2001)

Excess fluoride may also have detrimental neurologic effects. Rats given sodium fluoride in their drinking water — at a concentration producing a plasma level of fluoride equivalent to that found in humans consuming water with 4 ppm of fluoride — developed symptoms resembling Attention Deficit-Hyperactivity Disorder. (Mullenix et al., 1994)

Gerard F. Judd, PhD, lists 113 ailments reportedly caused by fluoride, all with literature citations to studies, of which 13 were double-blinded. One such was a double-blind study by 12 physicians establishing 13 side-effects in 50 patients. One effect is that fluoride causes pockets between gums and teeth; this is called periodontal disease. These can harbor infective bacteria that cause the condition known as gingivitis. (Judd, 1996)

So far, there are no known naturally occurring compounds of fluorine in the human body. Fluorine is not listed as even a trace element in whole body assays (Minoia et al., 1990), showing that there is no requirement for it at all. A popular Biochemistry text by Lehninger et al. does not list any naturally occurring fluorine compounds at all in animals. (Lehninger et al., 1993)

Barry Groves wrote that typical orange tea contains unsafe amounts of fluoride, and that he stopped drinking it. (Groves, 2001) This was surely an especially tough decision for an Englishman. I confess that I did not quite believe the data until a poignant case-study came to my attention accidentally in 2005. A 52-year-old white woman who was probably a resident of Missouri, USA, complained of spinal discomfort and stiffness, later worsening, with stiffness in the shoulders, neck, back and knees. A detailed case-study was published from four medical centers in St. Louis, MO. (Whyte et al., 2005) The presence of periodontal disease along with other evidence, including high urinary fluoride level, suggested skeletal fluorosis after a lengthy period for diagnosis. She had been using well water containing 2.8 ppm fluoride, which the MDs thought was OK, since it was below the 4 ppm said to be safe by the EPA. This well water provided 11-22 mg of fluoride daily. After relocating to where well water "filtration" cut the fluoride level to 0.24 ppm, her urinary fluoride level dropped somewhat, but her health continued downhill. The MDs looked for any possible source of fluoride with little success until she admitted to drinking 1-2 gallons (4-8 liters) of double-strength Lipton instant tea. An assay of her later decaffeinated instant tea allowed the calculation that she was drinking 26-52 mg of fluoride from her tea, for a total exposure of 37-74 mg per day. She was persuaded to switch to lemonade in 1999. By 2003 her urinary fluoride levels were normal and she felt completely well.

Should you be tempted to ignore this case-study and swill tea, the assays of fluoride level in a number of common teas that the St. Louis MDs had analytical labs do are shown in Table 11-1. Each fluoride level found is the mean of duplicate assays by each of 2 laboratories in St. Louis on tea prepared according to label instructions. The tea with the most fluoride, Lipton Instant made in 2003, with 6.5 mg per liter, would provide 52 mg of fluoride in 8 liters, and 104 mg if made double strength. (Whyte et al., 2005) You can see in Table 11-1 that all of the tea samples provided at least as much fluoride (1 ppm) as fluoridated water, and that the mean value was 2.6 ppm.

### Table 11-1: Fluoride Content of Typical Brands of Tea*

| Brand | Product Name | Fluoride** |
|-------|--------------|-----------|
| Lipton | Instant (1999) | 2.6 ppm or mg/L |
| | Instant (2003) | 6.5 |
| | Instant decaf | 2.7 |
| | Instant diet iced (decaf lemon) | 1.0 |
| | Naturally decaf flow-thru bags | 2.0 |
| Nestea | Instant | 2.3 |
| | Instant decaf | 2.3 |
| Schnucks | Instant | 1.3 |
| AriZona | Lemon iced tea mix | 2.2 |

* Prepared regular strength using distilled water (no fluoride) according to label directions.

** Mean of 2 assays from each of 2 labs. Method: fluoride ion-selective electrode. Modified from Whyte et al.,2005

Wine and beer drinkers should not get complacent. California wines contained 3-6 ppm of fluoride ion in one study. It comes from the cryolite ($Na_3AlF_6$) used as a pesticide for grapes. At 6 ppm a 175 mL (6 oz) glass contains as much fluoride a a liter of fluoridated water. Beer made with fluoridated water contains 0.7-1 ppm. (FAN, 2005)

Water fluoridated to 1 ppm fluoride is not safe in the general population. How much of the toxicity results from the arsenic and heavy metal contamination in the newer fluoridating agents is not yet known. Additionally, certain populations such as patients with diabetes or renal impairment are at increased risk, especially if they drink more than average amounts of water. (Connett, 2004) A study comparing 25 young adults with fluorosis against 25 matched controls showed very significant impairment of glucose tolerance in those with fluorosis, which, however, was reversible when water with low fluoride levels was given. (Connett, 2004)

Fully 17 accidents in water fluoridation have been reported. As a consequence, fluoride concentrations, assuming all fluoridating agent was hydrolyzed to fluoride ion, were as high as 23-1,041 ppm, at least for a while, causing injury to about 750 people, of whom about 10 died. (FAN2, 2005) For this reason alone, fluoridation should never have been approved. Accidents are inevitable.

### How Antifluoridationists Have Weakened Their Case

Groups such as the Fluoride Action Network, based in Vermont, USA, Parents for Fluoride Poisoned Children (PFPC), based in British Columbia, Canada, and the National Pure Water Association Ltd. (NPWA) in the UK justifiably attempt to prevent fluoridation of water. We have a lot for which to thank these groups. Without them all the municipal water supplies in the USA, Canada and the UK might be fluoridated. The push to fluoridate it all continues unabated 60 years from the first human experiments in Michigan and New York. As an example, New Jersey is now under pressure to mandate fluoridation of all its town water supplies, not just the 20% already unfit to drink.

Unfortunately, the PFPC and NPWA suffer from chemophobia, which is not only an unreasoned fear of all "chemicals," but a fear of consulting with chemists. As a result, they list any material that contains fluorine in any form as a danger by claiming that it contains "fluoride," and certain book authors and many website authors opposing fluoridation repeat this unsound assertion.

The list of "evils" includes Teflon and Tefal non-stick pan coatings, fluorocarbon propellants, and many drugs. Drugs that contain fluorine include: fluoxetine (Prozac), ciprofloxacin (Cipro), flunitrazepam (Rohypnol), fluconazole (Diflucon), fluticasone (Flixonase or Flixotide), trifluoperazine (Stelazine), flucoxacillin (Floxapen), cerivastatin (Baycol), cisapride (Propulsid), astemizole (Hismanal), and fenfluramine (Pondimin). In fact, none of these materials contain fluoride ion or are metabolized to generate any significant amount of fluoride ion. All contain the very stable carbon-fluorine bond in the form of trifluoromethyl ($CF_3$—), difluoromethylene (—$CF_2$—), fluoroalkane (—$CHF$—), or fluorophenyl ($FC_6H_4$—) groups. The fluoro groups are chosen for these drugs to retard their metabolism, increasing the duration of effective drug levels in the body. This allows lower doses to be used, leading to fewer side-effects and more even levels of the drug in our bodies, real benefits. Gerard F. Judd, a chemist, did not make this mistake in his book. (Judd, 1996)

For teflon the maximum continuous service temperature is listed as 260°C or 500°F in the *Chemical Rubber Co. Handbook* of 1976-7. Overheating Teflon may produce an irritant, perhaps perfluorooctanoic acid, perhaps the monomer of teflon (tetrafluoroethylene), or maybe even hydrogen fluoride, but the irritant is unlikely to be fluoride ion. Asked for evidence on the toxicity of Teflon, the scientific advisor to one of the antifluoridation groups sent me citations to four papers on the decomposition of Teflon by ionizing radiation. Clearly this is irrelevant to ordinary use in cooking. Above some concentration, perfluorooctanoic acid is toxic. Dupont is being investigated by the EPA, at least, on emissions from its Parkersburg, WV, plant. Dupont already has agreed to pay up to $345 million to settle one of several lawsuits. This one is on behalf of 60,000 WV and OH residents whose drinking water is contaminated by perfluorooctanoic acid. (Hawthorne et al., 2005) However, at this time, emissions near the plant seem much more of a menace than exposure to the useful products in which the perfluorooctanoic acid is solidly bonded in place. An experiment reported by the Fluoride Action Network in which fluoridated water is boiled in a teflon pan, concentration of fluoride ion, which does not evaporate, increased as expected; the teflon did not contribute any, contrary to the comments of the experimenters. (EWG, 2005)

Fluorocarbon refrigerants and propellants such as R12 or R134a, and general anesthetics such as halothane and methoxyflurane, are metabolized very slowly or not at all. However, some of the fluorine in the general anesthetics enflurane, desflurane, and isoflurane is metabolized to fluoride ion. (Williams, 1995)

Asked for evidence on the toxicity of fluorinated drugs, the scientific advisor to one of the antifluoridation groups provided citations to 13 papers. Ten of the 13 were published in 1952 or earlier. Some concerned analytical methods and methods of synthesis of fluorine-containing compounds. Citations from the 1930s showed the toxicity of sodium fluoride from its interference with thyroid hormone biosynthesis. (Kraft, 1937) Another from 1949 showed that that 3-fluoro-5-bromo(or iodo)tyrosine was toxic in mice, and five other fluorophenyl compounds less so. (Euler et al., 1949) The toxicity of 3-fluorotyrosine and 3,5-difluorotyrosine was confirmed, including in humans, (Litzka, 1936; 1937; 1937A) but this is a special case in which these amino acid derivatives interfere with thyroid hormone biosynthesis. So these particular fluoro compounds are really toxic because they fool the body into using them as thyroid hormones, not because they are converted to fluoride ion. This did not stop Big Pharma from making some fluoro compounds and fluorides available as drugs to counteract hyperthyroidism.

Nerve gases such as sarin are extremely toxic, to be sure. In this case the very reactive P—F bond is present.

Ciprofloxacin is associated with some toxicity. The scientific advisor to one of the antifluoridation groups raised an alarm by citing a report showing elevated serum and urine levels of fluoride in children after administration of this drug. (Pradhan et al., 1995) The actual elevation of fluoride in serum was from 0.08 to 0.21 ppm in 12 hours, and could not account for more than a fraction of the fluorine (23 mg) in the 400 mg doses used of ciprofloxacin; moreover, there was no follow-up measurement. The elevation of fluoride in urine from 0.97 to 1.12 ppm after a week was not statistically significant. The authors did not try to measure fluorinated metabolites or unchanged drug, and after MRI scans and about 2 years of follow-up by physical examinations, they pronounced short courses of ciprofloxacin safe in children. Although ciprofloxacin liberates fluoride under UVB illumination *in vitro,* it is metabolized in vivo mostly by hydroxylation and N-sulfation, not by loss of fluoride ion. (Williams, 1995)

The risk of rhabdomyolysis, the major toxicity of the statin drugs (see Myth 3), is about the same with atorvastatin and pravastatin, which contain fluoro groups, and simvastatin, which does not. (see Appendix D), (Graham et al., 2004) A group at Duke University Medical Center searched the literature from November 1997 to February 2002 to find 60 cases of statin-induced memory loss, of which 36 were due to simvastatin, 23 to atorvastatin and 1 to pravastatin. (Wagstaff et al., 2003) Clearly, there is no correlation of either side-effect with the presence of a fluoro group.

Thus the scientific evidence presented by members of certain antifluoridation groups and by others does not support their assertions that *all* fluorinated organic compounds are toxic because they contain fluorine or "fluoride". The case against fluoridation needs to be made solely on the basis of the effects of fluoride ions and their precursors in drinking water.


## Who Benefits from Fluoridation?

Groves's book does not explain how water fluoridation can be continued despite all the evidence against it. Bryson's book, however, suggested that many corporations benefit from the cheap disposal of toxic waste. In the 1940s these included: US Steel, DuPont, Alcoa, Alcan, Reynolds Metals, Kaiser Aluminum, Pennsalt Chemicals (now ELF Atochem), and Allied Chemical, among others.

Over the last 50 years the Florida phosphate fertilizer industry was the main beneficiary. The few surviving companies include Cargill, CF and IMC — not exactly household names. There are also phosphate fertilizer producers in North Carolina and Idaho. Morocco is said to have 5 times the reserves of phosphate rock as the USA does. According to Myron Coplan, PE, the small fraction of uranium in phosphate rock has been an important and domestic source. The gypsum board made from the calcium sulfate by-product of fertilizer production is slightly radioactive.

Philadelphia, Pa., obtains its hexafluorosilicic acid from Solvay Fluoride. A dozen other manufacturers of hexafluorosilicic acid were listed on an antifluoridation website sponsored by the Fluoride Action Network Pesticide Project. It is stated that industry is able to profit by selling 155,000 tons of fluoride byproducts per year for water fluoridation instead of having to dispose of them as toxic waste at great expense. (Bryson, 2004) Another consideration might be avoiding enormous tort liability that could be incurred if toxicity were officially recognized (especially if the EPA's "safe" level of 4 ppm were scaled back properly). Dr. J. William Hirzy, the current Senior Vice-President of the EPA Headquarters Union said in 2000:

"If this stuff gets out into the air, it's a pollutant; if it gets into the lake it's a pollutant; but if it goes right into your drinking water system, it's not a pollutant. That's amazing...There's got to be a better way to manage this stuff."

## How Can Fluoridation of Water Be Stopped?

Despite evidence for negligible benefit and considerable risk, the American Dental Association (ADA), the American Medical Association (AMA), the CDC, the NIDR, the British Fluoridation Society, the WHO and others have not retreated from their support for fluoridation. Because opposition has been marginalized, primarily by ignoring it, and by control of the mass media except for the internet, the only route to change appears to be through litigation.

A pro-fluoridation how-to kit by Michael Easley, DDS, MPH, Associate Professor, School of Dental Medicine, SUNY, calls all opposition to water fluoridation unprincipled. He also calls it "health terrorism". Every ailment pinned on fluoride is called a lie. The journal *Fluoride* is said not to be peer-reviewed (Easley, 1999), but the journal's website says that all papers are evaluated by qualified reviewers, much like *The Lancet.*

Had there been only one or two failed lawsuits over the years, one might conclude that the antifluoridation cause is hopeless. In fact, lawsuits have met with some success. Antifluoridation lawsuits were argued by attorney John Remington Graham in non-jury trials in Pittsburgh, Pa. (1978), Alton, Ill. (1980), and Houston, Tex. (1982). In all cases, the judges found for the plaintiffs and issued injunctions against fluoridation on the grounds that it caused cancer and other ailments in humans. Based on the injunction in the Pittsburgh case, the Province of Quebec, Canada, stopped fluoridating. However, all three cases were overturned on appeal on trivial legalistic grounds. In spite of the appellate actions, however, the judicial findings of fact, namely that fluoridation is an unreasonable risk to public health, remain on the record and unchallenged. After the Alton case, an attorney for the ADA, who was a member of the Rules Committee of the Illinois Supreme Court, told an audience that he was the one who had secured a stay of the execution of the nonfluoridation injunction. (Graham & Morin, 1999)

There have been five other lawsuits resulting in judgments against fluoridation: two in Pennsylvania and one each in Indiana, Ohio, and Missouri. None were ruled on the merits (or lack thereof) of fluoridation, only on legal technicalities. (PEN, 2001)

Bottled water in a local supermarket sports an FDA-style food label, making it a food under the law. The FDA position that fluoride is neither an essential nor probably essential nutrient and is not safe at any level does help the antifluoridation cause and puts the FDA in a vulnerable position. (Groves, 2001)

Since fluorides have been shown to increase the risk of cancer, addition of any of them in any amount to water violated the Delaney Clause of the 1958 Amendment to the Food, Drug, and Cosmetic Act of 1938. (Cornell, 2005) The Delaney Clause was repealed in 1996 with passage of the Food Quality Protection Act. A stronger argument based on the cancer issue is that adding fluoride violates the EPA policy on setting drinking water standards under the Safe Drinking Water Act. Under this provision, the Maximum Contaminant Level Goal (a pure health-based standard) for carcinogens is zero, so adding any fluoride should be banned. This is apparently why the 1990 National Toxicology Program bioassay on sodium fluoride was "revised" so that the findings went from "clear evidence of carcinogenicity" to "equivocal" evidence. Without that change, the fluoridation program would have been unsustainable under law.

Fluoride in water is also a medication that is forced upon people who do not want it. This is arguably a violation of law, because in the United States, people may not be medicated without their permission. Fluoridation is different from chlorination of water, because the chlorine is used to kill microbes, not to medicate people.

In India, the government constructed *defluoridation* plants and attempted to end sales of fluoridated toothpaste, based on Susheela's work on the toxicity of fluoride. (Groves, 2001) Unfortunately, in the United States, class-action lawsuits may be the only way to influence municipal authorities, who are operating on the basis of old, erroneous information on which legal precedent rests.

## Removal of Fluoride Ion from Tap Water

Since preventing or ending fluoridation of public water supplies is so difficult, you may wish to remove fluoride ion from your drinking water. Filters do not work because the diameter of a fluoride anion is too small at 0.064 nm. Activated carbon "filters" are not effective, nor are water-softeners based on cation exchange resins designed to take out calcium, magnesium, and iron, not anions. It might be possible to make effective anion exchangers for fluoride ion. Anion exchange resins have been sold in bulk for over 50 years.

There are three effective methods for removal of fluoride ion: use of a cartridge containing activated alumina adsorbent, the most expensive because the cartridge must be changed so often; reverse osmosis; and distillation, the least expensive method. The last costs about 7 cents per liter for electricity and about 2 cents per liter for depreciation of a distiller costing $135 at Sears, assuming a 5-year life. Distilled water is often passed through an activated carbon filter such as a Brita filter to remove volatile organics, and then aerated for flavor. (Franks, 2005; Letorney, 2005)

You will find that, by buying spring water in gallon or larger containers, the cost is higher than that of distillation, but it is convenient. One way you can find out whether there is fluoride in the spring water is to ask the vendor for an assay. I did this with Whole Foods, Inc., and they were kind enough to e-mail a very lengthy assay that showed no fluoride. If you know an analytical chemist or can pay one, you can have water samples assayed for fluoride ion. At present, use of an ion-selective electrode is the only common reliable method.

In buying beer or wine or distilled spirits (see Myth 5) you can make use of the knowledge that only Ireland in Europe is substantially fluoridated. You can therefore choose any of these beverages from anywhere else in Europe or from Japan with pretty good confidence that they will not be fluoridated.

## The Sad Conclusions

Artificial fluoridation of drinking water by municipalities at 1 ppm of fluoride ion probably does not reduce tooth decay, except for a minor effect on deciduous teeth. Hexafluorosilicic acid and its sodium salt, which contain other toxic substances because they are not purified, certainly have no significant benefit.

Proponents of fluoridation have censored most mass media, ignored intelligent discussion of fluoridation, slandered most opponents of fluoridation, and overturned legal judgments against fluoridation in a manner that demonstrates their political power. Many published studies that had conclusions favoring fluoridation were later found unsupported by their raw data. Three specific examples were given in this chapter. Such studies are still quoted regardless.

There is evidence that fluoridation increases the incidence of cancer, hip fractures, joint problems, and that it damages both teeth and bones by causing fluorosis. Other medical problems may also occur, including hypothyroidism, neurologic damage, and a tendency toward glucose intolerance.

Antifluoridationists compromise their credibility by unwarranted assertions that all stable fluorine-containing materials are harmful. Some are, not all. Antifluoridationists should maximize their valuable contributions by avoiding distractions and blanket condemnations.

The EPA should set the enforceable Maximum Contaminant Level at 0.4 ppm fluoride in drinking water.

The drug half of the FDA should reverse its position on permitting sale of products containing fluoride that claim dental benefit without proof of safety or effectiveness. The food half of the FDA should not permit foods to be sold which will provide more than 1 mg per day of fluoride ion in normal consumption.

Fluoridation of municipal water should cease. Defluoridation of naturally fluoridated water down to 0.4 ppm of fluoride should be mandated. Individuals should remove fluoride from their tap water until fluoridation is stopped, or use bottled spring water with under 0.4 ppm fluoride present.

Acknowledgements for Myth 11

Frances Eleanor Heckert Pane, MSLS, and Alayne Yates, MD, edited the manuscript and provided key references, as did Michael A. Pane, Jr., JD, LLM, and Leslie Ann Bowman, AMLS. Certain reviewers made important contributions, as did Myron Coplan, PE.


Potential conflicts of interest

The author has no financial interest in fluoridation or alternate treatments for public water supplies, or in any form of defluoridation.

References for Myth 11

Bryson C (2004) *The Fluoride Deception.* New York, NY: Seven Stories Press.
CDC (2000). Centers for Disease Control and Prevention. Recommendations for using fluoride to prevent and control dental caries in the United States. *MMWR* 50(RR14):1-42.
Cohn PD (1992). *An Epidemiologic Report on Drinking Water and Fluoridation,* New Jersey Department of Health, November 1992.
Colquhoun J (1997*).* Why I changed my mind about water fluoridation. *Perspectives in Biology and Medocone* 41(1):29-44.
Connett M (2004). Letter to *J Natl Cancer Inst. Fluoride* 37(3):231-232.
Cornell University (2005), Legal Information Institute, Food and drug law: an overview. No date. Available at: http://www.law.cornell.edu/topics/food_drugs.html Accessed Apr 21, 2005.
Cox GJ (1939). New knowledge of fluoride in relation to dental caries. *Journal of the American Water Works Association* 31:1926-30.
Danielson C, Lyon JL, Egger M, Goodenough GK (1992). Hip fractures and fluoridation in Utah's elderly population. *Journal of the American Medical Association* 268(6):746-748.
Easley MW (1999). Community Water Fluoridation in America: The Unprincipled Opposition. Available at: www.dentalwatch.org/fl/opposition.pdf Accessed 12 Jan 05.
Euler H, Eichler O, Hindemith H (1949). Über die Wirkung einiger organischer Fluoride bei chronischer Darreichung. *Naunyn-Schmiedeberg's Arch Pharmacol* 206:75-82
EWG (2005). Environmental Working Group. Available at: http://www.ewg.org/issues/fluoride/20050627/index.php      Accessed 20 Jul 05.
FAN (2005). Fluoride Action Network, Fluoride Sources. Available at: http://www.fluoridealert.org/f-sources.htm Accessed 27 Jul 05.
FAN2 (2005). Available at: http://www.fluoridealert.org/health/accidents/fluoridation.html Accessed 20 Jul 05.
Fejerskov O, Thylstrup A, Larsen MJ (1981). Rational use of fluorides in caries prevention: a concept based on possible cariostatic mechanisms. *Acta Odontologica Scandinavica* 39: 241-249.
Forbes B (1999). Prominent researcher apologizes for pushing fluoride. *The Tribune,* Mesa, Ariz., Dec 5, 1999. Available at: http://www.apfn.net/messageboard/10-17-04/discussion.cgi.5.htm Accessed Oct 17, 2004.

Featherstone JDB (2000). The science and practice of caries prevention. *Journal of the American Dental Association* 131:887-899.

Foulkes RG (2004) Editorial: Public deception on fluoride. *Fluoride* 37(2):55-57.

Franks G ( 2005). Fluoride in drinking water. Should you have it? How do you get rid of it if you don't want it? Denton, Tex.: Pure Water Products, LLC. Available at: http://www.purewatergazette.net/fluorideinwater.htm Accessed Jan 3, 2005.

Graham JR, Morin P (1999). Highlights in North American litigation during the twentieth century on artificial fluoridation of public water supplies. *J Land Use Environ Law* 14(spring):195-248. Available at: http://www.law.fsu.edu/journals/landuse/vol142/Graham-final2.pdf. Accessed Sept. 26, 2004.

Graham DJ, Staffa JA, Shatin D, et al. (2004). Incidence of hospitalized rhabdomyolysis in patients treated with lipid-lowering drugs. *Journal of the American Medical Association* 292:2585-2590.

Griffiths J (1992). Fluoride: Commie Plot or Capitalist Ploy. *Covert Action Quarterly,* Fall, 1992. Available at: http://www.fluoridealert.org/f-industry.htm Accessed 6 Jan 05.

Groves B ( 2001) *Fluoride: Drinking Ourselves to Death.* Dublin, Ireland: Newleaf.

Hawthorne M (2005) EPA charges Dupont hid Teflon's risks. U. S. orders study on health perils of key chemical. *Chicago Tribune Online Edition,* 18 Jan 05. Available at:
http://www.chicagotribune.com/news/nationworld/chi-0501180271jan18,1,1986717.story?coll Accessed 21 Jan 05.

Judd GF (1996). *Good Teeth Birth to Death.* Glendale, AZ: Research Publications Co; .

Kalsbeek H, Verrips GHW (1990). Dental caries and the use of fluorides in different European countries. *Journal of Dental Research* 69 (special issue):728-732.

Kauffman JM (2004) Bias in recent papers on diets and drugs in peer-reviewed medical journals. *Journal American Physicians & Surgeons* 9:11-14.

Kauffman JM (2005). Water Fluoridation: Review of Recent Research and Actions. *Journal of American Physicians & Surgeons* 10(2),38-44.

Kraft K (1937). Beiträge zur Biochemie des Fluors. I. Über den Antagonismus zwischen Fluor und Thyroxin. *Hoppe-Seyler's Zeitschrift der Physiol. Chemie* 245:58-65.

Krook LP, Connett P, Burgstrahler AW (2004). Misplaced Trust in Official Reports. *Fluoride* 37(3):147-150.

Lee JR (1990). Editorial: fluoride and osteoporosis. *Fluoride* 22(2):51-53.

Lehninger AL, Nelson DL, Cox MM (1993). *Principles of Biochemistry.* 2nd ed. New York, NY: Worth Publishing Group.

Letorney J, Jr (2005). Blowing the lid off of distilled water myths. Rockland, Mass.: Durastill Export, Inc. Available at: http://www.durastill.com/myths.html Accessed Jan 3, 2005.

Limeback H (1999). A re-examination of the pre-eruptive and post-eruptive mechanism of the anti-caries effects of fluoride: is there any anti-caries effect from swallowing fluoride? *Community Dental and Oral Epidemiology* 27(1):62-71.

Litzka G (1936). Die antithyreotoxische Wirkung des Fluotyrosins. *Nauyn-Schmiedeberg's Arch Pharmacol* 183:436-458.

Litzka G (1937). Erfolgskontrolle bei Behandlung der Schilddrüsenüberfunktion. *Zeitschrift für Klinische Medizin* 131:791-9.

Litzka G (1937A). Die experimentellen Grundlagen der Behandlung des Morbus/Basedow und der Hyperthyreose mittels Fluortyrosin. *Dtsch Med Wochenschr* 63:1037-1040.

Minoia C, Sabbioni E, Apostoli P, et al. (1990). Trace element reference values in tissues from inhabitants of the European Community I. A Study of 46 Elements in Urine, Blood and Serum of Italian Subjects. *The Science of the Total Environment* 95:89-105.

Mullenix PJ, Denbesten PK, Schunior A, Kernan WJ (1994). Neurotoxicity of sodium fluoride in rats. *Neurotoxicology & Teratology* 17(2):169-177.

PEN (2001). Pennsylvania Environmental Network, Aug 14, 2001. Available at:
www.penweb.org/fluoride/lawandcourts/#courtcases Accessed Sept 28, 2004.

Pradhan KM, Arora NK, Jena A, Susheela AK, Bhan MK (1995). Safety of ciprofloxacin therapy in children: magnetic resonance images, body fluid levels of fluoride and linear growth. *Acta Pediatrica* 84:555-560.

Shames RL, Shames KH (2001). *Thyroid Power,* New York, NY: HarperCollins.

Teotia SPS, Teotia M (1994*).* Dental caries: a disorder of high fluoride and low dietary calcium interactions. *Fluoride* 27(2):59-66.

Trivedi N, Mithal A, Gupta SK, Godbole MM (1993). Reversible impairment of glucose tolerance in patients with endemic fluorosis. *Diabetologia* 36:826-828.

Vanloveren C, Buijs JF, Tencate JM (1993). Protective effect of topically applied fluoride in relation to fluoride sensitivity of mutans streptococci. *Journal of Dental Research* 72:1184-1190.

Wagstaff LR, Mitton MW, McLendon Arvik B, Doraiswamy PM (2003). Statin-associated memory loss: analysis of 60 case reports and review of the literature. *Pharmacotherapy* 23(7):871-880.

Whyte MP, Essmyer K, Gannon FH, Reinus WR (2005). Skeletal fluorosis and instant tea. *The American Journal of Medicine* 118:78-82.

Williams DA (1995). Drug metabolism. In: Foye WO, Lemke TL, Williams DA, Eds. *Principles of Medicinal Chemistry*. 4th ed. Media, PA: Williams & Wilkins; 110-111.

Yiamouyiannis JA (1990) Water fluoridation and tooth decay: results from the 1986-1987 National Survey of U.S. Schoolchildren. *Fluoride* 23(2):55-67.

# Conclusion: Get the benefits of developing your own case of medical paranoia.

*"Just as there is an art to being a doctor, there is an art to being a patient. You must choose wisely when to submit and when to assert yourself. Even when patients decide not to decide, they should still question their physicians and insist on explanations."*
--Atul Gewande, MD, Surgeon (Gewande, 2002)

### Does the USA Have the Best Medical Care in the World?

With an $11 trillion annual gross domestic product, and 17% of this used for health care, the annual cost of medical care in the USA per person is about $7,000! This is more than the total annual gross domestic product per person in many countries! Do Americans live the longest? No! Are Americans the healthiest? No! If not, why not?

The poor performance of the USA was recently confirmed by the World Health Organization, ranking the USA 15th among 25 industrialized nations. Ranking was based on life expectancy, child survival up to age 5 years, individuals' experiences with the health care system, and equality of family out-of-pocket expenditures for health care regardless of the need for services.

In another report, the Institute of Medicine (IOM) of the National Academy of Sciences (USA) ranked the USA second worst of 13 countries on health. The rankings were: Japan > Sweden > Canada > France > Australia > Spain > Finland > the Netherlands > the United Kingdom > Denmark > Belgium > USA > Germany. Some of the indicators used were:

- 13th (last) for low-birth-weight percentage
- 13th for both neonatal and overall infant mortality
- 11th for postneonatal mortality
- 13th for years of potential life lost
- 10th for age-adjusted mortality
- 10th for life expectancy at 40 years for females, 9th for males
- 3rd for life expectancy at 80 years for females and males

This result cannot be blamed on excessive smoking or drinking, or entirely on motor vehicle collisions and violence. Though the writer of the article from which much of this data is taken, Barbara Stanfield, MD, MPH, was puzzled by the negative result of both the relatively low consumption of animal fats and the low serum cholesterol concentrations in American men, being unaware of the facts in Myths 2 and 3, even she could not blame diet entirely for the poor health of Americans.

She places the blame largely on over-medicalization, most of which is not due to errors, but to excessive testing and treatment. Her actual figures are:

- 7000 deaths/year from medication errors in hospitals
- 12000 deaths/year from unnecessary surgery
- 20000 deaths/year from other errors in hospitals
- 80000 deaths/year from from infections contracted in hospitals
- 106000 deaths/year from non-error, adverse effects of drugs

The total is 225,000 premature deaths/year in the USA from medical care! And these are from the lower estimates in the IOM report. Even so, mortality from treatment (iatrogenic) is the third biggest cause of death in the USA after cardiovascular disease (CVD) and cancer. Infant mortality in the USA, very poor for decades, has *not* been shown to result solely from the experience of Afro-Americans.

Stanfield's conclusions are that there is too much medical treatment in the USA, much more than in Japan, where diagnostic procedures are equally available, and which are equally utilized in both countries. She avoids a direct exposure of why there are so many prescription drugs with adverse effects (Stanfield, 2000). These two dangers are combined when a person is hospitalized for treatment of drug side effects. This is far from rare, since about 1 in 5 hospital admissions in both the USA and the UK are for adverse drug effects (Fulder, 1994, p42).

Mark Sircus Ac., OMD, Executive Director, International Medical Veritas Association (http://www.imva.info) provided the following:

"The number of people in the United States who die iatrogenic deaths was estimated by Dr. Barbara Stanfield to be approximately 225,000 to 284,000 a year, which included 106,000 deaths from properly prescribed medicine. These are considered avoidable deaths occurring at the hands of doctors in hospitals. Gary Null Ph.D. and his medical colleagues (Null, et al., 2003) estimate the iatrogenic death figures much higher – 786,000 by including outpatient deaths estimated at 199,000 (noted but not included by Stanfield), and other categories of iatrogenic deaths like malnutrition perpetuated in hospitals, bedsores and infections - 108,000, 115,000, and 88,000 respectively. The high end of these numbers represents 6 jumbo jets falling out of the sky each and every day and that is just for the population in America."

True, rich people do come to the USA from all over the world for some of the most difficult surgical operations, which are often performed magnificently, partially because there is no attempt whatever at cost-containment.

## Medicalization of Childbirth

With 58% of American women having children, childbirth is a great example of over-medicalization of a natural and common experience of healthy women. An anecdote from Dr. and Mrs. Stephen Fulder's experience in 1977 is just as appropriate now, 28 years later, as it was then:

"It was a windy Saturday afternoon in March 1977 when labour began. We were tremendously excited at the prospect of the birth of our first child. The contractions stopped as soon as we got to the hospital in North London, because, as my wife remarked, no one in their right mind would want to be born in such a place. Then the farce began. The contractions restarted while we fenced off a series of authoritative suggestions: 'You ought to have an epidural anesthetic now, it is much more difficult later on.' 'We want to see the baby's heart beat on the screen, don't you too?' which then turned into commands: 'Of course you must have a drip, we cannot help you any other way.' I refused the staff. A distraction was created so the birth could be induced... Under threat and in pain along with its mother, the baby was born... We were fine, but depressed by the 'loss' of our birth.

"Glaring lights, the monitor wheeled in and out, the nurses popping in at regular intervals 'to discuss the epidural'. Then: 'We must induce now, you have had long enough' and from a Sister: 'Come on, it's Sunday morning'.

"As one teacher of the Lamaze technique (which stresses psychological preparation for a fulfilling natural birth) told me: 'Your will is removed right from the prenatal checkups. Your baby is tested with equipment, you are introduced to pathology and the continuous feeling of risk: something may be wrong... No one will trust the mother right from the beginning, and soon she no longer trusts herself...

"'The bright-eyed, quiet, attentive newborn, who is the product of a birth in which the mother was relaxed, constantly supported, fully mobile, unmedicated, delivered gently and quietly...is not recognized in hospital obstetrics... The experts expect, instead, a sleepy neonate, one who does not focus the eyes or follow objects and mimic faces, one who feels poorly, is hard to "contain" or comfort and has few periods of "quiet alert" state...'

"Birth is different because it is not an illness...and birth is a risky moment... This is the expressed reason for all the medical procedures...and in an excess of zeal, this birth apparatus tends to encompass every birth, normal or not..."

The USA offers the most medicalized births in the world, yet 18-22 infants per 1000 die at birth. In Holland where half the births are at home without a doctor present, 11-14 infants per 1000 die at birth. A study in the *New England Journal of Medicine* (28 Dec 89) surveyed 12,000 women. Only 4.4 % had a Caesarean in non-hospital centers compared with 30% in general hospitals in the USA!

Fulder goes on to show the dangers of ultrasound, of electronic monitoring of fetal heartbeat, which leads to unnecessary Caesareans, of artificial induction, and even the drawbacks of the recumbent birth position. He shows the dangers of painkillers, anesthetics (including epidurals) and tranquilizers, all of which enter the baby, and of the episiotomy and Caesareans. Fulder's advice for the UK is to go to small hospitals staffed by general practitioners. In the USA, he recommends alternative birth centers. What was regarded as "interference with staff" in 1977 is seen as "parent's choice" at present, even in the UK. Knowing how difficult it can be, Fulder gives plenty of practical advice for dealing with large hospitals when undergoing childbirth (Fulder, 1994, pp215-226).

One organization for help in avoiding hospitals for childbirth is www.BabyCenter.com: http://www.babycenter.com/refcap/pregnancy/childbirth/2007.html A nationwide (USA) list of centers is available at: http://www.birthcenters.org/

### Medicalization of Age

There is some pervasive implication in the medical profession that no one is allowed to die a natural death free from the adverse effects of FDA approved, yet unproven treatment. Yes, the profession can and should deal with repairing injuries from trauma, rescusitating victims of heart attacks or sudden heart failure, and curing infections. Yes, some conditions may be treated to advantage with a drug or a drug combination; but this book has plenty of evidence to show how so many conditions are better treated with diet and supplements. The typical 70-year-old USA citizen takes about 7 prescription drugs daily, of which none are really a benefit in most cases, and 5 merely deal with the adverse effects of the other 2. Here is a quick review of how medical myths have made normal aging expensive, debilitating and depressing:

Myth 1 showed that daily aspirin does indeed prevent heart attacks, mostly non-fatal ones, yet does not reduce mortality in men, while typical doses increase mortality in women. Like Tylenol, Motrin, Vioxx and Celebrex, aspirin puts plenty of people in the hospital, with staggering costs we all pay for in endlessly increasing medical insurance premiums and in taxes for Medicaid and Medicare. Supplements such as omega-3 fish oils (EPA and DHA) and coenzyme Q10 can prevent many heart attacks and heart failures with no side-effects. Most people over age 40, regardless of diet, will benefit from vitamin C and magnesium supplementation, to name two more. Tailored to each individual, certain other supplements will increase quality of life and its duration.

Myth 2 showed that advice to eat low-fat diets, especially low in saturated fat and cholesterol, the ubiquitous advice from every governmental agency and most non-profit foundations, has no basis whatever, and results in immense suffering and costs. For people who are carb-sensitive, or who have gluten or grain allergies, low-carb high-fat diets with plenty of saturated fat and cholesterol, can stave off obesity, NIDDM, celiac disease, Crohn's disease, and even cancer.

Myth 3 showed that the basis for using cholesterol-lowering drugs was pure mythology. Low cholesterol levels are dangerous; high ones usually are not. Cholesterol levels increase naturally with age, probably as a defense mechanism against inflammation and cancer. Clinical trials (RCTs) of statin drugs indicate no worthwhile overall benefit for primary prevention of heart attacks, but high risk of debilitating side-effects. Trials on secondary prevention indicate very minor benefits on the order of what might have been obtained from Bufferin, and the benefits are unrelated to the achieved cholesterol levels. In hospitalized men with CVD or demonstrated cytomegalovirus or inflammation, possibly caused by nanobacteria, the minor benefits of statin drugs have nothing to do with lowering serum cholesterol levels. It is unlikely that the adverse-effect-prone statin drugs such as Lipitor are of any overall benefit in men, and certainly not in women. Any hype for *alternative* cholesterol-lowering treatments indicates a complete fraud since there is no reason for lowering cholesterol levels.

Myth 4 showed that blood pressure increases naturally with age, and is higher in women than in men of the same age. Very low blood pressure is dangerous. It was shown that only people in the 90% percentile of high blood pressure would obtain any benefit at all from antihypertensive drugs, and this would be minor as well as accompanied by severe side-effects. Broadening the fraction of the population taking these drugs was not supported by the results of clinical trials, quite the opposite.

Myth 5 showed that the slight protection from CVD conferred by 1-3 alcoholic drinks per day did not extend to other causes of death. The "special antioxidant" properties of red wine were inferior to those of a small dose of vitamin C, and no long-term trials exist on the effect of red wine specifically on all-cause mortality.

Myth 6 showed that extreme exercise *causes* heart failure and other injuries, quite the opposite of preventing them. Moderate exercise improves well-being, but there is the likelihood that we are seeing that well-being improves the ability and desire for moderate exercise.

Myth 7 showed that EDTA chelation does retard or reverse atherosclerosis with improvements in edema, wound healing and in walking distance before pain. This chapter also showed the first example that mainstream medicine does not "fight fair" in debunking alternative treatments any more than in promoting mainstream treatments.

Myth 8 showed that hysteria over low-dose ionizing radiation has been a costly excess of overzealous environmentalism. Not only is typical background radiation harmless, it is actually beneficial, and is usually less than the optimum amount. This means that small leaks from nuclear power plants, from radioisotopes in transit, from radon in homes, and from most medical exposures for imaging are harmless and probably beneficial.

Myth 9 showed that annual mammography to detect breast cancer is a needless expense and pain with no effect on all-cause mortality rates, and a reduction in RR for breast cancer death to 0.8 at best. Even this is likely to have been due to the beneficial effects of the low-dose Xrays used in mammography in the past. Other imaging methods have their advantages, especially when breast cancer is detected initially some other way, which can be by means of palpation or a simple AMAS test on a blood sample. The case is made that treatment of breast cancer does not change the all-cause death rate and may change the cause of death to heart failure or something else other than cancer.

Myth 10 showed that oncologists and others pretend that they can cure 60% of cancers when nothing of the sort is true. It was also shown how the 5-year survival rates have been manipulated and used to mislead, how poor mainstream treatment is, and how seriously patients are misled about its adverse effects. Mainstream opposition to alternative treatments, while often justified, has held up at least two useful treatments for decades.

Myth 11 showed that highly respected corporations and federal government agencies conspired to dispose of fluoridated waste products in our drinking water. A minor benefit to baby teeth was magnified out of proportion, and long-term side-effects were not even considered, then denied when found.

*****

Normal changes in our bodies as we age are considered abnormal, and treatment, typically by drugs, is often advised (Moynihan & Cassels, 2005). Discussion of clinical trial results on drugs throughout this book have shown that US FDA approval of a drug does not guarantee its safety or efficacy. Efficacy is often evaluated by surrogate endpoints of no real value, such as the lowering of moderately elevated blood pressures and cholesterol levels. Conversely, non-approval of a supplement or treatment by the FDA, as is the case for EDTA chelation for CVD, does not guarantee that the so-called alternative is either unsafe or ineffective. In the words of Moynihan & Cassels (p174): "The tough words of [an] FDA letter to [a] drug company might sit better in a script for a farce. Perhaps a tragedy. There is a bark, albeit a soft one, but no bite. It is the appearance of regulation without the substance. In this instance, as in so many others, there was no penalty even though the FDA had determined a violation of the rules on [drug] advertising."

General screening tests are often used to detect mythical "abnormalities" in people to make them candidates for drugs or treatments. When the treatments for the conditions sought are poor, or the condition is unusual, these screening tests and their scary results from false positives are a waste of resources and cause a lower quality-of-life for those caught by the system. (http://w3.aces.uiuc.edu/DLM/Liberty/Tales/Thalidomide.Html)

Patients should not have to protect themselves against the medical profession with all its financially conflicted members. Jerome P. Kassirer, M. D., former Editor of *The New England Journal of Medicine,* acknowledges that at present in the USA, patients must suspect self-serving bias in almost every recommendation for medical testing and treatment (Kassirer, 2005, p207).

Authoritarian Excesses

The Codex Alimentarius Commission was created in 1963 by the Food and Agriculture Organization and World Health Organization (FAO/WHO) of the United Nations to develop food standards, guidelines and related texts such as codes of practice under the Joint FAO/WHO Food Standards Programme. The main purposes of this program are protecting health of the consumers and ensuring fair trade practices in the food trade, and promoting coordination of all food standards work undertaken by international governmental and non-governmental organizations. This seems very sensible and humanitarian, but the Codex has a plan afoot to ban all non-prescription sales of vitamins and supplements.

Few Americans have heard of the Codex Alimentarius Commission partly because it meets in Europe and has not been publicized in the USA. This semi-secrecy is typical of the world government bureaucrats when they want to pass regulations with a minimum of fuss from the people being regulated. What supplements will Codex "allow" you to have? NONE that you can afford, and ALL by prescription only. The drug companies are licking their chops as they see the natural foods and health industry, (which has been eating into their profits) face wipe-out or take-over. The ruthlessness of the pharmaceutical industry is clearly evident in this move to monopolize the health food and nutrient business of the entire world. You think it will not happen here? A Codex-driven pharmaceutical takeover of the natural products industry in Canada is already in full swing. In fact, possession of DHEA, a harmless and valuable supplement, is now a felony in Canada, carrying the same penalty as possession of crack cocaine. Some foods are now being regulated as "drugs." (http://www.medicallibrary.net/sites/framer.html?/sites/_codex_alimentarius.html)

282

This book has shown that many supplements are of great value, despite their low cost, in preventing and treating some important conditions. Vitamins C, E, B6, B12, magnesium, coenzyme Q10 and others have been proven by experience and trials to have great benefits. The loss of these to consumer choice and restriction of them to prescription-only status, raising their prices, will be one of the great catastrophes of modern medicine, literally costing millions of lives. The Codex plot was concocted by the pharmaceutical industry: (http://www4.dr-rathfoundation.org/PHARMACEUTICAL_BUSINESS/ health_movement_against_codex/health_movement02.htm).

The European Court of Justice has made a decision, following the Codex, that will have 300 supplements off the shelves in the UK as of 1 Aug 05, with as many as 5000 to follow. Prime Minister Tony Blair criticized the decision, and 300 physicians and scientists plus 1 million others in the UK signed a petition for the UK to opt out. Thousands of vitamins are threatened by the ruling. (Laurance, 2005)

"As Codex continues its march, herbs are increasingly classed as drugs with restricted access. Germany has already complied fully by regulating all supplements and herbs as drugs. In a country with an age-old tradition of natural medicine, no one can freely access these products now. This is designed to assist drug companies in their technology of PharmaPrinting, which produces versions of herbs that will be standardised and patented by drug companies and approved by government regulators as drugs... There is a fortune to be made by multinational drug companies solely controlling the manufacture and sale of all life sustaining natural products. Many doctors and health freedom advocates are deeply disturbed by these events. Dr. Matthias Rath, a medical specialist in nutritional medicine demonstrated that nutritional supplements reversed many conditions including heart disease. He states: 'If the Codex Commission is allowed to obstruct the eradication of heart disease by restricting access to nutritional supplements, more than 12 million people world-wide will continue to die every year from premature heart attacks and strokes. Within the next generation alone, this would result in over 300 million premature deaths, more than in all the wars of mankind together...' One Scandinavian vitamin supplier was chased by the federal police for supplying vitamin C tablets that exceeded 200 mg. The amount of vitamin C contained in three oranges had made this man a criminal." (http://members.austarmetro.com.au/~hubbca/codex.htm)

According to Jamie Whyte, PhD in Philosophy, University of Cambridge, the British Medical Association has recommended that the UK tax the fat content of food. Aside from the scientific asininity of such a recommendation (see Myth 2), the arrogant challenge to civil liberties of such a tax is appalling (Else & Anderson, 2004).

Costs of Malignant Medical Myths

This book has shown that the prevailing medical myths on simple things, from daily aspirin to red wine consumption, to low fat diets and extreme exercise, provide few or no benefits, yet have serious costs. Many common classes of drugs are not only expensive, costing as much as $1,000,000 to prevent 1 heart attack for 1 year at best (Myth 3), but their adverse effects run up hospital expenses in the $billions. Many routine tests have no benefits, and lead to unnecessary biopsies and operations (see Myths 9 and 10). There is data that as many as 1/3 of all surgical operations in the USA are not necessary. Yet all this testing and treatment is reimbursed by medical insurance, Medicaid and Medicare.

Conversely, alternative treatments and supplements that actually do work, and which are often less costly than patented drugs or surgery, are usually not reimbursed by medical insurance and Medicare in the USA.

Medical insurers, including non-profits, have no incentive to keep claims down. They can always make a case for higher premiums based on claims. The officers then can obtain higher salaries and more perks based on the same percentage of the increased revenues from higher premiums.

As a medical insurer, Independence Blue Cross, to give one example, in its quarterly newsletter *Update* consistently gives ill-considered advice on diet and drugs, despite being fully informed by this author of what they are doing. Almost every issue of *Update* contains advice to fill up on carbohydrates with no exceptions for the obese or diabetics, to use whole grains with no exceptions for people with grain allergies (see Myth 2), and to do exercise in the absence of any evidence for its benefit (see Myth 6). Screening tests shown to be useless in Myths 3, 9 and 10 are routinely recommended. Like a broken 78-rpm record, a 1-page article in a recent issue actually manages to recommend very high-carb foods, frozen foods regardless of vitamin loss due to processing, and nonfat dry milk despite its oxycholesterol content. The article, addressing the elderly who live alone, laments that many have diets low in vitamin A, vitamin C, some B vitamins and calcium. The impossibility of taking in an *optimal* amount of vitamin C and some others from food, and the omission of magnesium as a generally deficient diet mineral, indicate an appalling lack of knowledge at best (Floria, 2004).

The socialized medicine or national health systems in other countries hold down the costs as much by denying beneficial treatments than by not paying for unnecessary tests, drugs and surgery. These systems are not the answer to skyrocketing costs. With 1/5 of hospitalizations occurring because of the adverse effects of drugs, and costing more than the drugs themselves, lower drug costs are not much of a saving compared with eliminating the use of drugs that do not extend or improve life. What is called "evidence-based medicine" is the answer, but, granted, it can be almost impossible to obtain or identify unbiased evidence.

The tendency of Big Pharma to publish only drug trial results which are positive is so pervasive and misleading that Spain mandated by law that the results of all clinical trials run in that country must be published. There is no reason to believe that Big Pharma is giving the FDA *all* trial results, rather than only the most positive ones. As this is being written, several influential medical journals have made it clear that they will not publish results of a trial unless the trial protocol was first registered in a public manner (website). However, the loophole is obvious — the drug sponsor does not have to report any results! An editor of the *Journal of the American Medical Association* stated in an interview on PBS on 10 Sep 04 that we have to trust them, the editors, to find any registered trials on a given drug with no results before they publish an article on a positive result. Only if they do this search in order to write an editorial on the missing data from trials with negative or missing results would we know there was a problem. Otherwise the article on the positive trial would be published as usual. The other journals involved in the registration requirement so far are *The New England Journal of Medicine* and *The Lancet.*

While there is plenty of malpractice in the USA, "...outsized jury awards for the plaintiffs and their attorneys is another major source of the outrageous costs of medical care. Among the low blows in the malpractice debate delivered by doctors, a Texas database accessible online to doctors effectively blacklisted past Lone Star State malpractice plaintiffs, their lawyers, and their expert witnesses within the medical community. The site was all but shut down in early 2004 after a barrage of criticism... Next, near-simultaneous instances of doctors refusing treatment to malpractice lawyers, sympathetic lawmakers, or their family members sprung up in South Carolina, New Hampshire, and Mississippi... And back in June, 2004, one brazen MD submitted a formal proposal to the American Medical Association suggesting that physicians should be officially allowed to *withhold care* from attorneys involved on the plaintiff side of medical malpractice cases." (Douglass, Jr., 2004)

Judges share blame for allowing frivolous malpractice suits and huge awards. Juries also get carried away. There is plenty of blame to go around. Outsize punitive awards must be curbed by federal law. Only by doing this is there any chance that malpractice insurance premiums will go down.

One of the reasons that malpractice has been overdone is the supposition that most medical errors are made by "bad" doctors, especially surgeons. Investigation has shown that this is not true — most surgical mistakes are the occasional ones of average surgeons. Destroying their careers does not help the rest of us at all, nor does it improve the self-confidence of the rest of them (Gawande, 2002). This is a tough concept to sell because we want to believe in small numbers of bad guys and eliminate them. Another case was exposed 40 years ago by Ralph Nader. Turns out that 9% of drivers have 48% of the collisions. Using the Poisson statistical distribution, one finds that *by chance alone* 9% of drivers would have 40% of the collisions (Nader, 1965, p290). That is why no-fault insurance was such a great idea. In most cases an average driver has a moment of inattention, or is debilitated by a drug, the situation suddenly deteriorates (night, fog, ice, mechanical failure) and crashes, or is simply crashed into. Average drivers who are victims of chance should not be slammed with above-average punishment. Same goes for surgeons.

Over promotion of tests, drugs, high-dose ionizing radiation and devices has been bared in this book and others (Moynihan & Cassels, 2005). Surgery should not be spared. There are too many operations. Why should you believe such a blanket statement? Because of the number of surgeries that fail to give a positive long-term result. More than 300,000 people have kidney shunts fitted per year; about 2/3 fail within a year. (Hooper, 2005) More than 500,000 coronary artery bypass grafts are done annually; about 1/2 fail in the first year (Hooper, 2005, Gawande, 2002). Bare metal stents for coronary arteries have proven equally useless (Katritsis et al., 2005).

For at least 10 years in the USA there have been claims that a national health service could hold down medical costs because it is a single payer with huge bargaining power. The subversion of the FDA, NIH, USDA and other federal agencies by some medical providers including Big Pharma is so extreme that there is no reason to believe that Medicare will be any more resistant to corruption. Arthur M. Evangelista, a former FDA investigator, reckoned that 80% of the top level FDA officials had some sort of financial conflict with the drug companies they are supposed to regulate (Evangelista, 2004). Corruption at the NIH was detailed in the Introduction, and of the USDA in Myth 2.

The solution is not to chip minor fractions off the cost of medical care. The problem is that too many screening tests, too many surgeries and too many drugs are promoted. Effective supplements and generic drugs are usually ignored as low-cost alternatives. Big Pharma has arranged a number of insidious disparagements to discourage the use of alternatives. In a free-enterprise economy, one can hardly blame businesses for trying every lawful method to raise profits. The corruption of physicians, hospitals, insurers and government administrators is another matter.

Sometimes good things happen. On 8 Jun 05 the US House of Representatives voted 218 to 210 to prohibit outside doctors and scientists who work for drug companies from sitting on Food and Drug Administration panels that pass judgment on those same companies' products. Will the US Senate confirm this?

Several suggestions come to mind to curb this intransigent set of problems.

(1) Since Big Pharma and others can hide behind FDA approval, which they influence, and our ultimate protection is from class-action lawsuits, the drug section of the FDA should be abolished, except for increasing the size of the tiny staff that collates reports on adverse effects from drugs and medical devices. Let Big Pharma sink or swim on its own judgment. As soon as an example is made in a class-action lawsuit, perhaps destroying one company, the others will become very careful. Our only real protection at present has been the threat of lawsuits.

(2) Government employees at NIH, etc., should be barred from any consulting agreements with businesses or any other form of compensation or gifts other than their already high salaries.

(3) All clinical trials of devices, tests, surgeries and drugs (including supplements) should be registered with the NIH or the surviving bit of the FDA. All results should have to be published before any of these interventions are permitted on the market. Results obtained after market introduction also would have to be published. An NIH observer pair would be assigned to each study to make sure it was not perverted or buried. Alternatively, the NIH should run all clinical trials intended to show that a proposed new drug is better than both a placebo and the best current drug for the same condition, including generics. Tests or devices need similarly open trials. All results should be required to be published. For more details on this and other machinations of Big Pharma, see *The Truth About the Drug Companies*, 2004, by Marcia Angell, MD, former Editor-in-Chief of *The New England Journal of Medicine.*

(4) Medical insurance ought to be for emergency care and catastrophic care only, say for claims over $20,000 for the latter. Free market efficiencies (smart shopping) would then bring down the cost of routine care in a hurry. Would you voluntarily pay $1,000 for annual medical examinations and tests if you had no symptoms? I doubt it. Losses to administrative overhead for medical insurance will be cut by 90%. The premiums for coverage against emergency and catastrophic care only would be a small fraction of what they are now.

(5) The Federal Trade Commission should require sponsors of medical websites, "educational" seminars for health providers, fake consumer lobbying groups and fake disease-specific self-help groups to disclose their identity and provide contact information.

## So What can *You* Do?

Using some of the books reviewed in Myth 2, see whether you are a candidate for a low-carb, high-fat diet. It is not healthful for most people to eat mostly carb or protein, or to be vegetarians.

Many health problems are caused by food allergies, typically to wheat gluten and gliadin or to milk proteins. These problems include eczema, frequent indigestion, celiac disease, Crohn's disease, colitis, cancers of the digestive system, multiple sclerosis, and lupus. Most physicians never consider food allergies for these problems. An alert allergist must be consulted.

If you are not sick, food will provide most of the vitamins and minerals you need; but there are some exceptions, for example, most people over 40 years old would benefit from supplemental vitamin C and magnesium. In areas with little sun, vitamin D would be added.

Find a physician who combines the best of mainstream and alternative treatments. Try to have a companion with you for evaluating the physician, preferably a medically knowledgeable companion, who will also be present for examinations. Avoid physicians whose office areas are completely polluted by pens, pads, mugs, wall hangings and brochures that are entirely gifts of drug companies. Explain to your physician that you will avoid screening tests and drugs whenever possible. Put your physician's fears of lawsuit to rest by writing a letter absolving her of any liability for a missed diagnosis from any test you refused to accept (Welch, 2004, pp 177-190).

Check the Institute of Physician Evaluation (http://ipe.nbme.org/) and otherwise search the internet or contact your State Medical Board to find how many complaints your medical providers have been subjected to. If you cannot be assigned a satisfactory physician by an HMO, change to a PPO. A physician who is a member of ACAM (see Myth 7) is more likely to have patient welfare as a high priority.

Find a registered pharmacist who will check drug doses, choice of drugs, drug interactions, and which supplements are needed to counteract nutritional deficiencies caused by drugs. Some pharmacists are unusually helpful and not afraid of the physician (Hogan, 2004).

Find a hospital by asking friends and relatives about their hospital experiences. Check out the emergency room. Check reports on the performance of the hospital provided by Solucient (http://solucient.ecnext.com/coms2/page_ush2002_description?referid=1850), or search the internet for State Medical Board evaluations of hospitals. If you must go to a hospital for an emergency or a planned operation, or if you are stuck with one for childbirth, try to have a companion with you, preferably a medically knowledgeable one. Hospitals can provide a cot for your companion to stay overnight or until you are stable. A companion may be needed to bring in healthful food, since most hospitals serve sugary, or otherwise high-carb meals with *trans* fat. Do not ask the hospital dietitian for a diabetic diet, or the results will be even worse.

Do not take any drug, even over-the-counter or generic prescription drugs, unless you check on their safety, at the least in *Worst Pills, Best Pills* and its *Companion* (See Appendix A), and in *Prescription for Disaster* by Moore. Check the dose in *Overdose* by Cohen. Check the Family PDR (http://www.pdrhealth.com/drug_info/rxdrugprofiles/alphaindexa.shtml). Check *Dr. Atkins' Vita-Nutrient Solution* (Appendix A) for possible vitamin and supplement use instead of drugs for a specific condition. Information on internet sites had better be backed up by references to peer-reviewed papers on trials or studies. You can, at least, read the abstracts of these trials on PubMed (http://www.ncbi.nih.gov/entrez/query.fcgi). From any source, watch out for clinical trials with no control or placebo groups, relative risks with no absolute risks, or changes in death rates from a particular condition with no all-cause death rates. Another favorite trick is testing drugs on healthy male adults, then using the results to prescribe for women, children and the elderly as well.

If you do experience unexpected adverse effects from drugs, see whether others have by going to www.DrugIntel.com. Do not expect your physician to reveal all or even any side-effects of any drug. Look them up in *Worst Pills Best Pills* or the Public Citizen website: http://www.publiccitizen.org/hrg/ and http://www.prodigy.nhs.uk/PILs/index.asp. Both sources are, nevertheless, too sanguine about chemotherapy, cholesterol and blood pressure drugs.

Antibiotics usually kill beneficial bacteria along with the targeted invaders. Swallowing yogurt does not replace all the main beneficial bacteria. For dealing with this problem, there is a good source of information on probiotics, the friendly and essential bacteria: *Bacteria for Breakfast* by Kelly Dowhower Karpa, PhD, 2003.

Summing Up

The USA may have some of the best trauma care in the world. Emergency medical technicians with defibrillators and oxygen, etc., may arrive within minutes of a request, may perform heroically, and may get the patient to a hospital in minutes, often by helicopter.

Major surgical operations can be among the best-performed in the world, as well they should be, because price is no object, due to the third-party-payer norm, or rich patients. On the other hand, there is too much surgery, and too often it is too extensive.

The USA certainly has the most expensive medical care in the world, yet this has not led to the longest-lived population, the best survival for newborns or almost any other population group, or the lowest obesity and diabetes rates in the world. Natural events such as childbirth are medicalized to the detriment of mother and child alike.

Too many screening tests are run, and many should be refused. Among them are those for TC, LDL, the PSA test, mammograms and most other tests for cancer in people with no symptoms. If there is no satisfactory treatment for a condition, as is the case for most cancers, there is little point in having a test done.

Too many drugs are prescribed, including many of the best-sellers such as antiinflammatories (NSAIDS or steroids), anti-cholesterol, antihypertensive, and antidepressant drugs. Too many antibiotics are prescribed for non-bacterial infections. Too many drugs are prescribed at too high a dose. Most are prescribed with no instructions for dealing with the nutritional problems drugs cause.

Medical errors were estimated to have caused 225,000 premature deaths in the USA alone in a recent year, half from FDA-approved drugs used according to instructions.

Approval of drugs, tests and devices by the USA FDA, too often merely copied by other countries, does not guarantee either safety or efficacy. Conversely, non-approval by the FDA does not guarantee lack of either safety or efficacy, especially of non-patentable alternatives.

Vitamins and other supplements are required by the FDA to have uninformative labels which may make users overlook benefits. Certain of these supplements shown to be both safe and effective by evidence given throughout this book would have been banned by the FDA but for a congressional intervention in 1994.

Food labeling required by the FDA wrongly focused on calorie content, cholesterol and saturated fat content, and even sodium ion content. At present new FDA plans are said to address *trans* fat content, misleading serving sizes, and other errors in food labels. Sadly, we may anticipate that the most useful part of a food label will remain the list of Ingredients.

According to Stephen Fulder, physician-patient relations are changing for the better:

> "You can use alternative medicine to look after yourself during [or instead] of medical treatment... Now there is a range of new options and choices available to all of us, options having nothing to do with physicians and hospitals and which the medical staff often do not know anything about [and often disparage].
>
> "Doctors used to be more distant, superior and unapproachable. They expected patients to beg treatment, and dutifully swallow whatever was decided for them without a murmur. The patient was not part of his treatment — it was done to him. Although medicine today is still today highly technical and confusing, patients often feel freer to take part [perhaps because of information so easy to obtain on the internet]. They are becoming more active. There is today a growing mood that a patient is a consumer who should be free to choose, to question, and to select the treatment that is in his *own* interest rather than the physician's. In the new age of patient power, physicians are learning to listen. It is now up to you to take advantage of this and ask the right questions." (Fulder, 1994, p4).

There are some wise and helpful medical providers out there, including pharmacists, physicians, nurse practitioners, physician assistants, midwives and doulas. Find the good ones and give them a chance.

Acknowledgment for Conclusion

Frances Eleanor Heckert Pane, MSLS, edited this chapter and provided many suggestions.

References for Conclusion

Douglass, Jr., WC (2004) *Daily Dose,* August 31, 2004 <realheath@healthiernews.com>
Else L, Anderson A (2004). Get it Right! *New Scientist* 4 Sep 04, pp60-63.
Evangelista AM (2004). Government and Regulatory Malfeasance and Its Impact on Public Health. Talk at The Weston A. Price Foundation Fifth Annual Conference, *Wise Traditions 2004,* Arlington, VA 1-3 Oct 04.
Floria B (2004). Improving Your Nutrition If You Eat Alone. *Update* 4(3):17.
Fulder SM (1994). *How to Survive Medical Treatment,* New York, NY: Barnes & Noble.
Gawande A (2002). *Complications: A Surgeon's Notes on an Imperfect Science,* New York, NY: Metropolitan Books, Henry Holt.
Hogan B (2004). The Pharmacist Who Says No to Drugs. *AARP Bulletin* 45(8):3,12-14.
Hooper R (2005). Bypass surgery with a twist. *New Scientist,* 11 Jun, p28.

Kassirer JP (2005). On The Take: How Medicine's Complicity with Big Business Can Endanger Your Health. New York, NY: Oxford University Press.

Katritsis DG, Ioannidis JPA (2005). Percutaneous Coronary Intervention Versus Conservative Therapy in Nonacute Coronary Artery Disease, A Meta-Analysis. *Circulation* 111:2906-2912.

Laurance J (2005). From *The Independent,* 13 July 05: http://news.independent.co.uk/uk/health_medical/article298799.ece

Moynihan R, Cassels A (2005). *Selling Sickness: How the World's Biggest Pharmaceutical companies are Turning Us All into Patients,* New York, NY: Nation Books.

Nader R (1965). *Unsafe at any Speed,* New York, NY: Grossman.

Null G, Dean C, Feldman M, Rasio D, Smith D (2003). *Death by Medicine.* Nov 2003 – Nutrition Institute of America.

Stanfield B (2000). Is US Health Really the Best in the World? *Journal of the American Medical Association,* 284(4):483-485.

Welch HG (2004). *Should I Be Tested for Cancer? Maybe Not and Here's Why,* Berkeley, CA, USA, University of California Press.

# Appendix A: Recommended Books and Websites

A recommendation does not mean that *all* information in a book or website is accurate, but most of it is believed to be. Out-of-print books may be found used or in libraries.

## General Medical Topics

Angell, Marcia, MD, *The Truth About the Drug Companies,* New York, NY: Random House, 2004.

Cohen, Jay S., *Over Dose. The Case Against the drug Companies.* New York, NY: Tarcher/Putnam, 2001.

Gawande, Atul (2002). *Complications: A Surgeon's Notes on an Imperfect Science,* New York, NY: Metropolitan Books, Henry Holt. Also covers pain, obesity, sudden infant death.

Gigerenzer, Gerd, *Calculated Risks: How to Know When the Numbers Deceive You.* New York, N.Y: Simon & Schuster, 2002.

Kassirer JP (2005). *On The Take: How Medicine's Complicity with Big Business Can Endanger Your Health.* New York, NY: Oxford University Press.

Lomborg, Bjørn,*The Skeptical Environmentalist.* Cambridge, England, UK: Cambridge University Press, 2001.

Levy TE (2002). *Vitamin C, Infectious Diseases, and Toxins*, Xlibris.com, Xlibris.

McGee, Charles T., *Heart Frauds: Uncovering the Biggest Health Scam in History,* Colorado Springs, CO: HealthWise Pubs., 2001.

Moore, Thomas J., *Heart Failure,* New York, NY: Random House, 1989.

Moore, Thomas J., *Prescription for Disaster. The Hidden Dangers in Your Medicine Cabinet.* New York, NY: Simon & Schuster, 1998.

Moynihan R, Cassels A (2005). *Selling Sickness: How the World's Biggest Pharmaceutical Companies are Turning Us All into Patients,* New York, NY: Nation Books.

Pelton, Ross & LaValle, James B., *The Nutritional Cost of Prescription Drugs,* Englewood, CO: Perspective/Morton, 2000.

Pert, Candace B., *Molecules of Emotion,* New York, NY: Scribner, 1997.

Robin, Eugene D., *Matters of Life & Death: Risks and Benefits of Medical Care,* Stanford, CA: Stanford Alumni Assoc., 1984. Shocking revelations of the arbitrary and capricious nature of the adoption of medical tests and procedures that become dogma.

Robinson, J., *Prescription Games. Money, Ego, and Power Inside the Global Pharmaceutical Industry.* Toronto, Ontario: McClelland & Stewart, 2001.

Skrabanek, P. & McCormick, J., *Follies and Fallacies in Medicine,* Glasgow, Scotland, UK: Tarragon Press, 1989. Exposes logical flaws in clinical trials on tests as common as mammography and in diagnosing hypertension or recommending alteration of "lifestyle" factors.

Wolfe Sidney, Sasich Larry D.,*Worst Pills Best Pills.* New York, N.Y.: Pocket Books, 1999.

Wolfe Sidney, Sasich Larry D.,*Worst Pills, Best Pills, Companion for Use with the 1999 Edition,* Washington, DC: Public Citizen Health Research Group, 2002.

www.drugintel.com
www.health-heart.org
www.jrussellshealth.com/

## Aspirin and Nutritional Supplements

Atkins, Robert C., *Dr Atkins Vita-Nutrient Solution,* London, England: Pocket Books, Simon & Schuster, 1998. The best referenced book on vitamins and supplements I have found is also backed by Atkins' clinical experience.

Feinman, Susan E., Ed., *Beneficial and Toxic Effects of Aspirin,* CRC Press, Boca Raton, FL, 1993.

Hickey, Steve, Roberts, Hilary, *Ascorbate. The Science of Vitamin C.* Napa, CA; Lulu.com, Inc.., 2004.

Holick MF and Jenkins M, *The UV Advantage,* New York, NY:Simon & Schuster, 2003. Excellent on vitamin D, but ignore the diet advice.

Levy TE (2002). *Vitamin C, Infectious Diseases, and Toxins*, Xlibris.com, Xlibris.

## Low-Carbohydrate Diets

deMan, John M., *Princples of Food Chemistry,* 3rd ed., Gaithersburg, MD: Aspen, 1999.

Bernstein, Richard K., *Dr. Bernstein's Diabetes Solution,* Rev., Boston, MA: Little, Brown & Co., 2003.

Enig, Mary G., *Know Your Fats,* Silver Spring, MD: Bethesda Press, 2000.

Enig, Mary G., Fallon, Sally, *Eat Fat, Lose Fat,* New York, NY: Hudson Street Press, 2005.

Fallon S (2001). *Nourishing Traditions,* 2nd ed., Washington, DC: New Trends Publishing.

Ravnskov, Uffe., *The Cholesterol Myths: Exposing the Fallacy that Saturated Fat and Cholesterol Cause Heart Disease,* Washington, DC: New Trends Publishing, 2000.

Reading, Chris & Meillon, Ross, *Trace Your Genes to Health,* Ridgefield, CT: Vital Health Press, 1999.

www.THINCS.org
www.PowerHealth.net/nutrition.htm
www.westonaprice.org/
www.drbralyallergyrelief.com/
www.LowCarbEating.com/

## Statin Drugs

Graveline, Duane, *Lipitor, Thief of Memory, Statin Drugs and the Misguided War on Cholesterol,* 2004. www.buybooksontheweb.com
www.THINCS.org
www.health-heart.org
www.thenhf.com/articles_08.htm
www.vitamincfoundation.org/statinalert/

## Exercise

Solomon, Henry A., *The Exercise Myth.* Orlando, FL: Harcourt Brace Jovanovich, 1984.

## EDTA Chelation

Carter, James P., *Racketeering in Medicine: The Suppression of Alternatives.* Norfolk, VA: Hampton Roads Press, 1992.

Cranton, Elmer M., *A Textbook on EDTA Chelation Therapy,* 2nd ed. Charlottesville, VA: Hampton Roads Publ. Co., 2001.

## Radiation Hormesis

Luckey, Thomas D., *Radiation Hormesis,* Boca Raton, FL: CRC Press, 1991.

Ottoboni, M. Alice, *The Dose Makes the Poison,* 2nd ed., New York, NY:Van Nostrand Reinhold, 1991.

Rockwell, Theodore, *Creating the New World: Stories and Images from the Dawn of the Atomic World,* Bloomington, IN: 1st Books Library, 2004.

## Cancer

Bognar, David, *Cancer. Increasing Your Odds for Survival.* Alameda, CA: Hunter House, Inc., 1998.

Elias, Thomas D., *The Burzynski Breakthrough*, Rev. Ed., 40% New Content with Clinical Trial Statistics. Nevada City, CA: Lexikos, 2001.

Gearin-Tosh, Michael, *Living Proof : A Medical Mutiny,* Scribner, 2002. See Introduction or Myth #10 for descrption.

Haley, Daniel, *Politics in Healing: The Suppression and Manipulation of American Medicine.* Washington, DC: Potomac Valley Press, 2000.

Holick MF and Jenkins M, *The UV Advantage,* New York, NY:Simon & Schuster, 2003. Excellent on vitamin D, but ignore the diet advice.

Lee, John R., Zava, D. & Hopkins, V.,. *What Your Doctor May* Not *Tell You About Breast Cancer — How Hormone Balance Can Save Your Life,* New York, NY: Warner Books, 2002.

McTaggart L, Ed. (2001). *The Cancer Handbook. What's Really Working.* 2nd ed., Bloomington, IL: Vital Health Publishing, 2001.

Moss, Ralph W., *The Cancer Industry.* Brooklyn, NY: Equinox Press, 1999.

Moss, Ralph W., *Questioning Chemotherapy,* Brooklyn, NY: Equinox Press, 2000.

Welch, H. Gilbert, *Should I Be Tested for Cancer? Maybe Not and Here's Why,* Berkeley, CA, USA, University of California Press, 2004.

www.cancerdecisions.com/

www.breathing.com/articles/brassieres.htm

## Appendix B: Individual Reviews of a Dozen Books on Low-Carb Diets

Drafts of all reviews except those on Atkins' and Mercola's books were sent to the authors or their associates for criticism; responses were received from all but Eades and McCully.

Most of the authors make recommendations on aspects of diet that have nothing to do with carbohydrates. Often there are no supporting studies for these positions on food items as diverse as how much water, coffee, tea, and wine to drink; how much and what types of fat to eat; as well whether complex carbohydrates are generally superior to simple carbohydrates, and what supplements to take. Sometimes there is scientific support for their positions, but just as often there is not. Many recommendations are made on seemingly logical but actually unsupported theoretical grounds, but some of the authors have years of clinical experience to draw upon, and did. As Winston S. Churchill once said, "Logic is a poor guide compared with custom."

References cited in Myth 2 or here as being in Appendix B are the ones without dates, and refer to one of the 12 books reviewed here.

**Dr. Atkins' *New* Diet Revolution**, 3rd ed., by Robert C. Atkins, MD.
New York, NY: Evans, 2002. 442 pp. $24.95 (hardcover). ISBN 1-59077-002-1.

Brash, immodest by admission, self-promoting, Atkins' tome is, nevertheless, solidly backed scientifically by individual citations to about 400 peer-reviewed papers. Explanations are given as to why all calories in the diet are not equal, and why people will lose weight on a low-carb diet even if it contains more calories than a high-carb diet. The relation of hyperinsulinemia to a high diet load of carbs is clearly explained, as is the reality that insulin is the primary fat-building enzyme. A large number of diet trials and epidemiological data are quoted in support. Some were described in Myth 2. Atkins also has the advantage of about 30 years of clinical experience in his own practice, which comprised "tens of thousands" of patients. However, one of the greatest gaps in Atkins' work was his failure to use clinical assay data from his own patients before and after they tried his low-carb diet, and other aspects of his overall weight-loss plan, to show what fraction really were improved, or not, or had dropped out. His excuse (p65) was that his responsibility to his patients would not allow him to use any of them as controls; but that did not prevent Lutz from citing assay data from his patients, anonymously, as described in Myth 2.

Atkins shows the progression from high-carb diets to higher insulin levels to insulin resistance, to NIDDM (Type 2) with high insulin to later Type 2 with low insulin levels. He also shows the relation of obesity with NIDDM, and of NIDDM with heart disease, amputations, blindness, kidney failure and collagen problems, many due to glycation of proteins (p277).

Atkins' actual program demands not only a low-carb diet, but also at least moderate exercise (distinguishing aerobic from anaerobic, p252-3), use of supplements including fiber, and some standard blood work to follow progress. He reports an over 90% success rate with people who began the program at his Center, but did not define success or provide a dropout rate. The Atkins program diet begins with a few days to weeks eating a low-carb diet with only 20g of net metabolizable energy (NME) from carbs per day (Induction), and to help with the count, there is an extensive table of "digestible carbohydrate" per serving in the book, as well as advice on how to determine a rough NME from an FDA food label. Since the carbs recommended in all phases are mostly of low GI, this is not as restrictive as it seems, since 40-50 g of carbs according to Atkins' interpretation of FDA food labels can be used. The object, from the beginning, is to stop glycolysis (metabolizing glucose for energy) as the prime source of energy, and replace it partially by lipolysis, burning one's own fat for energy, so the weight loss is mostly to be from one's own fat. This phase is carried to ketosis, monitored with test strips for ketones in the urine, and the patient is to remain just short of ketosis until most of the desired weight loss occurs. Atkins clearly distinguishes the non-threatening ketosis of low serum glucose from the potentially lethal ketoacidosis due to the high serum glucose of Type I diabetics (p82ff). Ongoing Weight Loss is the next phase with 20-30g of NME from carb daily, and the amount is individualized based on testing, symptoms and weighing. Pre-Maintenance is next with 25-60 g, then finally Lifetime Maintenance with 25-100g. Use of certain low-caloric sweeteners is included, but not aspartame (p164). Atkins' favorite is sucralose, but stevia is not mentioned. Eating at least every 6 hours when awake is highlighted. Atkins emphasizes that people with the metabolic problem with carbs (carb-sensitivity) will never be cured, so an appetizing, varied and nutritious diet must be followed for life. Food allergies are addressed briefly (pp295-9).

Warnings against "twisted" (p308) *trans* fats are copious. See Figure 2-1 for the structure of a common *toxic trans* fatty acid. There are 87 pages of recipes for which preparation times are given (many very short). A daily 100 mL of wine is permitted when it does not hinder weight loss. Coffee is forbidden (p164); however, in a recent clinical trial, coffee consumption was inversely and strongly associated with lower risk of NIDDM (van Dam et al., 2002), so there were no grounds (pun intended) to forbid coffee.

Almost every objection to the program has been countered. The weight lost includes 2-4 kg of water at the beginning, but is then truly fat loss (p84-5). Higher protein consumption does not cause kidney damage (p86). Higher fat consumption does not cause gallstone formation (p87) or heart disease (p88). A great variety of related conditions are considered: excessive insulin from use of oral diabetic drugs or injected insulin, to the interference of many types of prescription drugs on weight loss, thyroid problems, food allergies and candida infections. Much criticism has been leveled at the unlimited amounts of fat and protein supposedly allowed, and Atkins indeed ballyhoos "no calorie counting" (pp1, 14, 83, 107, 124). However, his actual instructions are to eat fat and protein until one is satisfied, not stuffed; to pause when unsure to see whether one can stop eating. One of his major points is that food cravings disappear when carb intakes go down. The low-carb diet usually *lowers* LDL, and especially TG, and may raise HDL. He also notes that one can lose fat and gain lean body mass (LBM; all but fat), so body measurements for the very active can be more important than weight loss.

Among the few minor deviations from best nutritional science are the doubtful recommendations for liberal use of oils containing large amounts of omega-6 fatty acids (Ottoboni, pp37, 123-6, 193), too much concern about saturated fats (Ottoboni, pp54, 122, 129; Ravnskov, 2000, pp15-46), a recommendation for use of soy flour (p207) despite its phytate content that interferes with mineral absorption (Lentner, 1981, p265), and a recommendation to eat 10-20 olives to alleviate hunger, despite their salt content of 8.6 - 17.3 g! Atkins appears to accept the conventional (but incorrect) view that high total cholesterol or LDL levels predict cardiovascular problems. This is mitigated by his preference for the use of high serum HDL levels and also a low ratio of TG to HDL as desirable (p304). He admits that some people will not lower their total cholesterol levels on his program, while not quite understanding that it does not matter (Ottoboni, p119ff; Ravnskov, 2000, pp47-93).

**Life Without Bread: How a Low-Carbohydrate Diet Can Save Your Life,**
by Christian B. Allan, PhD & Wolfgang Lutz, MD. Los Angeles, CA:Keats, 2000. xiv + 240 pp.
$16.95 (paperback). ISBN 0-658-00170-1.

Easy to read, very clear, Allan & Lutz state their main message at the beginning and repeat it many times: Without exception, a low-carbohydrate diet will improve health by reversing many common conditions from insulin resistance to Crohn's disease to cancer. "The true fad diet of today is, in fact, eating too many carbohydrates." (p49) The distinction between good and bad carbs is made by christening the bad ones "utilizable" (instead of Atkins' "digestible"). Rather than burden the reader with GI and GL, the old unit of utilizable carb, the bread unit (BU), is adopted. This is 12 g of digestible carb per BU. A short table of foods with their BU per serving is given at the beginning and a long one is given at the end of the book. The main message is simple: Restrict carbs to 6 BU (72 g) per day. Eat any desired non-carbs without restriction. There is no individualization in contrast with Atkins, Eades and others. The specific benefits of the low-carb diet, oddly, are not given early, but much later.

Another unique feature of this book is that results of clinical assays on Lutz's patients before and after initiation of the low-carb diet are presented (see Myth 2 for examples).

The history of low-carb nutrition is given, beginning with a possibly apocryphal story from antiquity and leading to modern trials. There are citations in the text to about 100 peer-reviewed papers.

The metabolic balance between insulin and glucagon is given with diagrams showing how hyperinsulinemia can affect growth, sex drive, alertness and irritability. The special folly of feeding children high-carb diets is presented. It was noted that there is no requirement for any carb in the human diet, but that bacteria prefer glucose for energy. The DHT is demolished with evidence including the preference of the heart for fat over carb for energy. A history of the demonization of cholesterol and the discovery of the effects of the undesirable homocysteine (see McCully & McCully book review below) in CVD are presented. The need for fat in the diet is emphasized. The lack of evidence for kidney damage on a low-carb diet is noted (pp100-1). Quite a number of gastrointestinal conditions are alleviated with a low-carb diet. The authors note that the use of oral diabetes drugs, insulin and the use of other drugs may be diminished or eliminated by means of a low-carb diet. Finally obesity is addressed (pp131-146) with the evidence that low-fat diets have caused the present epidemics of obesity, insulin resistance or full-blown NIDDM. Then the adequacy of micronutrients in a low-carb diet is presented. An entire chapter on diet and cancer gives examples and evidence that low-carb (high-fat) diets do not increase cancer rates and may reduce them (pp172-7). The non-dangers of saturated fat are noted. Then the authors go back to the history of diets and make several main and unusual points: (1) The reduction of carb intake to nearly zero is not necessary to obtain the benefits of low-carb diets; (2) The 40% carb diet commonly promoted for athletes is not low enough (8-12% energy from carb is what 12 BU/day represents); and (3) Too rapid reduction in carb % can cause severe problems in the elderly or ill, and the reduction should be slow (just opposite to Atkins and Eades).

Some final helpful hints are to limit fruit and especially fruit juice consumption because of the high carb content and fast absorption: "The USDA Food Pyramid that advocates eating 5 to 9 servings of fruits and vegetables per day is dangerously imprudent." This is because many fruits have high carbohydrate content and/or high GI. Oddly, 1-2 bottles of beer or "several glasses of wine" daily are said not to be harmful. A typical 350 ml bottle of beer contains over 1 BU of carb and stout 1.5 BU. Several 180 mL glasses of a typical low-sugar ("dry") wine (merlot) would contain 1.5 BU. The alcohol content would not be a problem (Theobald et al., 2001), except for those with IDDM, in whom these amounts would cause hypoglycemia (Bernstein, 118-120).

The program is not at all punishing, and this book is recommended for its clarity, lack of errors, and unique clinical findings.

**Dr. Bernstein's Diabetes Solution**, rev. ed. by Richard K. Bernstein, MD.
Boston, MA:Little, Brown, 2003.  xxiii + 391 pp.  $28 (hard bound).  ISBN 0-316-09906-6.

Based on 20 years of clinical experience and 57 years of suffering from IDDM himself (see Myth 2 for more biographical data), Dr. Bernstein brings a unique background to this book, which is aimed primarily at persons with IDDM or NIDDM. He estimates that 1/4 of all adult Americans have impaired glucose tolerance, and that 80% of these are overweight (pp65-74). The non-diet aspects of his treatment will be given less emphasis in this review than they would deserve in a more general one for diagnosed diabetics.

"The evidence is now simply overwhelming that elevated blood sugar is the major cause of the high serum lipid levels among diabetics and, more significantly, [is] the major factor in the high rates of various heart and vascular diseases associated with diabetes... My personal experience with diabetic patients is very simple. When we reduce dietary carbohydrate, blood sugars improve dramatically...[and in a few months lipid profiles do also]" (p434-5). He notes that excess insulin, produced in response to excess glucose, causes atherosclerosis (p40), and that normalizing glucose levels can reverse neuropathy, retinopathy, kidney damage, erectile dysfunction, hypertension, CVD, vision impairments and mental problems (p41). High TG and low HDL, rather than high TC, are associated with insulin resistance and CVD.

Focusing on diet at this point, it may be seen that Bernstein recommends 3-5 meals per day (or 3 meals and 2-3 snacks), eaten 3.5-4 hours apart for those not taking insulin, and 5 hours apart for those who do (pp168-9, 360). The main meals may contain just 6g, 12 g and 12 g of low-GI carb, a total of 30 g/day, about the same as in the initial diets of Atkins or of Eades & Eades. Since fat has no glycemic response, the amount eaten is not controlled. Diet contents (but not the variety of foods) are to be constant from day to day to maintain even blood glucose levels, because most of Bernstein's patients are taking oral hypoglycemic drugs and/or insulin, which must be balanced with food intake, and the results are to be checked frequently by self-determination of blood glucose levels. Individualization is highly encouraged within these parameters (pp187-9). Eating just enough to feel satisfied but not stuffed is a goal.

Bernstein is mindful that cooking raises GI (p144). Low GI caloric sweeteners such as sorbitol and fructose, so prominent in so-called "sugar-free" foods for diabetics, are shown to raise blood glucose too much over time, thus they are not suitable (p139-40). Of the non-caloric sweeteners, aspartame is acceptable if not cooked, along with saccharin and cyclamate, all in tablet, not powdered form with added sugars (p124). Fruit and honey are not recommended by Bernstein because of their fructose content, which raises blood glucose levels faster than any treatment can bring it down (p140). Alcohol in any form does not alter blood glucose, except lowering it at mealtimes for those with IDDM because it prevents the liver from converting protein to glucose. Bernstein is the only author to specify *dry* wine, limited to 1 glass (3 oz, 90 mL) (p132-3, 159, 173). [The "driest" (least sugary) of the common red wines, by the way, is pinot noir.] Some brands of soybean milk and flour are acceptable, as are bran-only crispbreads and toasted nori (pp152-4).

Unlike many authors in this group, Bernstein is not excited by many supplements, recommending vitamins C at 500 mg/day and E (400-1200 IU/day as gamma or mixed tocopherols) as well as B-complex and calcium only when needed, and the latter with vitamin D, magnesium, and manganese (p161, 175-6). As an insulin-mimetic agent, slow-release alpha-lipoic acid is recommended with evening primrose oil; both reduce insulin requirements (pp227-8).

The book begins with some biographical data, followed by 14 testimonials from patients before and after treatment, which demonstrate the appalling failure of conventional treatment of diabetes with concomitant complications, then descriptions of IDDM and NIDDM (with the little-known observation that no amount of injected insulin of the most rapid-acting type can control blood glucose from a high GL meal), then medical tests to determine the condition of individual patients, a compendium of the supplies needed, then a description of measuring and recording one's own blood sugar levels (with the revelation that only a few models of glucometer available at publication time were acceptably accurate, and that one should telephone Bernstein to find which ones); the virtue of small inputs of food, insulin or oral hypoglycemic drugs as leading to no or small mistakes, and establishing an overall treatment plan; all this is given in great detail. As noted above, a low-carb diet is a key part of the plan, so the basic food groups are described, 3 days of initial meal plans are given, and, in a later chapter, recipes for low-carb meals, with grams of carb and protein for each food and individual serving. Some history of the safety of low-carb diets, and conversely, the often devastating effects of high-carb diets (in Pima Indians, etc.) are given. A method of self-hypnosis is described for control of appetite, as is also the use of small doses of naltrexone, a drug used originally to curb narcotic addiction (p196-9). A whole chapter on exercise has the best distinction between aerobic and anaerobic exercise in this whole group of books, with the desirability of regressive anaerobic to build muscle mass in order to reduce insulin resistance. Consideration is given to those who must begin exercise very slowly, and many hints on how to avoid exercise damage are presented.

Oral hypoglycemic drugs are discussed (p224-6). The flaw in the concept behind the old sulfonylurea types is exposed. Among insulin-sensitizing agents in the glitazone class, it was noted that troglitzone (Rezulin™), was withdrawn from the market in May, 2002, because of side-effects. Metformin (Glucophage™), rosiglitazone (Avandia™) and pioglitazone (Actos™) are favored. The former now has an FDA "black box" warning for similar side-effects to those of Rezulin, and is known to increase homocysteine levels (Pelton et al., 2000, pp125, 136, 204). Avandia has new labeling, since it also has sometimes fatal side-effects (Wolfe, 2001, 2001a).

Next there is a chapter on where and how to inject insulin and on the characteristics of slow- and fast-acting insulins, followed by great detail on how to compensate for skipping meals, eating out, crossing time zones and hypoglycemia (and not confusing it with alcohol intoxication or autonomic neuropathy or postural hypotension, which may be caused by diuretics and antihypertensive drugs). Then there is a chapter on how to deal with erratic blood sugars caused by gastroparesis (delayed stomach emptying) and another chapter on how to deal with vomiting and diarrhea, in which an excellent discussion of ketoacidosis is given (p334-5). Advice on consideration for relatives, and tagging oneself as a diabetic is provided.

Appendix A is more technical. It gives the scientific basis for ignoring the nonsense on dietary cholesterol, fat, protein, carbohydrate, salt and the current high-fiber fad. Appendix B shows how to inform a hospital that food will be chosen by the patient, since "diabetic" diets in hospitals (as well as on airliners) are hyperglycemic, that the blood sugar measurement kit and the insulin supplies should not be confiscated, and that dextrose will not be used for re-hydration. Appendix C gives a long list of drugs that may affect blood sugar levels. Appendix D is about the all-important (to avoid amputation) foot care for diabetics. A glossary defines many terms for diabetics. In it, polyunsaturated fats, and to a lesser degree, monounsaturated fats, are given lukewarm mentions for virtues whose existence is doubtful (Ravnskov, 2000, pp15-97). There is a recipe index and an excellent general index.

There are a few footnotes to original medical papers with citations in the text; more would have been welcome. The tone of the book is simultaneously learned, determined, relentless, caring, and considerate, except for utter contempt for the American Diabetes Association. Limitations of time, money and insurance that may exist for patients are given consideration. Compared with several other books for diabetics your reviewer has seen, all of which recommended high-carb diets (for example, Whitaker, 1987), Bernstein's book is in a class by itself — the highest..

**Dangerous Grains: Why Gluten Cereal Grains May be Hazardous to Your Health,**
by James Braly, MD & Ron Hoggan, MA. New York, NY:Avery/Penguin Putnam, 2002. xx + 490 pp. $28 (hardcover). ISBN 1-58333-129-8.

Almost alone of the books in this group, *Dangerous Grains* recommends low-gluten diets, rather than generally low-carb diets, for the many sufferers from the "leaky gut" syndrome. Grossly under-diagnosed, this is a serious condition affecting 15-42% of humans for whom wheat products are a large portion of the diet (p30). Gluten is a protein fraction of wheat and other grains, and the toxic sub-fractions are called gliadin and glutenin. Perhaps initiated by preliminary damage to the lining of the GI tract by infection, gluten consumption in people sensitive to it leads to damage of the lining, allowing leaks of partially digested materials into the blood stream. These materials, often peptides, either create havoc directly, or the antibodies generated against them are damaging. Addictions to gluten-containing foods develop because of the presence of "feel-good" exorphins in them. These have similar effects to the endorphins produced inside your brain.

What is actually a sensitivity to gluten may be manifested initially as autism, ADHD (but see Ottoboni et al., 2003), depression, constipation, bloating or diarrhea, often treated only symptomatically, and may lead to irritable bowel syndrome, colitis, or enteritis. There may be progression to celiac disease in people genetically disposed to it, leading to an almost unbelievable set of dismal conditions, from IDDM, osteomyelitis, periodontal disease, and Crohn's disease into gastrointestinal cancer (evidence on p109), schizophrenia, multiple sclerosis, autism and even epilepsy; more are given in Appendix C. Victims may be under- or overweight; more are overweight. There are 187 symptoms of gluten sensitivity listed in Appendices A and D. So diagnosis is difficult and often delayed for decades of suffering until one of the terminal stages becomes obvious. The former best method of diagnosis, an intestinal biopsy, even the recently improved version, is deemed not as valuable or as safe as a number of new tests on blood (pp61-76, 177). Broad population screening beginning in childhood is strongly recommended (pp177-9). Cancer treatment by radiation or chemotherapy, both considered worthwhile in most cases by these authors, causes intestinal damage that often leads to gluten sensitivity (pp107-9).

The obvious treatment, often reversing serious symptoms, is avoiding gluten in the diet for the remainder of life. This is the basis for the recommendation of low-carb diets which are actually almost no-grain diets. A 1-day sample menu is given (p89-90) in which high-GI treats are kept separate from the other non-gluten-containing foods. Organic foods are recommended on theoretical grounds. Avoidance of *trans* and omega-6 fats and obtaining enough omega-3 fats are stressed (p86-7). Sources of gluten to avoid are given in Appendix B. As part of the diet, advice is given to supplement with quite a number of well-chosen vitamins and minerals (pp92-9). New evidence for supplementation by L-glutamine is given (pp176-7). Cautions are given on iron and calcium supplements, with a well-written explanation that calcium supplements are the last choice for prevention of osteoporosis, which is better prevented by magnesium, boron, zinc, and vitamins D and K. Supplements to lower homocysteine levels are also emphasized (p53-4, 97-8). Alcohol is said to cause or worsen a "leaky gut". Water is recommended at 8-12 glasses/day (p89). Drugs may contain gluten in formulations, which should be avoided (p84).

Of course, the USDA Food Pyramid receives well-deserved ridicule for making no exceptions for the gluten-sensitive (pp6,135,169). So also does the DHT, and the dangers of *low* cholesterol levels are laid out (p87). Widespread recommendations for whole grains are shown to be a disaster for the gluten-sensitive. Appendix E gives biographical data on prescient scientists who identified these sensitivities.

NIDDM is clearly described as a result of excessive carbohydrate (not necessarily containing gluten) consumption, which leads to excessive insulin production, leading to obesity, inflammation, cancer, allergy, CVD, and the overproduction of the undesirable prostaglandin E2 series of prostaglandins (p126). This agrees with all the other authors. However, people with NIDDM and its earlier manifestations get short shrift, unlike in Smith's book (see below). A great deal of fruit and other high-GI foods are recommended (p86). It is not clear how increased insulin levels, which are supposed to lower glucose levels, accelerate tumor growth (p115). Also, probably an oversight in writing, it does not make sense that removal of L-glutamine from the diet may reverse damage from a "leaky gut" (p177). A 200-item bibliography does not have citations in the text, a lack that is particularly annoying in this book, in which so many non-mainstream claims are made. One of the contact websites, www.cerealkillers.com, does not work; it is now info@drbralyallergyrelief.com.

This book is extremely valuable, nevertheless. One must ponder how much of the benefit of low-carb diets is from lower insulin levels, and how much is from avoiding gluten or other grain sensitivities.

**The ProteinPower LifePlan**, by Michael R. Eades, MD & Mary Dan Eades, MD.
New York, NY:Warner Books, 2000. xxviii + 434 pp. $10 (paperback). ISBN 0-446-52576-6.

Perhaps the title *The Protein Power LifePlan* and the authors' website: <www.eatprotein.com> are the least fortunate aspects of this encyclopedic work, since the Eades's are realistic about the amount and type of fats to be eaten as part of a low-carb diet. The actual diets are near the end of the book, which focuses on obesity and insulin resistance, leading to all the modern nutritional diseases, with attention given to gluten and other food sensitivities. The authors have a clinical practice in which "thousands" of patients are using their low-carb diet, and about 3,000,000 adopted the diet based on the sales of this and other books by the Eades' on diet.

There are 3 phases of diet: Intervention, Transition and Maintenance, in the manner of Atkins and Mercola. There are 3 levels of restriction, called Purist, Dilettante and Hedonist, in the manner of Mercola (see review below). Individualization is strongly encouraged. GI and GL and their limitations are discussed earlier, and the non-fiber carbs in foods, called effective carbohydrate content (ECC) and shown in a table (pp326-31) are used for the guidelines (p355), in which Intervention begins at a level of <40 ECC/day, Transition utilizes <60 ECC/day, and Maintenance allows levels of <80, <100 and <120 ECC/day depending on what each individual can tolerate. The minimum amount of protein to maintain one's lean body mass is readily determined from a table; one must know only one's height and weight (p312-3). The amount of fat to eat is said to take care of itself, and said not to matter if weight loss is not a goal, or the goal has been reached; otherwise, if one is consuming the correct ECC/day and not losing weight, the fat quantity must come down. Since more fat may be eaten than using the Eades' LifePlan diet than formerly, the type of fat is considered important, meaning, for the Eades, no *trans,* very little omega-6, at least the minimum few g of omega-3 to obtain or make DHA and EPA, no oxidized fats, and no restrictions on saturated fat or cholesterol intake. There are moderate numbers of menus and recipes, and advice for buying and cooking foods, eating out, and packing lunches including those for children. Organic food is recommended for the more restrictive plans, with the usual theoretical reasons; but neither this nor any of the food choices are fanatical or impractical in any way. Wasa™ crispbread is recommended as a bread substitute. Nuts and canola oil are seen as healthful (pp119-20). Among non-caloric sweeteners, aspartame is banned (pp165-7, 206, 332, 341) because of its effects on the brains of some people. Sucralose and stevia are favored (pp341, 356-7). Sorbitol is considered OK, contrary to Bernstein (pp124-6). Two liters of liquids are to be drunk daily. Water is preferred, coffee is acceptable, as is alcohol (liquor, beer or wine containing 15 mL of alcohol/day) (pp342-3). A drink called Paleolithic Punch made from blended fruits is suggested (p366), and some recipes for drinks made with protein powders and fruit are given also.

The USDA Food Pyramid is thoroughly ridiculed (pp xv-xxiii, 321-3), and the ADbA gets an equally well-deserved drubbing (pp35-6). It is made clear that people are a wide range of metabolic types of whom 1/4 will not benefit much from the LifePlan diet, 1/2 will derive a significant benefit, and 1/4 will have their lives resurrected by it. There is a fine discussion of pre-farming diets, of insulin resistance and all the conditions it leads to, the best description of how to measure it, and of the best types of fats. Of all the books I have reviewed, this one has the best discussion on the sub-fractions of cholesterol, leading to the conclusion that one of the best indicators of ill-health is a low TG/HDL ratio (pp95-6). Low cholesterol levels are linked to higher rates of accidents and violent death (p263). Very few supplements are recommended, but those that are were very well-chosen, including ones to lower homocysteine levels (p98), and this selection, too, is to be tailored to the needs of each individual. The discussion of the leaky-gut syndrome and grain sensitivities rates third after Braly & Hoggan's and Smith's, which are more narrowly focused. An entire chapter is devoted to sweeteners of all kinds, including their GIs. The Eades recognize that the degree of cooking as well as particle size influence the GI of foods. Iron overload receives an entire chapter with advice to have one's ferritin level measured, and, if it is too high, to reduce iron load by giving blood. [It is odd that EDTA chelation for this purpose was not mentioned (Cranton, 2001, p34-5)]. Magnesium is considered the single most valuable supplement and is the subject of an entire chapter. Exposure to the sun to make one's own vitamin D and the false claims on sunblock preparations are discussed at length. More details may be seen in Myth 10. Psychological aids to health also rate a chapter, as does exercise, which is presented in a realistic manner — to be approached for real benefits without self-damage. The distinction between aerobic and anaerobic exercise is given clearly.

This book had few problems beyond misspelling linolenic (pp69,70,77) and tocopherols (p351), and abusing some transitive verbs. The dangers of toxins in large fish were not quantified (p74), so one cannot be certain of how much is safe to eat, and actually PCBs are biodegradable and not very toxic to humans (Ray, 1990, pp86-8). As good as the discussion on cholesterol is, the Eades recommend levels of TC of 160-220 mg/dL (pp100-1), not realizing that the levels go up naturally with age, that women and men over 60 with the highest levels live the longest, and that high levels are strongly protective against cancer, infections, and other conditions (Ravnskov, 2002a). A cup (235 mL) of almonds (no shells) does not contain 167 g of fat (p216), but only 73g. The fiber on US FDA food labels is crude fiber and omits soluble fiber, which is 2-16 times greater (de Man, 1999, pp203-206), so the ECCs are a bit high since soluble fiber has an NME of 0-2 kcal/g (Livesy, 2001). Figure 10.2 (p230) has incorrect wavelengths for UV and several colors of light, and Fig. 40.3 (p251) has mislabeled path-lengths for summer sunlight.

Overall this book is very accurate and helpful. At first it seemed that a mere two dozen references (as footnotes) with citations in the text was inadequate referencing; but the Eades make available on their website their complete bibliography, or will mail copies of it for a fee of $3. Outside sources of information are carefully chosen and cited. Between clear writing, the use of a plethora of American colloquialisms and many doses of humor, this book comes closest to being literature in this group, as well as one of the most scientifically solid and useful.

**Eat Fat Get Thin!**, by Barry Groves.
London, England:Vermilion, 1999.  220 pp.  £6.99 (paperback).  ISBN 0-09-182593-8.

With beautifully written reasoning in a compact form, Groves used his own low-carb diet experience of decades (see Myth 2) to promote a low-carb diet. He has an excellent literature review (pp15-26), with about 170 references, but no numbered citations in the text. Obesity is his main focus, with cancer, CVD and diabetes receiving attention as well. The diet industry receives a well-deserved drubbing; just one example: "...the many commercial interests that rely on overweight people to make a living compound today's weight epidemic" (p5). "Low calorie dietary regimes inevitably fail. More importantly they damage your health, engender a feeling of disillusion and failure, lower morale and increase mental as well as physical stress" (p54). An entire chapter: "Are You Really Overweight?" shows how to determine your BMI, and points out what is not obvious to many young women — dieting when not fat is dangerous. "If you are not overweight, don't diet."

The Eat Fat, Get Thin diet is simply a matter of reducing the digestible carb content of meals to 60-67 g/day until an acceptable weight is achieved, then the carb weight may be increased, or "...indulge yourself in chocolate once a week.", but only with high cocoa butter chocolate (pp118-120). There is a BMI table (pp96-7). The "Rules" are set out with the wonderful clarity characteristic of this book: "Reduce your intake of refined (but see p36) carbohydrates (pp112-3); exercise only if you want to; don't try to lose more than 1 kg per week; leave the fat on meat; eat a high-protein breakfast."

However, Groves has failed to note, as other authors have (Bernstein, Mercola, Smith, etc.), that unrefined grains have about the same glycemic response and most of the carb content of refined grains. The other advice is fine, except that some people who are not overweight may still have IDDM or grain allergies. There are no limits to protein or fat intake. The 60 g/day limit for carbs may not be low enough for some people, and there is no individualization except noting that the time for people to reach the desired weight will differ. Groves wrote that 20 g/day of carb (Atkins' lowest amount) is too low and will cause ketosis, which he does not clearly differentiate from ketoacidosis (pp110-1). Mild ketosis is not a problem.

While other authors wrote that exercise is mandatory, Groves gives very persuasive evidence that it does not aid weight loss, and could be dangerous for the obese (pp85-90).

There are tables of *digestible* carb content per 100 g of many foods, a glossary of nutritional terms with unusual detail, including a table of the fatty acid content of various foods, but lacking *trans* fat and the omega types. There are 54 pages of recipes with carb content, but not preparation times, and an unusual "extra", a recipe index. There is nothing punishing about Groves' recommendations. Small amounts of sugar, bread and other treats are allowed.

"Fats are essential for health. Cut them out and you will shorten your life." (pp9-10). Since high fat intake is justifiably promoted, it is interesting that an old RCT on heart attack survivors is noted by Groves, in which those people given corn oil (polyunsaturated) had the poorest survival rates, those given olive oil (monounsaturated) did a little better, and those given animal fats (about half of which were saturated) did much better (Rose et al., 1965). The link between low cholesterol levels and cancer incidence was made very clear, and the cholesterol mania exposed unmercifully. The anti-cancer properties of conjugated linoleic acid (CLA, 18:2,c9,t11) found only in the fat and milk of ruminant animals (Enig, 2000, p46) was noted (pp56-84), [not to be confused with the dangerous 18:2,t10,c12 linoleic acid found in partially hydrogenated vegetable oils and shown in Fig. 2-1 (Risérus et al., 2002a, 2002b)]. "The low-fat, high-carbohydrate slimming diets of today will inevitably be deficient in protein." (p45) and may lead to gallstones (p102). Polyunsaturated and *trans* fats are revealed as the true fatty villains.

The fallback position of so many diet "authorities", that one must cut out sugar and that complex carbs are safe, is demolished by pointing out that all carbohydrates are converted to glucose on digestion (p36). This is oversimplified, since fiber, often a carbohydrate — cellulose — is not digested by humans, and fructose is not converted to glucose directly. The use of non-caloric sweeteners is discouraged on the grounds that one's craving for sweets is exacerbated (p39). Water (not juice or sweet soda) intake is to be *ad libitum,* not forced at 6-8 glasses per day. Alcohol, wrongly called a carbohydrate, without sugar, is considered acceptable at the level of 1 drink at lunch (p140), contrary to other authors. Many helpful hints are provided for bag lunches at work, dining out, and at dinner parties. It was odd that crispbreads such as Ryvita™ (made in the UK) were not recommended, nor were sensitivities to wheat covered. A low-carb breakfast was said to be the most important meal of the day, and this was well-supported by research (pp123-31).

Where he differs from other authors, Groves may well be correct. This book is easy to read and follow, being 1/4 the size of Atkins, Eades, or Mercola's books, and, if followed, would probably cut the UK's National Health Service costs in half for a while.

**Homo Optimus**, by Jan Kwasniewski, M. D. & Marek Chylinski, Engl. transl. by Bogdan Sikorski, PhD, Warszawa, Poland:Wydawnictwo WGP, 2000. 374 pp. $28 (paperback). ISBN 83-87534-16-1.

Jan Kwasniewski, M.D., lives and worked in Ciechocinek, a health resort in central Poland. He started his medical career in the 1960s as a specialist in helping people recuperate. After accumulating years of clinical experience, he was able to conclude that the wide variety of ailments in his patients was not the product of a great many pathogenic factors, as other doctors would claim, but the result of one underlying cause - bad nutrition via specific effects on the sympathetic and parasympathetic nervous systems. He also observed that different diseases are caused by different forms of malnutrition. After discovering this, Dr. Kwasniewski embarked on a search for a nutritional model that would not give rise to any detrimental effects and, moreover, would ensure a body's health and proper functioning. The fruit of this search is a dietary model he calls "optimal nutrition" by means of the Optimal Diet, developed around 1965-7, because he found that it represents the "best" possible way for a human to feed himself.

Its basic premise is that a person should take care to keep proper proportions among the three fundamental nutrients in food - carbohydrates, fat and protein. He found that the ideal proportions by mass are anywhere from 0.3-0.5 to 2.5-3.5 to 1, meaning that every gram of protein consumed should be accompanied with between 2.5 and 3.5 grams of fat and about half a gram of carbohydrates (p51). In short, optimal nutrition is a high-fat, very low carbohydrate diet, not to exceed 50 g of protein and 2,000 kcal/day for an average adult. Using the fuel values for food groups, the lower-fat regimen corresponds to 11% energy from carb, 76% from fat and 13% from protein (p235). The Optimal Diet is not only the highest in fat and saturated fat content of all the books in this review; it also recommends substantial amounts of collagen, well-cooked for palatability, and organ meats for certain conditions. Eating apples (and fruits in general) is discouraged, contrary to the Ottobonis, who specifically recommended them several times. Potato is recommended as fries on p234 and not recommended on p235. Water is to be *ad libitum*. Recipes list many foods high in GI, but since they are allowed in such small amounts, and accompanied by huge amounts of fats, the effects on insulin response are low. Nutrition needs of infants and children and pregnant women are all addressed.

This book was included in this review to obtain both diversity and the findings of another unorthodox clinician with long experience. Written in 17th century style, it has no bibliography, no index, and is replete with testimonials and single-case reports in order to appeal to semi-educated general readers. A dozen or so published findings of other researchers were quoted, but never with enough data to allow a citation to be found easily. The first 135 pp are an interview of JK with himself, and this section is a mixture of philosophy with many supposed quotations from biblical, ancient and medieval sources, and some modern ones, with occasional dabs of diet wisdom. Uninhibited, the authors describe 16-year-old, physically well-developed Polish girls as having "...heads full of garbage soaked in Coca Cola" (p128). In contrast, the next section (pp137-238) gives actual clinical findings with a much smaller proportion of philosophy, which includes the advice not to vote for the obese for political office because their brains are adversely affected (p204). This is followed by recipes with calorie content (pp207-307), menus for 2 weeks, tables with the nutritional value of food products (also using fuel values), and more testimonials. GI, GL and NME are not addressed. Exercise is addressed realistically: those who are not in condition for it should not damage themselves until and unless the Optimal Diet improves their condition and allows safe exercise (p104).

The specific conditions that were stabilized or cured with the Optimal Diet were said to include Bürgers disease, Bechterew's disease, multiple sclerosis (in agreement with Braly, pp157-8), rheumatoid arthritis (in agreement with Ottoboni, pp152-3), liver cirrhosis, neurasthenia, IDDM [said to be caused by sugar (not in agreement with Bernstein, p36) and in which not all pancreatic beta cells are destroyed (in agreement with Bernstein, p36)], NIDDM (in agreement with all the other authors), atherosclerosis (in which the DHT is demolished, pp72-5, 102ff), hypertension, CVD, obesity (in which lean body mass improved, even if weight did not go down, in agreement with Atkins and Sears), colitis, stomach ulcers, bronchial asthma, migraines and certain infectious diseases. Clinical findings with results of blood work are given in a believable manner, with the numbers and proportions of patients who recovered. But complicating these findings were simultaneous treatments with electric currents of patients who had a number of these afflictions! Other than noting that the current was limited to 20 mA for safety, no voltage, frequency or duration was given, let alone a description of the apparatus. So naturally, a modern scientific view is that one cannot be certain whether the diet or the currents were responsible for healing when both were used. Moreover there is no recognition that some cures could have been for gluten or grain allergies, not excess carbs.

Many of the theoretical examples in support of actual clinical findings were not good science. For example, "By increasing the weight of the unsaturated fat molecule by 1% through hydrogenation we can expect an increase in the caloric value by as much as 18%" (pp31-3). In fact, the NME of fats made from saturated long-chain fatty acids is lower than that of their unsaturated analogues because of indigestibility (see Appendix C), and the saturates certainly do not yield "10 cal/g" (actually meant 10 kcal/g) when partially metabolized. The "10 kcal/g" value may be the fuel value of a saturated hydrocarbon. Formation of *trans* fats during hydrogenation is totally misunderstood, as is the relative metabolic need for oxygen, for which hydrogen is said to require much less than carbon (p35). The facts are that 1 g of hydrogen requires 8 g of oxygen to form water, and 1 g of carbon requires 2.7 g of oxygen to form carbon dioxide. Perhaps Kwasniewski & Chylinski meant the atomic ratios in $H_2O$ and $CO_2$. Margarine is said to be better than the oil from which it is made because margarine contains more hydrogen (pp35, 234), contrary to all the other authors in this group, and is clearly wrong. "Carboxylic" (actually carbonic) acid will *not* react with salt to give hydrochloric acid and sodium carbonate (p67); the reverse reaction is the correct one. Apes were said to be plant eaters (p162), contrary to the findings of Jane Goodall, who found that animal and insect prey were avidly sought after and eaten.

While this book meets most of the present criteria for junk science, this reviewer is convinced that the clinical findings are genuine, nevertheless, and that these support the use of low-carb diets for treating many afflictions. Subjective findings were often confirmed by clinical assays of blood as done elsewhere in the world. It is revealing that the negative attitude of the Medical Science Therapy Committee of the Polish Academy of Science towards Kwasniewski's evidence (pp9-15) exactly parallels those of the US government agencies towards Atkins, Eades, etc.

**The Heart Revolution: The Extraordinary Discovery that Finally Laid the Cholesterol Myth to Rest**, by Kilmer S. McCully, PhD, MD & Martha McCully, New York, NY: Perennial/Harper Collins, 2000. xxii + 257 pp. $13 (paperback). ISBN 0-06-092973-1.

The USDA Food Pyramid, in perpetuating the anti-cholesterol mania, "...wildly exaggerates the importance of carbohydrates, which erroneously have become known as health foods" (p33). "Obesity is another consequence of the [USDA Food] pyramid's push toward carbohydrates...But fat is not the demon...*a high fat intake does not lead to obesity* if the diet contains unprocessed whole foods...when the diet includes a high proportion of calories from refined carbohydrates — as does the American diet — the population develops diabetes, hypertension, tooth decay, obesity and heart disease." (pp39-41) The progression from carb in the diet to serum glucose to insulin resistance, obesity and NIDDM is presented. However, this book is unusual for this group in that its focus is on heart disease, but is relevant with its discussions on cholesterol and oxycholesterol, as well as on nutrient losses during processing and cooking food, as well as limiting carb intake somewhat.

The McCullys recommend a diet with a typical energy contribution of 45% from carb (all unrefined), 30% from fat and 25% from protein; this is a medium-carb diet — about 250 g per day. A detailed program for the first 6 weeks of the Heart Revolution Diet is given (pp191-232) with many suggestions and recipes, but without carb or calorie content. Red wine is recommended at 1-2 glasses per day as the only permitted alcohol. Chocolate of 70% or more cocoa butter is recommended (p91), as is fruit juice (p92). Rye crisp bread is recommended, as are meat, fish, eggs, butter and other dairy foods with fat; and coffee in moderation but with tea preferred, as well as many vegetables and fruits. There is a half-hearted recommendation for organic food (p125). Eating canned and frozen food is discouraged because of vitamin loss as a result of processing, for which actual % losses are given (pp55-70). Irradiated foods are said to have the same fraction of vitamins destroyed as in canning or sterilization, and to contain free radicals (pp67,157). (The free radicals seem unlikely to persist, given the high reactivity of free radicals.) Use of powdered egg and powdered milk is strongly discouraged because the processing forms oxycholesterol, said to be a bad actor, unlike cholesterol (p167). One reason to avoid fried foods in restaurants is the presence of oxycholesterol in old frying oil. Both an excess of omega-6 and any *trans* fats are banned (pp85-7, 163), while omega-3 fats are promoted, with a brave recommendation of canola oil, contrary to many diet "experts". Fake fat, such as olestra, prevents the absorption of the fat-soluble vitamins A, E and D, as well as coenzyme Q10 and essential fatty acids (p123). There is very little individualization, and no special emphasis on diabetics as the ones most likely to benefit from this diet; indeed, diabetics are counseled to seek medical care. A week of sample menus is given (pp97-102) and a whole section with helpful hints and recipes (no GI or GL or NME of carbs), (pp191-232). Drinking 8 glasses of water/day is recommended (p196).

Kilmer S. McCully received his PhD in Biochemistry from Harvard University under the nobelist Konrad Bloch, and his MD from Harvard Medical School. There he discovered, beginning in 1968, that one of the main causes of atherosclerosis and the resulting CVD is high levels of homocysteine in the blood. Further tests on animals confirmed that homocysteine is a true cause, not cholesterol, of arterial plaque formation. He worked out that low levels of either vitamins B6 or B12 or folic acid led to high levels of homocysteine, and that supplementation with them brought homocysteine levels down. Current work from other researchers (some cited on his pp21-7) has confirmed that higher homocysteine levels are associated with both CVD and all-cause mortality (Vollset et al., 2001), congestive heart failure (Vasan, et al., 2003), dementia and Alzheimer's Disease (Seshadri et al., 2002). Supplementation with folic acid (Stanger et al., 2002) and with vitamin B6 as well (Mark et al., 2002) lowered homocysteine levels and reversed arterial stenosis (blockage). Far from receiving a well-deserved Nobel Prize for his work, McCully was eased out of Harvard Medical School and the Massachusetts General Hospital in 1979, prevented from receiving grant funding, and ostracized for 20 years by the Cholesterol Mafia. Only a threatened lawsuit against the pair of "prestigious" institutions allowed McCully to obtain employment anywhere. Happily, beginning around 1998, the confirmation of his work being so overwhelming, McCully is now back in good graces.

So understandably, much of the book is devoted to exposing all the activities that can raise homocysteine levels, and what to eat to lower them (pp81-102), and there is a table on what to supplement at each measured serum level of homocysteine (p117). If diet alone does not suffice, there is vitamin advice (p161-3). Each of the following activities are discouraged because they raise homocysteine levels: eating processed foods (p10), smoking, or taking the drugs methotrexate, azaribine, Dilantin™, phenobarbital, primidone, carbamazepine, valproic acid and some diuretics (thiazides). Statin drugs come in for well-deserved criticism in several places (see Ravnskov, 2000, pp198-211).

Exercise at a moderate level, at least, is considered mandatory. Tables are given of the calories expended in common activities (pp146-50); none of the other books have this.

There are a few inconsistencies. The proscription on beer (pp140, 204) because it "...is filled with carbohydrates..." is not reasonable, since diet beer contains only 2.5-9 g of carbs per 366 mL bottle, far less than the recommended apple, and less than the recommended 1-2 glasses/day of many types of red wine (p131-3). The recommendation for tea was ill-advised because of the fluoride content of most tea (see Myth 11). Saturated fat is to be limited (p44), but is acceptable if eaten in meat or fish (pp83, 187), and is perfectly fine on p86. Whole eggs are recommended (pp79, 102), but then avoiding yolks is suggested (p91, 199). Low-fat yogurt is unhealthful on p96, but recommended on p102 and p203. Both Häagen-Dazs and Ben & Jerry's ice creams, recommended on his p96, because they did not containi corn syrup, *now* contain corn syrup instead of sugar.

McCully has made an extremely valuable discovery of the origins and bad health effects of homocysteine, and his book is a great effort to make it accessible to the non-specialist. A revised edition with a simpler arrangement and more consistency would be appreciated. A 45% energy intake from carb is far too high for many carb-sensitive people.

**The No-Grain Diet**, by Joseph Mercola, DO, with Alison Rose Levy,
New York, NY:Dutton, 2003. vii + 312 pp. $25 (hardcover). ISBN 0-525-94733-7.

The sub-title gives the emphasis: "Conquer Carbohydrate Addiction and Stay Slim for Life". Obesity is partially attributed to the effects of government recommendations, especially the USDA Food Pyramid, which is called a possible product of lobbying and special interests, not science (pp22,34). Recent U. S. Supreme Court rulings were said to reveal conflicts of interest in 6 of the 11 members of the Pyramid committee (p10).

The Mercola program is summarized on a single page (vii). Like Atkins and Eades there are 3 phases, Start-Up (first 3 days), Stabilize (next 50+ days), and Sustain (lifelong). Like Eades there are 3 levels of diet severity, Booster, Core and Advanced, so there are 9 variations in all, the other extreme from Allen & Lutz, Groves or McCully & McCully, each of whom have a simple single plan, as does Smith for each of the 3 food sensitivities in her book. There is a quiz to determine which level of severity to adopt (pp90-5). Mercola does not address GI, GL, carb grams or NME directly, or have tables of them, but he achieves his results by the choices of foods recommended for each phase of each diet. The permitted foods, a wide variety of non-starchy vegetables, fruits, dairy (resumed after a few weeks of abstinence to detect sensitivity) and meat may be eaten *ad libitum.* Many fish, all shellfish and most pork products are to be avoided in most versions of the diets. There are sample menus for all phases and levels, including a 2-week menu, because Dr. Mercola recognizes that most people have only about 10 types of meals in their diets. There are 48 pages of recipes (pp199-247); but with no preparation times, including Dr. Mercola's Green Juice Drink [celery, cucumber and fennel subjected to a juicer (p200)]. Of course, nearly all sweets and sweeteners, even stevia (contrary to Bernstein and Smith) and sucralose (contrary to Atkins and Smith) are out. Soy products are out. The main drink is to be purified (not distilled) water, and red wine is permitted without limit (except for alcoholics) once one's target weight level is reached (pp120-1). Omega-3 fats are in (albeit mainly as supplements, because so much sea food is out), as are monounsaturated and saturated fats and small amounts of omega-6. Great individualization is encouraged with advice to try eating more or less of this or that food group to see what happens, and to increase carb consumption only until weight gain reappears, with daily weighing (opposite to Atkins who suggests it be done once a week or less). Another check is waist size using a tape or tight-fitting slacks. The claimed success rate is 85% of people who tried this plan.

Digestible carbs, usually called grains, are identified by Mercola and Levy as the main culprits in weight gain because of the insulin response (leading to heart disease) and suppression of glucagon and human growth hormone, hypertension, NIDDM, osteoporosis and a number of autoimmune diseases. Stopping grains prevents celiac disease and irritable bowel syndrome (pp25-7), but there are no methods given to determine who has these specific conditions. The mainstream myths surrounding cholesterol and saturated fat are demolished (pp18-32). For those with profound insulin resistance a diet with 75-90% of calories from fat at 1,000 kcal/day is recommended, at least for a short period. A number of standard tests on blood are recommended (pp69-72) with a special Appendix (pp264-270) with emphasis on thyroid testing, but homocysteine, an important risk factor for heart disease, is conspicuously missing. Mercola has years of clinical experience with about 15,000 patients, and feedback from many others via his websites, www.drmercola.com and www.nograindiet.com. About a dozen each of other websites and books are given as sources, but there are no dates, editions, or publishers for the latter. About 120 articles are listed in a bibliography, but with no citations in the text.

To distinguish these diets from those of the other authors, especially Atkins', which is said to have many weaknesses, and can fail (p6), organically grown food is strongly recommended for the usual plausible (theoretical), but unproven reasons (pp6, 102, 249). Very high vegetable consumption, with as much raw as possible, is recommended (p6). A better transition from the Stabilize to Sustain phases than in the corresponding Weight-Watchers or Atkins plans is claimed, but no evidence for the superiority of Mercola's plan is given (pp80-1). Metabolic typing to find who should eat what is promoted (pp125, 292), but one must go to outside sources to do this. The one really unusual feature of this book (of the ones in this review) is that 20% of the text is on psychological approaches to hunger and food addictions. The scheme is called the Emotional Freedom Technique (EFT), which is a combination of acupressure according to traditional Chinese medicine, and use of mantras, which the client may individualize, but the final part of the mantra is to be "I deeply and completely accept myself" (pp8-9, 13, 45-6, 80, 85-6, 145-7, 165-95, 258-63). So far EFT has worked more than half the times tried by this reviewer, but there is no evidence for its effectiveness in this book by comparing results from clients who do or do not use it, or from trials.

There were a few inconsistencies and omissions. Some of the times Mercola uses the term "grains" they include simple sugars. The most confusing error is his definition of simple and complex carbohydrates. The former are the ones said to be present in potatoes and grains, as well as in sugars and sweeteners, and the latter in fruits and vegetables (pp11, 28, 39, 42, 103). This is at odds with the definitions used by nearly all others, and is bound to lead to confusion for many readers (deMan, 1999, pp183-206). Macro- and micronutrients were confused (p74). Ketosis and ketoacidosis were confused (p29). Fructose is among the sweeteners to avoid, yet Mercola recommends raw honey, which contains 39% fructose (p118). After the fine endorsement of dietary cholesterol and fat (pp18-32), bison and ostrich were recommended over beef, pork and chicken because the former contain less fat and cholesterol (p255), a paradox. While no limits on protein and fat quantities eaten was the story in the earlier parts of the book, there is an admonition not to eat too much protein, without explaining how much is too much, because doing so is said to damage kidneys and bones, contrary to Atkins, Bernstein and others. Coffee is to be eliminated because it "...worsens your insulin levels..." (pp120, 131); however, in a recent clinical trial, coffee consumption was inversely and strongly associated with lower risk of NIDDM (van Dam et al., 2002a). Evidence in Myth 10 showed it cut liver cancer significantly. Figures of food amounts of 60 lbs, 30 lbs and costs of $1.5 trillion were given with no time frame (p4); all should have had "per year" or whatever applied. Temperatures were given without the C or F (pp118-9). Salt was said to change in composition at 1200° (no C or F), but actually it can be distilled at 1413°C with no change. In the calculation of HDL/TC the decimal point was omitted, making the values 100x too high (p69). Unrefined sea salt is recommended without evidence; see the review of Smith's book below for the likely fallacy. The "chemical additives" to be avoided in common salt are calcium silicate to prevent caking and sodium or potassium iodide to prevent goiter; no actual evidence is given against their reasonable use (p119). Fish were claimed to be highly contaminated with PCBs, DDT and mercury (pp110-1). Actually PCBs are biodegradable and not very toxic to humans (Ray, 1990, pp86-8). The usual metabolite of DDT found in humans is DDE, which has never been shown to have had toxic effects (Lieberman, 1997; Lagomasini, 2002, p149-177). Listed among fish to avoid because of mercury content are lobster, shrimp and tuna; but common tables list these as among the lowest in mercury content. Using the FDA's limit of 0.3 µg/kg body weight daily, one could eat 100 g of tuna or lobster daily without exceeding this limit, which is 1/10 that of the WHO. The Chicago Western Electric Study followed the effects of fish consumption on 2107 men 40-55 years old for 30 years; those who ate the most fish lived the longest (Daviglus et al., 1997). The Nurses' Health Study on 84,688 women aged 34-59 years and followed for 16 years showed that those who ate the most fish lived the longest (Hu et al., 2002). If fish and pork (p114) were toxic, some of the longest-lived populations in the world (Crete, Japan, Okinawa before 1986) would not be. Eating fiber is strongly recommended (p19) but the use of juicers, which separate fiber for disposal, contradicts this.

There are a number of issues addressed in this book that are either not deemed important by the authors of the other books, or on which a different position is taken. Most nuts are not recommended due to high omega-6 content (pp111-2); while omega-6 oils are unhealthful in large amounts, this is greatly at odds with the highly significantly lower risks of CHD and all-cause deaths in the oldest-old in The Adventist Health Study who consumed the most nuts (Fraser et al., 1997). No consideration is given to extent of cooking on GI for carrots or pasta (p105). Microwaves were said to cause the greatest nutrient losses of all cooking methods (p161-2). There was no support given for this, and it is hard to see how baking, broiling and grilling could be any gentler (see Introduction). A literature search for nutrient damage by microwaves turned up nothing beyond the effects of hot water (McCully, 2003). Eggs, said to be high in omega-6 fats, are to be eaten raw, or, if cooked, not scrambled (pp107-8, 251-3); there is no evidence whatever given for the benefits of doing this, or of the dangers to people who react badly to raw eggs. Canola oil was lumped in with safflower and other oils with high omega-6 content despite the fact that the USDA assays show the -6:-3 ratio as 2:1, by far the best of any vegetable oil, and the omega-3 content is the highest (in non-hydrogenated form). Advice not to drink or swim in chlorinated water (pp150-1) is not backed by any evidence. Storing water in poly(ethylene) containers is recommended over poly(vinyl chloride) (PVC) ones to avoid the "dangerous chemicals" leached from the latter; there is no evidence given for this. Use of reverse osmosis to purify drinking water rather than distillation, where both remove valuable minerals, has no epidemiological support either. Exercise is recommended for everyone because it "guarantee[s]...weight loss" (contrary to Banting, see Myth 2, and Groves, pp88-90, and Myth 6), and "prevents heart disease"; this latter is contradicted by a clinical trial (Dorn et al., 1999).

Except for the criticisms of the Atkins diet, the main messages in this book are the excellent ones, with the same excellent reasons for eating low-carb diets, as are used by the other authors for treatment of obesity. There is *almost* no nonsense about eating cholesterol and saturated fat. The diets are good, if unnecessarily limited in fish, pork and nuts; and the support of the EFT scheme may be worthwhile. The devil is in the details on a variety of side-issues, as exposed above.

**The Modern Nutritional Diseases: heart disease, stroke, type-2 diabetes, obesity, cancer, and how to prevent them**, by Alice Ottoboni, PhD & Fred Ottoboni, MPH, PhD, Sparks, NV: Vincente Books, 2002, 2nd printing, rev., 2/03. vi + 218 pp. $30 (paperback). ISBN 0-915241-03-X.

"The American diet over the last hundred years seems to be a story of the triumph of junk science over real science. This is the situation today despite the fact the biochemical pathways that nutrients follow in the body are reasonably well known and competent studies relating diet to human health have scientifically validated the detrimental effects of high-glycemic diets and essential fatty acid imbalances" (p199).

Determined to have non-biochemists follow the scientific evidence for the effect of diet, supplements, and drugs on health, the Ottobonis have provided informative word diagrams of metabolic pathways on digestion and beyond, along with clear descriptions. There are citations in the text to references at the end of each chapter to books, medical journals, and other sources. And all of this is done and without using a single chemical structure, certainly a welcome feature to most lay readers. The Ottobonis have shown how common supplements and drugs influence these metabolic pathways, and they expose the biggest fraud in the history of medicine and diet without restraint — the diet-heart theory (DHT). Since their interpretation of the science differs so much from that of the dictatorial directives by the deceptive defenders of diet dogma, the Ottobonis call their recommendations "alternative nutrition". The authors' advice, which encompasses lifestyle, diet, supplements and drugs is given with solid citations and great clarity.

For most people their recommendation is for a low GI diet with energy from carb:fat:protein of 40:30:30%. With due homage to Barry Sears, they note that the human body has no requirement for any carbohydrate at all (pp85,90). Not worrying about saturated fats, minimizing omega-6 fats, maximizing omega-3 fats, and eliminating *trans* fats are other important parts of the message, based both on published studies, and backed by those biochemical diagrams showing how the best food leads to low serum insulin levels and the most beneficial eicosanoids, those 20-carbon signaling compounds. The biochemical path from high glycemic index carbohydrates to high insulin to undesirable eicosanoids (prostaglandins, etc.) is presented in the clearest manner I have yet seen. For those who cannot accept experimental evidence without a plausible theory, the Ottoboni's provide both. One of the most hard-headed and accurate sections on nutritional supplements among all these books is found here, with recommendations. This book was informational, and the Ottobonis recommend other books for menus and recipes, and give general guidelines for evaluating sources of medical advice (pp184-6). Further recommendations include an *ad libitum* intake of water based on thirst (p138), 1-2 drinks per day of alcoholic beverages (p189), special recognition of homocysteine control (p146), the unproven benefits of organic food (p185), and the doubtful benefits of non-caloric sweeteners (p92). The effect of cooking time on GI was given special attention (p85). There was no specific recommendation for individualization of diets, or to adjust carb consumption to weight loss or to incipient ketosis, but there was an excellent distinction drawn between ketosis and ketoacidosis (pp114-5).

Dozens of their paragraphs are gems of clear, truthful and practical correlations or conclusions, which should be prize verbatim quotations for many years to come. For example, here are just a few of their accurate observations, all of which are presented with ample evidence:

- Acetaminophen is not innocuous.
- Fats made from the 12-carbon lauric acid (12:0) are very beneficial.
- Children on low-fat diets can be harmed seriously.
- Certain vitamins and supplements, (but relatively few herbs) can be very beneficial.
- The vegetarian diet can be perilous.
- Anticholesterol drugs are dangerous.
- A good cholesterol supply in the human body is a vital necessity .

The Ottobonis correctly expose the National Cholesterol Education Program (NCEP) Guidelines on diet as an attempt by those with ulterior motives to use the US government umbrella of the NHLBI of the NIH to make it appear that the guidelines have government sanction.The process of generating them was not the open and complete process we have a right to expect, which would have included public hearings and publication in the Federal Register, and not just in *JAMA*. "Although the New Cholesterol Guidelines will be a windfall for drug companies and some agricultural interests, they will adversely impact both the practice of medicine and the long-term health of Americans" (pp179-82).

Flaws in dietary studies connecting consumption of saturated fats with the chronic Western diseases are explained. Many examples of better studies are provided, and the contradiction with the Unified Dietary Guidelines of the AHA and other groups still in the Dark Ages regarding GI is exposed fearlessly.

Perhaps the Ottoboni's homage to Barry Sears, author of Into The Zone, should have been qualified, based on findings in my review of his book which follows. The first edition of the Ottoboni's book (9/02) had less-than-perfect proof-reading and some minor errors in chemistry, nearly all of which were eliminated in the second printing of 2/03, an exception being the meaning of l- and d- prefixes in naming amino acids (p95). The recommendation for drinking 1 quart of milk per day (p194) is surprising in view of the 44 g of high-GI lactose therein contained (Lentner, 1981, p255). However, these minor complaints do not alter the validity of the conclusions and advice in this marvelous book.

**Enter the Zone**, by Barry Sears, PhD, and Bill Lawren.
New York, NY:Regan/HarperCollins, 1995. xviii + 328 pp. $25 (hardcover). ISBN 0-06-039150-2.

Brilliant and fearless in debunking the desperate dons of diet dogma: "No cholesterol-lowering diet study has ever decreased total mortality" (pp141-3), Barry Sears provides a number of insights in the oldest of the books reviewed here (1995), and he reported on a number of small RCTs he initiated without outside funding. The "Zone" refers to periods of the highest exhilaration and performance experienced by athletes. Sears' theme is to show how 3/4 of us can reach our Zone by eating a low-carb diet. (The other 1/4 are either in their Zone or not harmed by their present diets.)

One of Sears' main themes is that essential fatty acids are converted into good eicosanoids (such as prostaglandin $E_1$, a vasodilator that lowers blood pressure) in the presence of glucagon, the fat-metabolizing hormone; and into bad eicosanoids (such as thromboxane $A_2$, a vasoconstrictor that raises blood pressure) in the presence of insulin, the fat-building hormone (p35ff). This is elaborated by noting that thromboxane $A_2$ stimulates the growth of cells in arterial walls to form the lesions of atherosclerosis (p149). An interesting offshoot is that insulin activates HMG-CoA reductase, one of the catalysts for cholesterol synthesis. Another is that the poor results in RCTs of antihypertensive drugs may be due to the tendency of the drugs to raise insulin levels (pp140-1).

Before and after some history and literature examples supporting his theses, Sears points out that many chronic conditions in aging, obesity, chronic fatigue and others can be alleviated by entering the Zone by means of a low-carb diet, because this is the only way to minimize blood glucose and insulin levels. He calls hyperinsulinemia the single most important risk factor for CVD (p136-8). He is careful to note that about 1/4 of people will not obtain a benefit from a low-carb diet; that 1/4, including diabetics and the obese, will respond very well; and 1/2 will respond well enough to justify maintaining the low-carb diet (pp30, 102-3).

The Zone diet — 40% carb calories, 30% fat, 30% protein, using the fuel values — is individualized by determining one's lean body mass, setting the amount of protein high enough to prevent muscle loss (80 g/day for a 70 kg human), matching the protein calories with fat calories (34 g/day), and fixing the calories from carbs at 4/3 those of protein (thus 107 g/day of digestible carb), (pp69-76). Since low-GI and high-fiber carbs are strongly recommended, the total carb intake could be 200 g/day. Major supplementation is not needed (pp105-112). One glass of red wine per day is recommended. A reasonable number of recipes are given (without preparation times), as well as tables for determining lean-body-mass, equi-caloric servings of food, rough GI values, and ideal body weights.

In a 1-patient anecdote modestly referred to as an Aunt Millie tale, a CVD patient on a high-carb diet had TG = 650 mg/dl, TC = 229 and HDL = 34. The patient started simvastatin and the Zone diet, which changed TG = 108, TC = 152 and HDL = 49. Dropping the drug, but not the diet changed TG = 101, TC = 175 and HDL = 52. "This...is a dramatic indication that cholesterol levels are ultimately determined by eicosanoid balance, which is controlled by the food you eat" (pp144-5).

A trial of the Zone diet on 6 college football and 3 professional basketball players in which all meals in a camp setting were checked by the coach (who was already converted to a Zone diet) was checked against the high-carb diet to which many nutritionists commit athletes. After just 6 weeks the low-carb diet increased weight 5%, decreased fat 20%, increased LBM 8%, and improved several performance parameters 2-30% (all $p < 0.005$), (p41-4).

An RCT of 15 NIDDM patients was done comparing 8 weeks of ADbA diet of 60% high-GI carb or the Zone diet (40% low-GI carb) with typical American diets to give the following results: ADbA diet: No significant changes occurred in weight loss, fat loss, fasting serum glucose, or the levels of serum TG (up 20%, but ns), fasting insulin, or blood pressure. Of significance: glycosylated hemoglobin went down 4% and TC up 8%. Zone diet: No significant change in fasting glucose, fasting insulin, diastolic blood pressure. Significant drops occurred in weight, fat, glycosylated hemoglobin (down 14%), TG and systolic blood pressure. Another 8 weeks brought diastolic blood pressure down significantly as well. This showed that the ADbA diet was no better than an average American diet, but the Zone diet was far better.

Sears noted the benefits of the Zone diet in obesity, diabetes, cancer, AIDS, arthritis, MS PMS, lupus, chronic fatigue, depression and others. Fair to excellent evidence is given for every claim of benefit of the Zone diet.

However, Sears did some things that are at odds with other authors and the medical literature. He understood that aspirin has its side-effects, and that the male Physician Health Group Study (PHS), after 4 years, found no change in all-cause death rates, and Sears thought a longer period would change the outcome, but was oddly ignorant of the 7-year results which had been reported in 1989 (Kauffman, 2000) and, of course, of a newer report (reported in 2001) that found in a 3.1-year study that more women died on aspirin than on placebo (Kauffman, 2002a). Sears actually calculated the expected death rates based on non-fatal heart attacks in the PHG study rather than using the actual ones! He sent mixed messages on aspirin, the "miracle drug" of eicosanoid control, yet noting some of its long-term problems (pp113-8, 138, 151-2, 161).

He recommended avoiding saturated fats, egg yolks, accentuating this for cancer patients, for whom he emphasized seafood and sea vegetables. There is good evidence that saturated fat and meat do *not* cause cancer or CVD (Malhotra, 1967; Allen & Lutz, pp172-7; Ottoboni, p192), nor do whole eggs (see Atkins, p96; Hu et al., 1999). Your reviewer cannot help noting that the Japanese eat sea food and sea vegetables, and in the past little red meat, and have had a high cancer rate.

In one place Sears wrote that omega-6 fatty acids in the diet lead to good eicosanoids and are more important than omega-3s (p120), then later wrote that he had tried to grow a source of a "good" omega-6 fatty acid (gamma-linolenic acid), borage oil, in Canada; but he eventually realized that most people obtained enough omega-6 from their normal diets (pp129-131). It is puzzling that he did not recommend canola oil, an excellent source of alpha-linolenic acid, an omega-3 that the body converts to good eicosanoids (Enig, 2000, p29; Lemaitre et al., 2003). In his newer book, *The Omega Rx Zone,*

2002, the omega-3 and -6 fatty acid message is greatly improved, but the message on saturated fats was not.

Sears wrote that all mammals have the same responses to food (p12), and that rabbits, which are both mammals and vegetarians, develop atherosclerosis when fed saturated fat. That this is true or is relevant to humans is strongly disputed (Ravnskov, 2000, pp137-8).

While very conscious of the benefits of the Zone diet for diabetics, Sears does not address those who cannot tolerate diets as high as 40% carb (pp152-60), or those who are grain-sensitive.

There is a bibliography with about 400 entries, but there are no citations in the text. Despite the many errors and rigidities in this book, the important insights based on the biochemistry of eicosanoids and the striking results of Sears' diet trials have made this book a benefit to over 4 million readers.

**Going Against the Grain: How Reducing and Avoiding Grains Can Revitalize Your Health,** by Melissa Diane Smith, Chicago, IL:Contemporary Books, 2002. xv + 304 pp. $15 (paperback). ISBN 0-658-01722-5.

In *Going Against the Grain,* Smith has tackled 3 serious diet-related problems: (1) diabetes-related carbohydrate sensitivity, which is also addressed by most of the other books in this review, and about which she has written a book (Challem et al., 2000); (2), gluten sensitivity; and (3) wheat sensitivity. No indication was given of the fraction of people afflicted with carbohydrate sensitivity, but gluten sensitivity was put at 10-50%, and other food allergies at 10-60%. A small US study was described in which 221 adults in a shopping mall who did not admit to having a GI disease were tested for an antibody that indicates gluten sensitivity; 10% had the antibody; 20 of these 22 were further tested, and 1 had celiac disease (p77), which is in line with other studies on prevalence (p69). The appalling number of health conditions that can result from persisting with a poor, and even addictive high-grain diet are given, from cancer to arthritis to osteoporosis, and many more. A good historical review was provided.

The USDA Food Pyramid comes in for a well-deserved condemnation (p5ff). A history of long-term human diet changes is given. "Grains aren't the holier-than-thou health foods that people think they are" (p277). "Grains may seem the staff of life, but they're really scythes that whittle away most people's health... To stay fit and free of disease, all of us should eat fewer grains. Some of us should eat no grains at all" (p ix). Smith found, with difficulty, that she herself was gluten-sensitive (pp xi-xiii).

Quizzes are given to diagnose each of the 3 conditions, with points for certain answers, so the reader may diagnose herself. Other medical tests, with emphasis on accurate and non-invasive ones, are recommended for confirmation. The concepts of GI and GL are covered, but the effect of cooking on the GI of carrot or pasta is not given. The presence of undesirable antinutrients (phytate, etc.) in whole grains is cited (pp47-65). Diets are given for each condition with great emphasis on observing one's own reactions to food, and thus to individualize each diet. A week of sample menus is provided, and a number of recipes, which clearly indicate whether they are for the carb-, gluten-, or wheat-sensitive. These do not have the NME or digestible carb content, or GI, or GL or preparation times. The major problem with this otherwise very useful and enlightening book is not that the recommended diets are either low-carb, low-gluten, or low-wheat, or all 3, which are all fine; but that the diets also appear to be low in fat, certainly in land animal fat, with a heavy emphasis on the use of olive oil as shown by a week of sample menus (pp209-212, 219-222, 228-233). In fact, an RCT of 2 years duration showed that olive oil was inferior to animal fat in protection from cardiac events (Rose et al., 1965). Lean cuts of meat are recommended, as well as coconut oil; the latter is called "...a source of saturated fat that does not contribute to heart disease..." (p174). Coconut oil contains 30% of the same longer-chain (14-18 carbon atoms) saturated fats as animal fat; none of these fats is a cause of CVD

(Ravnskov, 2000). A "high" TC (pp xiv, 27, 42, 180, 207-8, 263) is not a cause of CVD either (Ravnskov, 2000). Oddly, the 18-carbon stearic acid, the main saturated one in animal fat, is called nonatherogenic on p11, and said not to be as prevalent in the fat of today's grain-fed animals (but see p22), yet fat is to be removed from meat when cooking it (pp239-40)! Surviving eating out, unsympathetic associates and feeding children are nicely addressed except for the fat issue. Asthma symptoms in children who consumed milk fat were much rarer than in children who did not (see Wijga et al., 2003). Smith addressed the GI of protein for the very carb-sensitive by recommending replacement of some protein by fat, but it is all plant fat (p213), except for omega-3 fish oil supplements, despite recent evidence that neither saturated nor total fat intake increases the risk for NIDDM (van Dam et al., 2002). Coffee, tea and nuts are considered acceptable, with an unusual warning against coffee substitutes that contain gluten (p164), and no notice on the fluoride content of tea (see Myth 11). Genetically engineered foods are disparaged (p101) and organic foods are promoted, both on theoretical grounds with no scientific support.

Other chemistry-related issues disappoint: Unrefined Real Salt™ is recommended (pp 174, 200) on theoretical grounds. In fact, this salt contains 98.3% sodium chloride and negligible amounts of anything beneficial (http://waltonfeed.com/self/labels/saltreal.html). In a generally good chapter on supplements, homocysteine is not even mentioned in connection with the B vitamins (p261), and is marginalized elsewhere. Vitamin C made from beets or sago palm is recommended rather than from the usual source, corn, for people very sensitive to corn (p261).This assumes that allergens (proteins in this case) would survive a multi-step synthesis with crystalline intermediates, because some of Smith's corn-sensitive clients told her they reacted badly (e-mail from Smith, 29 Jul 03). Egg powder is mentioned, along with the other refined protein powders, as alternate protein sources (p139), but with caveats, and see McCully's proscription, above. Distilled vinegar and alcohol, made from gluten-containing grains, are condemned as though the gliadin fraction of gluten of minimum molecular weight 11,000 daltons (deMan, 1999, 153-6) of such a protein could vaporize during distillation of the fermented grains. Smith also notes that alcohol increases intestinal permeability, increasing allergic reactions, which she urges individuals to watch for (pp100, 149, 166, 173, 178). Use of DDT was damned (p101) despite lack of evidence for harm (Lagomasini, 2002, p149-177). Unrefined grains are noted to be higher in fiber than refined, but no mention is made of their protein and fat content (pp32, 47ff), which is significant (11% protein is present in one whole-wheat pasta). Cramps are said to be due to a calcium deficiency (p58); but other more reliable sources indicate that low magnesium may be another or additional culprit (Atkins, 1998, p121-31); however, it is true that magnesium is recommended by Smith for other conditions (pp261, 266). Exorphins are said to have similar amino acid sequences to those in morphine (p95); but morphine actually contains no amino acids.

There are about 150 references with citations in the text; more would have been welcomed to back many of the unsupported statements. Other books, magazines, websites, and connections to enlightened nutritionists or nutrition-oriented physicians are cited; this is an especially valuable feature of Smith's book. The lack of knowledge about food allergies and nutrition of conventionally educated MDs that Smith notes is all too true. In this reviewer's opinion, such victims of food allergies would be much better off consulting with Smith than with typical MDs, who typically recommend low-fat diets, but rarely low-carb, or low-grain. The main messages of this book are extremely valuable and apply to the broadest variety of food problems. A rewrite with more reasonable diets and the help of a biochemist would make it even more valuable.

### Overall Book Recommendations

The two books in this group which do not contain menus or recipes, those by Braly & Hoggan on grain allergies and by Ottoboni & Ottoboni on the realities of diet and diet politics, are both excellent and complementary. The portions of McCully & McCully on homocysteine and oxycholesterol, subjects on which Kilmer S. McCully, PhD, MD, is an expert, are excellent and complementary to both of the others. These are the ones to read for general information.

For diagnosed diabetics, Bernstein's book is in a class by itself — outstanding.

For people who are not sure which diet-based affliction they might have, Smith's book has the best tests for self-diagnosis, and the newest, least invasive, most accurate blood tests to confirm the diagnosis, as well as the best suggestions on how to find medical providers who do not merely repeat the diet dogma of the agencies and foundations named above. Her diet advice is not the best.

For overweight people who want minimal reading and a simple plan to follow, Allan & Lutz's and Groves' books are the best.

For overweight people who want more information and more diet plans, the book by Eades & Eades is superior, followed closely by Atkins'.

Because conditions in Eastern Europe are so different from those in the USA and UK, people there might do best following Kwasniewski and Chylinski.

For any coach, trainer or athlete who thinks "carb-loading" is a great benefit, Sears' book will nullify that notion.


## Books on Low-Carb Diets Not Reviewed

The authors of the following books, which will not be reviewed, also favor low-carb diets:

Cleave, T. L. *The Saccharine Disease: The Master Disease of Our Time.* New Canaan, CT: Keats, 1975.

Tarnower, H. & Baker, S. *The Complete Scarsdale Medical Diet.* New York, NY: Bantam Books, 1995.

Steward, H. L., Bethea, M., Andres, S. & Balart, L. *Sugar Busters.* New York, NY:Ballantine Books, 1995.

Ezrin, C., Kowalski, R. E. & Kowalski, R. E. *Your Fat Can Make You Thin.* New York, NY: McGraw-Hill/Contemporary Books, 2nd ed,1997.

Gittleman, A. L. *Eat Fat, Lose Weight.* Los Angeles, CA: Keats Publ., 1999.

Cordain, L. *The Paleo Diet: Lose Weight and Get Healthy by Eating the Food You Were Designed to Eat .* New York, NY:John Wiley & Sons, 2001.

Price, W. A. *Nutrition and Physical Degeneration.* New York, NY: McGraw Hill - NTC; 6th ed., 2002.

By no means is this list an exhaustive one. Cursory examination of books on the Weight-Watchers, South Beach and Glycemic Index diets indicate a lack of understanding by their authors of the facts in Myths 2 and 3.

## Acknowledgment for Appendix B

Sally Fallon and Frances Pane, MSLS, edited this section.

## References

Atkins RC (1998). *Dr Atkins Vita-Nutrient Solution,* London, England: Pocket Books, Simon & Schuster.

Challem J, Berkson B, Smith MD (2000). *Syndrome X: The Complete Nutritional Program to Prevent and Reverse Insulin Resistance,* New York, NY: John Wiley & Sons.

Cranton EM (2001). *A Textbook on EDTA Chelation Therapy,* 2nd ed., Charlottesville, VA: Hampton Roads Publ. Co.

van Dam RM, Feskens JM (2002a). Coffee consumption and risk of type 2 diabetes. *The Lancet* 360:1477-1478.

Dorn J, Naughton J, Imamura D, Trevisan M (1999). Results of a Multicenter Randomized Clinical Trial of Exercise and Long-Term Survival in Myocardial Infarction Patients. *Circulation* 100:1764-1769.

Enig MG (2000). *Know Your Fats,* Silver Spring, MD: Bethesda Press.

Fraser GE, Shavlik DJ (1997). Risk factors for all-cause and coronary heart disease mortality in the oldest-old. The Adventist Health Study. *Archives of Internal Medicine* 157:2249-58.

Hu FB, Stampfer MJ, Rimm EB, Manson JE, Ascherio A, Colditz GA, Rosner BA, Spiegelman D, Speizer FE, Sacks FM, Hennekens CH Willett WC (1999). A Prospective Study of Egg Consumption and Risk of Cardiovascular Disease in Men and Women. *Journal of the American Medical Association* 281(15):1387-1394.

Hu FB, Bronner L, Willett WC, Stampfer MJ, Rexrode KM, Albert CN, Hunter D, Manson J-AE (2002). Fish and Omega-3 Fatty Acid Intake and Risk of Coronary Heart Disease in Women. *Journal of the American Medical Association* 287(14):1815-1821.

Kauffman JM (2000). Should You Take Aspirin to Prevent Heart Attack? *J. Scientific Exploration* 14(4):623-41 (2000).

Kauffman JM 2002a). Aspirin Study Flawed, Letter to Editor, *J. Scientific Exploration* 16(2):247-249 (2002).

Lagomasini A (2002). Chemical Warfare: Ideological Environmentalism's Quixotic Campaign Against Synthetic Chemicals in *Global Warming and Other Eco-Myths,* Bailey, R., Ed., New York, NY: Forum Random House Prima.

Lemaitre RN, King IB, Mozaffarian D, Luller LH, Tracy RP, Siscovick DS (2003). n-3 Polyunsaturated fatty acids, fatal ischemic heart disease, and nonfatal myocardial infarction in older adults: the Cardiovascular Health Study. *American Journal of Clinical Nutrition* 77:319-325.

Lentner C, Ed. (1981). *Geigy Scientific Tables,* Excerpts, 8th ed., West Caldwell, NJ: CIBA-Geigy.

Lieberman AJ (1997). Facts versus Fears: A Review of the 20 Greatest Unfounded Health Scares of Recent Times. *American Council on Science and Health Report,* pp3-4. http://www.acsh.org/publications/reports/factsfears.html

Livesy G (2001). A perspective on food energy standards for nutrition labeling. *British Journal of Nutrition* 85:271-287.

Malhotra SL (1967). Serum lipids, dietary factors and ischemic heart disease. *American Journal of Clinical Nutrition* 20:462-474.

deMan JM (1999). *Principles of Food Chemistry,* 3rd ed., Gaithersburg, MD: Aspen.

Mark L, Erdei F, Markizay J, Kondacs A, Katona A (2002). Effect of Treatment with Folic Acid and Vitamin B6 on Lipid and Homocysteine Concentrations in Patients with Coronary Artery Disease. *Nutrition,* 18(5):428-429.

McCully KS (2003). E-mail of 17 Dec 03.

Ottoboni, F. & Ottoboni, A. (2003). Can Attention Deficit-Hyperactivity Disorder Result from Nutritional Deficiency? *Journal of American Physicians and Surgeons* 8(2):58-60.

Pelton R, LaValle JB (2000). *The Nutritional Cost of Prescription Drugs,* Englewood, CO:Perspective/Morton.

Ravnskov U (2000). *The Cholesterol Myths: Exposing the Fallacy that Saturated Fat and Cholesterol Cause Heart Disease,* Washington, DC: New Trends Publishing, pp15-46.

Ray DL, Guzzo L (1990). *Trashing the Planet,* Washington, DC: Regnery Gateway.

Risérus U, Abner P, BrismarK, Vessby B (2002a). Treatment with Dietary *trans*10*cis*12 Conjugated Linoleic Acid Causes Isomer-Specific Insulin Resistance in Obese Men with the Metabolic Syndrome. *Diabetes Care* 25(9):1516-1521.

Risérus U, Basu S, Jovinge S, Fredrikson GN, Ärnlov J, Vessby B (2002b). Supplementation with Conjugated Linoleic Acid Causes Isomer-Dependent Oxidative Stress and Elevated C-Reactive Protein. A Potential Link to Fatty Acid-Induced Insulin Resistance. *Circulation* 106:1825-1929.

Rose GA, Thomson WB, Williams RT (1965). Corn Oil in Treatment of Ischaemic Heart Disease. *British Medical Journal* 12 Jun:1531-1533.

Seshadri S, Beiser A, Selhub J, Jacques PF, Rosenberg IH, D'Agostino RB, Wilson PWF, Wolf PA (2002). Plasma Homocysteine as a Risk Factor for Dementia and Alzheimer's Disease. *The New England Journal of Medicine,* 348:2074-2081.

Stanger O, Semmelrock H.-G, Wonisch W, Bös U, Pabst E, Wascher TC (2002). Effects of Folate Treatment and Homocysteine Lowering on Resistance Vessel Reactivity in Atherosclerotic Subjects. *The Journal of Pharmacology and Experimental Therapeutics* 303:158-162.

Theobald H, Johansson S, Bygren L, Engfeldt P (2001). The Effects of Alcohol Consumption on Mortality and Morbidity: A 26-Year Follow-Up Study. *The Journal of Studies on Alcohol* 62(6):783-789.

Vasan RS, Reiser A, D'Agostino RB, Levy D, Selhub J, Jacques PF, Rosenberg IH, Wilson PWF (2003). Plasma Homocysteine and Risk for Congestive Heart Failure in Adults Without Prior Myocardial Infarction. *Journal of the American Medical Association* 289(10):1251-1257.

Vollset SE, Refsum H, Tverdal A, Nygård O, Nordrehaug JE, Tell GS, Ueland P (2001). Plasma total homocysteine and cardiovascular and noncardiovascular mortality: the Hordaland Homocysteine Study. *American Journal of Clinical Nutrition* 74:130-136.

Whitaker JM (1987). *Reversing Diabetes,* New York, NY: Warner Books.

Wijga AH, Smit HA, Kerkhof M, de Jongste JC, Gerritsen J, Neijens HJ, Boshuizen HC, Brunekreef B (2003). Association of consumption of products containing milk fat with reduced asthma risk in pre-school children: the PIAMA birth cohort study. *Thorax* 58:567-572.

Wolfe SM, Ed (2001). The Diabetes Drug Metformin (Glucophage) and Lactic Acidosis. A Reminder About a Potentially Fatal Adverse Drug Reaction. *Worst Pills Best Pills News* 7(7):49-51.

Wolfe SM, Ed (2001a). Warning! GlaxoSmithKline's Disregard for the Safety of Diabetics Taking Rosiglitazone (Avandia). *Worst Pills Best Pills News* 7(9):68-69.

# Appendix C: Calculated[a] Fuel Value (9 kcal/g) vs. Actual Caloric Availability of Fats in Rodents or Other Animals

| Type of Fat or Oil | Caloric Availability |
|---|---|
| cocoa butter | 5.7[b] (rats) |
| | 5.5[c] (rats) |
| | 6.5[d] |
| | 6.8[e] |
| coconut oil | 7.8[l] (humans) |
| corn oil | 8.5[l] (humans) |
| lard | 8.3[e] |
| | 8.4[f] (pigs) |
| | 8.5[g] (turkeys) |
| | 7.9[h] (chickens) |
| | 8.4[i] (chickens) |
| tallow | 7.3[e] |
| | 5.9[f] (pigs) |
| | 6.5[g] (turkeys) |
| | 7.1[h] (chickens) |
| | 7.4[j] (chickens) |
| | 7.7[l] (humans) |

[a]CRC Handbook, 35th ed., 1953-4, p1794.

[b]Chen IS, Subramanian S, Vahouny GV, Cassidy MM, Ikeda I, Kritchevsky D. A Comparison of the Digestion and Absorption of Cocoa Butter and Palm Kernel Oil and Their Effects on Cholesterol Absorption in Rats. J Nutr 1989:119:1569-1573.

[c]Apgar JL, Shively CA, Tarka SM. Digestibility of Cocoa Butter and Corn Oil and Their Influence on Fatty Acid Distribution in Rats. J Nutr 1987:117:660-665.

[d]Hoagland R, Snider GG. Digestibility of Some Animal and Vegetable Fats. J Nutr 1942;25:295-302.

[e]Finley JW, Leveille GA, Klemann LP, Sourby JC, Ayres PH, Appleton S. Growth Method for Estimating the Caloric Availability of Fats and Oils. J Agric Food Chem 1994:42:489-494.

[f]Carlson WE, Bayley HS. Utilization of Fat by Young Pigs: Fatty Acid Composition of Ingesta in Different Regions of the Digestive Tractand Apparent and Corrected Digestibilities of Corn Oil, Lard and Tallow. Can J Anim Sci 1968:48:315-322.

[g]Whitehead CC, Fisher C. The Utilization of Various Fats by Turkeys of Different Ages. Br J Poult Sci 1975:16:481-485.

[h]Peterson CB, Vik-Mo L. Determination of Digestibility and Metabolizable Energy in Pure Fats and Discussion of Analytical Methods Employed in Experiments with GRowing Chickens. Acta Agric Scand 1968:18:42-48.

[i]Crick DC, Nwokolo EN, Sim JS. Effect of Blending Dietary Oils on Growth Performance, Total and Individual Fatty Acid Absorption by the Growing Chick. Nutr Res 1988:8:643-651.

[j]De Schrijver R, Vermeulen D, Viaene E. Lipid Metabolism Responses in Rats Fed Beef Tallow, Native or Randomized Fish Oil and Native or Randomized Peanut Oil. J Nutr 1991:121:948-955.

[l]Calc. from data in Finley JW, Klemann LP, Leveille GA, Otterburn MS, Walchak CG. J Agric Food Chem 1994:42:495-499.

## Appendix D. The "shorthand" chemical structures of the statin drugs

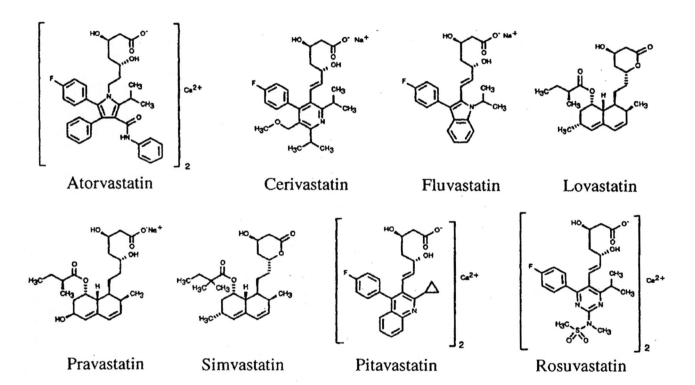

Atorvastatin  Cerivastatin  Fluvastatin  Lovastatin

Pravastatin  Simvastatin  Pitavastatin  Rosuvastatin

# Useful Medical Terms

*Absolute risk (AR) reduction.* If a treatment reduces the number of people who die of some specific disease from 6 per 1,000 to 3 per 1,000, the AR reduction is 3 per 1,000 or 0.3%.

*Anecdote.* A case study that has not been published, and therefore has low credibility.

*Average.* An arithmetic mean. The mean of 4 and 2 is 3.

*Baseline.* The condition of the subjects at the beginning of a clinical trial or observational study.

*Cardiovascular disease* (CVD or CHD). Gradual blockage of coronary arteries by plaque.

*Case study.* An anecdote on an experience with a single patient that has been published and gains credibility thereby.

*Clinical Trial.* An experiment on humans, who may be confined or free-living, to determine to effect of some treatment or diet.

*Congestive heart failure* (CHF or CF). Gradual reduction of the pumping ability of the heart. Accompanied by enlargement of the heart and low blood pressure.

*Crossover trial.* The treatment group of subjects and the placebo group are exchanged at intervals. Compensates for poor randomization, especially in trials with few subjects.

*Dose rate.* Effects of drugs depend on the amount of drug *and* the weight of the person or animal. The convention is to list how many milligrams of drug were given to the animal per kilogram of mass. Usually expressed as "mg/kg".

*Double-blind trial.* Neither the medical providers or the subjects know who is getting the treatment or the placebo.

*End point.* Criteria by which outcomes of trials are judged, such as risk of stroke or death.

*Evidence-based medicine.* Treating patients according to the best scientific evidence available while still considering the values of the patient. Not synonymous with reported findings in prestigious journals when the findings are biased or incomplete.

*False negative.* A test result that says "no" when the true result is "yes".

*False positive.* A test result that says "yes" when the true result is "no". Also called a "false alarm".

*Glycemic index* (GI). Ratio of how much a given food raises blood serum glucose level compared with the same mass of glucose.

*Glycemic load* (GL). The glycemic index multiplied by the mass of food.

*Incidence.* The proportion of individuals who develop some condition within a specific time interval, such as between ages 50 and 60. Often given as number per 100,000.

*In vitro.* Experiment carried out in glassware, not in whole living organisms.

*In vivo.* Experiment carried out in whole living organisms.

*Median.* A value such that half the data is above and half below it.

*Meta-analysis.* Combination of the results of many trials of the same type with more weight given to the trials with the most subjects.

*Mortality reduction.* The most important measure of treatment benefit — preventing early death from any cause. Often called all-cause mortality to emphasize "any cause" as opposed to death from a single cause.

*Myocardial infarction* (MI). Heart attack from loss of blood supply to heart muscle, usually because of a clot in a coronary artery. Can be fatal or non fatal.

*Non-fatal myocardial infarction* (NFMI). A non fatal MI.

*Number needed to treat* (NNT). If 5,000 people take a drug for 4 years and 1 heart attack is prevented, the NNT is 5,000.

*Observational study.* Examination of many free-living subjects, or their medical records, to find the effects of some lifestyle habits or medical treatment on the subjects.

*Placebo.* A dummy treatment or test or drug. Works on the mind well enough so that the result in a placebo group must be compared with the treatment group to see how much difference there really is.

*Prevalence.* The proportion of individuals who already have some condition at a certain time. Often given as number per 100,000.

*Prospective study.* An observational trial whose methods are planned before the trial starts, and which goes forward in time. Considered less biased than a retrospective trial.

*Randomization.* Selection of subjects or patients for a trial in which the treatment group and the placebo group are made as similar as possible.

*Randomized clinical trial* (RCT). An experiment in which participants are assigned to treatment or to a control group. The latter may have no treatment or a placebo.

*Relative risk* (RR) *reduction.* If a treatment reduces the number of people who die from some specific disease from 6 per 1,000 to 3 per 1,000, the RR reduction is 0.5 or 50%.

*Retrospective study.* An observational trial that looks back in time to find the effects of some lifestyle habits or medical treatment on the subjects. Considered more likely to be biased than a prospective trial.

*Screening.* Testing a symptomless population in order to detect disease at an early stage. The value of screening is often overrated.

*Sensitivity.* The percentage of individuals with a disease who test positive, say 90%. When added to the false negative rate, say 10%, the total is 100%.

*Single blind trial.* The subjects do not know whether they are getting the treatment or the placebo.

*Specificity.* The percentage of individuals with a disease who test negative, say 80%. When added to the false positive rate, say 20%, the total is 100%.

*Surrogate end point.* Measured trial results that may or may not be significant to a patient, such as serum triglyceride level or thyroid hormone level.

# Abbreviations

**ACAM** American College for Advancement in Medicine

**ADbA** American Diabetes Association

**ADtA** American Dietetic Association

**AHA** American Heart Association

**ASA** acetylsalicylic acid (aspirin)

**ATC** Antiplatelet Trialists Collaboration

**BMI** body mass index

**BMJ** British Medical Journal

**BP** blood pressure

**BU** Bread Unit (12 g of digestible carb)

**carb** carbohydrate

**CFIA** Canadian Food Inspection Agency

**CHD** coronary heart disease (same as CVD)

**CHF** congestive heart failure

**CI** confidence index

**CLA** conjugated linoleic acid

**CVD** cardiovascular disease (same as CHD)

**DDT** dichlorodiphenyl-trichloroethane

**DHA** Docosahexaenoic acid

**DHT** Diet-Heart Theory

**ECC** Effective Carbohydrate content

**EDTA** ethylenediamine-tetraacetic acid

**EFT** Emotional Freedom Technique

**EPA** Environmental Protection Agency or eicosapentaenoic acid

**FDA** Food & Drug Administration (US)

**GI** glycemic index

**GL** glycemic load

**HDL** high-density lipoprotein

**IDDM** insulin-dependent diabetes mellitus (Type 1, juvenile-onset)

**JAMA** Journal of the American Medical Association

**LBM** Lean Body Mass

**LDL** low-density lipoprotein

**LRC** Lipid Research Clinics

**MI** Myocardial Infarction (heart attack)

**MRFIT** Multiple Risk Factor Intervention Trial

**NFMI** non-fatal myocardial infarction

**NHLBI** National Heart, Lung and Blood Institute

**NIDDM** Non-insulin- dependent diabetes mellitus (Type 2, adult-onset)

**NIH** National Institutes of Health (US)

**NME** net metabolizable energy

**NNT** number (of patients) needed (to be) treated (to prevent 1 undesired outcome)

**PCBs** Polychlorinated biphenyls

**PDR** Physicians' Desk Reference

**PHS** Physicians Health Study Research Group

**PSA** prostate-specific antigen

**PVC** poly(vinyl chloride)

**RCT** Randomized controlled trial

**RR** relative risk

**TC** total cholesterol

**TG** Triglycerides (fats or oils)

**USDA** United States Department of Agriculture

**WHO** World Health Organization of the United Nations

# Index

324